D1526788

Handbook of Experimental Pharmacology

Volume 181

Yuti Chernajovsky · Ahuva Nissim

Editors

Therapeutic Antibodies

Contributors

L. Chatenoud, Y. Chernajovsky, A.L. Epstein, Z. Eshhar, F. Goldblatt, I.S. Grewal, A. Honegger, P. Hu, D. Isenberg, A. Jakobovits, P. Jin, L.A. Khawli, T. Kishimoto, M. Kraft, S. Lien, A.S.-Y. Lo, N. Lonberg, H. Lowman, C.M. Lynch, D.C. Maneval, W.A. Marasco, N. Nishimoto, A. Nissim, Z. Pirot, D.J. Shealy, M. Shepard, J. Singh, X.R. Song, S. Visvanathan, Q. Zhu

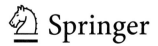 Springer

Yuti Chernajovsky
ARC Chair of Rheumatology, Centre Lead
Bone & Joint Research Unit
Queen Mary's School of Medicine & Dentistry
John Vane Science Centre
Charterhouse Square
London, EC1M 6BQ, United Kingdom
y.chernajovsky@qmul.ac.uk

Ahuva Nissim
Bone & Joint Research Unit
Queen Mary's School of Medicine & Dentistry
John Vane Science Centre
Charterhouse Square
London, EC1M 6BQ, United Kingdom
a.nissim@qmul.ac.uk

ISBN 978-3-540-73258-7   e-ISBN 978-3-540-73259-4

Handbook of Experimental Pharmacology ISSN 0171-2004

Library of Congress Control Number: 2007931735

Cover Design: WMX Design GmbH, Heidelberg

Printed on acid-free paper

9 8 7 6 5 4 3 2 1

springer.com

Preface

Antibodies are natural inhibitors of pathogens produced by B lymphocytes. The in vivo biological process involving antigen presenting cells, T and B lymphocytes necessary for their production are not addressed in this book, but can be found on any immunology text book.

The breakthrough study by Kohler and Milstein was the ability to produce in vitro antibodies by cell fusion. This finding catapulted the use of antibodies as therapeutic agents. With the emergence of recombinant DNA technology and the innovative ingenuity of scientists, these magic bullets are now continuously being developed both for research and therapeutic purposes by a myriad of techniques and their use in many clinical conditions are a testimony of their importance. This book provides examples of these developments and the current areas of further research and improvements.

We have in this book the contribution of scientists that have been involved in the development of these therapeutic antibodies from their conception and preclinical testing to their use in the clinic. We believe that each chapter contributes to our understanding of this process. In no case the path from discovery to application was simple and is through perseverance and further improvements that each therapeutic moiety reached its final marketed form.

Engineering of antibodies takes place allowing their use as targeting devices of both other immunomodulators such as cytokines or cells themselves by the use of chimeric receptors. The combination with gene transfer technologies to express some of these moieties directly by the cells of the patient and thus achieve long-term delivery is also being investigated. As always there is room for improvement in this field and we expect that in the years to come more of these biologicals will become available in more diverse therapeutic fields. Better understanding of molecular mechanisms and the function of targeted molecules will lead to the production of more specific targeted agents.

The science of pharmacology has been redrawn with the entrance of these biological agents in clinical practice. We need to consider introducing the term "biopharmacology" when dealing with naturally occurring compounds that have been modified by recombinant DNA technology. It is especially relevant in cases where two or more different targets are found in the same molecule such as in bi-specific antibodies or immunocytokines. We are actually witnessing a revolution in medicine and this book summarises it very well.

We dedicate this book to Kohler and Milstein for their seminal work on antibody production.

We thank Professor Gustav Born who gave us the opportunity to edit this book; Nathan Fox and Lin Wells for secretarial assistance, all the authors and Susanne Dathe from Springer Verlag for their commitment and help to bring this book to light.

London, United Kingdom   Ahuva Nissim
London, United Kingdom   Yuti Chernajovsky

Contents

Contributors   ix

Part I Introduction

Historical Development of Monoclonal Antibody Therapeutics   3
A. Nissim and Y. Chernajovsky

Preclinical Safety Evaluation of Monoclonal Antibodies   19
C.M. Lynch and I.S. Grewal

Part II Molecular Developments in Antibody Production

Engineering Antibodies for Stability and Efficient Folding   47
A. Honegger

Human Monoclonal Antibodies from Transgenic Mice   69
N. Lonberg

Part III Antibodies to Cytokines

Anti-TNF Antibodies: Lessons from the Past, Roadmap for the Future . . .   101
D.J. Shealy and S. Visvanathan

Therapeutic Anti-VEGF Antibodies   131
S. Lien and H.B. Lowman

Humanized Antihuman IL-6 Receptor Antibody, Tocilizumab   151
N. Nishimoto and T. Kishimoto

Part IV Antibodies to Cell Markers

**Anti-CD20 Monoclonal Antibody in Rheumatoid Arthritis and Systemic
Lupus Erythematosus** 163
F. Goldblatt and D.A. Isenberg

Herceptin 183
H.M. Shepard, P. Jin, D.J. Slamon, Z. Pirot, and D.C. Maneval

**The Use of CD3-Specific Antibodies in Autoimmune Diabetes: A Step
Toward the Induction of Immune Tolerance in the Clinic** 221
L. Chatenoud

Monoclonal Antibody Therapy for Prostate Cancer 237
A. Jakobovits

Anti-IgE and Other Antibody Targets in Asthma 257
J. Singh and M. Kraft

Part V Development of Antibody-Based Cellular and Molecular Therapies

**Cytokine, Chemokine, and Co-Stimulatory Fusion Proteins for the
Immunotherapy of Solid Tumors** 291
L.A. Khawli, P. Hu, and A.L. Epstein

The T-Body Approach: Redirecting T Cells with Antibody Specificity 329
Z. Eshhar

Intracellular Antibodies (Intrabodies) and Their Therapeutic Potential . . 343
A.S.-Y. Lo, Q. Zhu, and W.A. Marasco

Index 375

Contributors

L. Chatenoud
Université René Descartes, Paris, France, Institut National de la Santé et de la Recherche Médicale, Unité 580, Paris, France, chatenoud@necker.fr

Y. Chernajovsky
Bone and Joint Research Unit, William Harvey Research Institute, Barts and The London, Queen Mary's School of Medicine and Dentistry, University of London, Charterhouse Square, London EC1M 6BQ, UK

A.L. Epstein
Department of Pathology, Keck School of Medicine at the University of Southern California, Los Angeles, CA, USA

Z. Eshhar
Department of Immunology, The Weizmann Institute of Science, P.O. Box 26, Rehovot 76100, Israel, zelig.eshhar@weizmann.ac.il

F. Goldblatt
Centre for Rheumatology, Department of Medicine, University College London Hospital, 3rd Floor Central, 250 Euston Road, London NW1 2PQ, UK, Fiona.goldblatt@uclh.nhs.uk

I.S. Grewal
Department of Preclinical Therapeutics, Seattle Genetics, Bothell, WA 98021, USA, igrewal@seagen.com

A. Honegger
Biochemisches Institut, Universität Zürich, Winterthurerstrasse 190, CH-8057 Zürich, Switzerland, honegger@bioc.uzh.ch

P. Hu
Department of Pathology, Keck School of Medicine at the University of Southern California, Los Angeles, CA, USA

D.A. Isenberg
Centre for Rheumatology, Department of Medicine, University College London
Hospital, 3rd Floor Central, 250 Euston Road, London NW1 2PQ, UK

A. Jakobovits
Agensys, Inc., 1545 17th Street, Santa Monica, CA 90404, USA,
ajakobovits@agensys.com

P. Jin
Receptor BioLogix, Inc., 3350 W. Bayshore Rd., Suite 150, Palo Alto, CA 94303,
USA

L.A. Khawli
Department of Pathology, Keck School of Medicine at the University of Southern
California, Los Angeles, CA, USA
Genentech, Inc., One DNA Way, South San Francisco, CA 94080, USA,
aepstein@usc.edu

T. Kishimoto
Laboratory of Immune Regulation, Graduate School of Frontier Biosciences, Osaka
University, 1–3 Yamadaoka, Suita City, Osaka 565-0871, Japan

M. Kraft
Duke Asthma, Allergy and Airway Center Duke University Medical Center,
Durham, NC 27710, USA

S. Lien
Antibody Engineering, Protein Engineering, and Immunology Departments,
Genentech, Inc., 1 DNA Way, South San Francisco, CA 94080, USA

A.S.-Y. Lo
Dana-Farber Cancer Institute, Harvard Medical School, 44 Binney Street, Boston
MA 02115, USA

N. Lonberg
Medarex, 521 Cottonwood Drive, Milpitas, CA 95035, USA,
nlonberg@medarex.com

H.B. Lowman
Antibody Engineering, Protein Engineering, and Immunology Departments,
Genentech, Inc., 1 DNA Way, South San Francisco, CA 94080, USA,
hbl@gene.com

C.M. Lynch
Department of Preclinical Therapeutics, Seattle Genetics, Bothell, WA 98021, USA

D.C. Maneval
Receptor BioLogix, Inc., 3350 W. Bayshore Rd., Suite 150, Palo Alto, CA 94303,
USA

W.A. Marasco
Dana-Farber Cancer Institute, Harvard Medical School, 44 Binney Street, Boston
MA 02115, USA, Wayne_Marasco@dfci.harvard.edu

N. Nishimoto
Laboratory of Immune Regulation, Graduate School of Frontier Biosciences,
Osaka University, 1–3 Yamadaoka, Suita City, Osaka 565-0871, Japan,
norihiro@fbs.osaka-u.ac.jp

A. Nissim
Bone and Joint Research Unit, William Harvey Research Institute, Barts and The
London, Queen Mary's School of Medicine and Dentistry, University of London,
Charterhouse Square, London EC1M 6BQ, UK, a.nissim@qmul.ac.uk

Z. Pirot
Receptor BioLogix, Inc., 3350 W. Bayshore Rd., Suite 150, Palo Alto, CA 94303,
USA

D.J. Shealy
Centocor Research and Development Inc., 145 King of Prussia Road, Radnor,
PA 19087, USA, dshealy@cntus.jnj.com

H.M. Shepard
Receptor BioLogix, Inc., 3350 W. Bayshore Rd., Suite 150, Palo Alto, CA 94303,
USA, hms@rblx.com

J. Singh
Duke Asthma, Allergy and Airway Center Duke University Medical Center,
Durham, NC 27710, USA, Jaspal.Singh@duke.edu

D.J. Slamon
Division of Hematology and Oncology, University of California Los Angeles
School of Medicine, 10945 Le Conte Avenue, Suite 3360, Los Angeles, CA 90095,
USA

S. Visvanathan
Centocor Research and Development, Inc., 145 King of Prussia Road, Radnor,
PA 19087, USA, svisvana@cntus.jnj.com

Q. Zhu
Dana-Farber Cancer Institute, Harvard Medical School, 44 Binney Street, Boston
MA 02115, USA

Part I
Introduction

Historical Development of Monoclonal Antibody Therapeutics

A. Nissim(✉) and Y. Chernajovsky

1 Development of Monoclonal Antibodies by Mouse Hybridoma Technology 4
2 Display Technologies 7
3 Development of Technologies to Tailor the Properties
   Determining the Clinical Potential of Antibodies 10
   3.1 Affinity 10
   3.2 Effector Function 10
4 Pharmacokinetics 12
5 Conclusions 14
References 15

Abstract Since the first publication by Kohler and Milstein on the production of mouse monoclonal antibodies (mAbs) by hybridoma technology, mAbs have had a profound impact on medicine by providing an almost limitless source of therapeutic and diagnostic reagents. Therapeutic use of mAbs has become a major part of treatments in various diseases including transplantation, oncology, autoimmune, cardiovascular, and infectious diseases. The limitation of murine mAbs due to immunogenicity was overcome by replacement of the murine sequences with their human counterpart leading to the development of chimeric, humanized, and human therapeutic antibodies. Remarkable progress has also been made following the development of the display technologies, enabling of engineering antibodies with modified properties such as molecular size, affinity, specificity, and valency. Moreover, antibody engineering technologies are constantly advancing to enable further tuning of the effector function and serum half life. Optimal delivery to the target tissue still remains to be addressed to avoid unwanted side effects as a result of systemic treatment while achieving meaningful therapeutic effect.

A. Nissim

Bone and Joint Research Unit, William Harvey Research Institute, Barts and The London, Queen Mary's School of Medicine and Dentistry, University of London, Charterhouse Square, London EC1M 6BQ, United Kingdom
e-mail: a.nissim@qmul.ac.uk

Y. Chernajovsky, A. Nissim (eds.) *Therapeutic Antibodies. Handbook of Experimental Pharmacology 181.*
© Springer-Verlag Berlin Heidelberg 2008

1 Development of Monoclonal Antibodies by Mouse Hybridoma Technology

The development of mouse hybridoma technology by Kohler and Milstein in 1975 initiated high hopes for the production of antibodies for therapy (Kohler and Milstein 1975). Mouse hybridomas were the first reliable source of monoclonal antibodies and were developed for a number of in vivo therapeutic applications (Meeker et al. 1985; Cosimi et al. 1981). Clinical studies have, however, been disappointing due to the fact that the monoclonal antibodies (mAbs) were of murine origin and therefore triggered human immune responses (Shawler et al. 1985). Understanding the structure–function of antibody was the key element to address this problem. At the amino terminus, immunoglobulins have two identical target-binding variable domains (Fv portions), each of which forms a pocket where two polypeptide chains – the heavy and light chain – come together. Two heavy chains are linked to two light chains by disulfide bonds, and the two heavy chains are linked to each other by disulfide bonds in a flexible hinge region. The effector function of immunoglobulin encompass the Fc portion composed of constant region at the carboxyl termini of both heavy chains (Fig. 1). To reduce the potential human anti-mouse antibody (HAMA) responses, chimeric antibodies containing mouse variable domain regions fused to human constant regions were developed (Boulianne et al. 1984). Studies by Hwang and Foote (2005) have demonstrated that substitution of mouse with human Fc dramatically reduce the anti-antibody response (AAR). While with mAb 84% had marked, 7% tolerable and 9% negligible HAMA responses with chimeric Abs there were only 40% marked, 27% tolerable, and 33% negligible human antichimeric antibodies (HACA) responses. To counteract both HAMA and HACA responses associated with murine and chimeric antibodies, humanization was done by grafting mouse complementarity-determining regions (CDRs), the hypervariable regions that bind to the specific antigen, into human antibody backbone (Fig. 1 inset and Jones et al. 1986). In terms of immunogenicity of humanized mAbs, there is a dramatic decrease in marked anti-humanized antibody (HAHA) responses to only 9%. Nevertheless, the tolerable and negligible responses are similar to the chimeric mAbs with 36% and 55% incidence, respectively (Hwang and Foote 2005). Another problem arising from using the humanization approach was that the antibody variant in which only CDRs had been replaced had reduced affinity (Reichmann 1988). This was overcome by the conversion of human amino acids in framework region to their corresponding mouse sequences. This was followed by a "resurfacing" approach in which only the surface exposed mouse residues are replaced by human amino acids (Padlan 1991; Zhang 2005)

The number of chimeric and humanized antibodies approved by the American Food and Drug Administration (FDA) is constantly growing. The chimeric antibody is still dominating the therapeutic mAbs with four FDA approved products, led by Remicade (anti-TNFα) for the treatment of autoimmune diseases such as rheumatoid arthritis (Elliott et al. 1993) and Rituxan (anti-CD20) to treat B cell lymphoma (Coiffier et al. 1998) and rheumatoid arthritis (Cambridge et al. 2003).

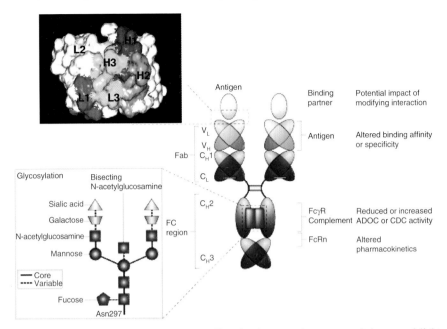

Fig. 1 Antibody parts and their functions: IgG molecules comprise a two each heavy and light chains linked by disulphide bonds (*green bars*). Each chain contain a variable (V) domain (the V_H domain, green; and VL, orange) and constant (s) domains (C_H1, C_H2, and C_H3 or one C_L domain; purple). Binding to antigen (*light blue*) is mediated by direct interaction of complementarity-determining regions (CDRs). CDRs are shown at the top left. VH-CDRs are indicated as H3, H2, and H1 for VH-CDR3, VH-CDR2, and VH-CDR1, respectively. VL-CDR1, VL-CDR2, and VL-CDR3 are L3, L2, and L1, respectively. The Fc region of IgG interacts with Fc receptors expressed by effector cells or with complement, leading to destruction of the target pathogen. The Fc also binds the salvage receptor FcRn to extend the half-life of human IgG. Glycosylation is needed to the FcR interaction and is attached to the conserved asparagine (Asn) residue at position 297. Part of the image is reproduced, with permission, from Nature (Carter, 2006)

The first humanized antibody has been Campath, which binds human CD52 and is used to treat patients with B cell chronic lymphocytic leukaemia (Dyer 1999) and acute transplant rejection (Morris and Russell 2006). Additional prominent example is humanized antireceptor tyrosine kinase ERB2, Herceptin to treat breast cancer (Eiermann 2001). Currently, there are nine approved humanized mAbs (Table 1).

Transgenic animals superseded the mouse hybridoma technology for the production of human mAbs. By transgenic technology human antibody genes were introduced into mice lacking their own immunoglobulin loci. These mice can be immunized with specific antigens and their B cells used for generating hybridomas as for the generation of mouse mAbs, but in this case producing intact human antibodies (Jakobovits et al. 1993). The immune response in transgenic mice is sometimes less robust and thus there is a need for an increased number of immunizations. The main advantage is that mAbs from transgenic mice often have high affinity reflecting in vivo affinity maturation and thus obviate the need of in vitro

Table 1 Mabs approved for therapy

Name (USAN)	Target	Isotype	Species	Indication Class
Synagis (*palivizumab*)	RSV F prot	IgG1K	Humanized	Antiinfective
Amevive (*alefacept*)	CD2	IgG1 fusion		Immunomodulatory
Enbrel (*etanercept*)	TNF alpha	IgG1 fusion		Immunomodulatory
Humira (*adalimumab*)	TNF alpha	IgG1K	Human	Immunomodulatory
OKT3 (*muromonab-CD3*)	CD3	IgG2a	Murine	Immunomodulatory
Raptiva (*efalizumab*)	CD11a	IgG1kappa	Humanized	Immunomodulatory
Remicade (*infliximab*)	TNF alpha	IgG1K	Chimeric	Immunomodulatory
ReoPro (*abciximab*)	GP 2b/3a	IgG1K Fab	Chimeric	Immunomodulatory
Simulect (*basiliximab*)	CD25	IgG1	Humanized	Immunomodulatory
Xolair (*omalizumab*)	IgE	IgG1 kappa	Humanized	Immunomodulatory
Zenapax (*daclizumab*)	CD25	IgG1	Humanized	Immunomodulatory
Tysabri (natalizumab)	a4 integrin	IgG4	Humanized	Immunomodulatory
Orencia (abatacept)	CTLA4-Ig	IgG1	Human	Immunomodulatory
Avastin (*bevacizumab*)	VEGF	IgG1 kappa	Humanized	Oncology
Bexxar (*tositumaomb*)	CD20	IgG2a	Murine	Oncology
Campath (*alemtuzumab*)	hu CD52	IgG1	Humanized	Oncology
Erbitux (*cetuximab*)	hu EGFr	IgG1kappa	Chimeric	Oncology
Herceptin (*trastuzumab*)	Her2	IgG1K	Humanized	Oncology
Vectabix (panitumumab)	EGFR	IgG2	Humanized	Oncologic
Mylotarg (*gemtuzumab ozogamicin*)	hu CD33	IgG4kappa	Humanized	Oncology
Rituxan (*rituximab*)	CD20	IgG1K	Chimeric	Oncology
Zevalin (*ibritumomab tiuxetan*)	hu CD20	IgG1kappa	murine	Oncology

Table 1 (continued)

Name (USAN)	Target	Isotype	Species	Indication Class
CEA-Scan *(arcitumomab)*	CEA	IgG1 (Fab′)2	Murine	Radiotherapy and imaging
Myoscint *(imciromab)*	Myosin	IgG2aK Fab	Murine	Radiotherapy and Imaging
NeutroSpec *(fanolesomab)*	CD15	IgM	Murine	Radiotherapy and imaging
Oncoscint *(satumomab)*	hu tu-assoc gp 72	IgG1K	Murine	Radiotherapy and Imaging
Prostascint *(capromab)*	PSMA	IgG1K	murine	Radiotherapy and imaging
Verluma *(nofetumomab)*	40kDa GP	IgG2b Fab	Murine	Radiotherapy and imaging
Lucentis (ranibizumab)	VEGF	IgG1	Humanized	Ocular

Sources are www.fda.gov/cder/rdmt web sites and (Carter 2006) with permission from Nature. Products are grouped according to their therapeutic application. Further details and references are listed in (Carter 2006). Rnibizumab and panitumumab have been approved last year. Ranibizumab developed by Genentech is a humanized, Fab directed against VEGF. It was derived from the full-length bevacizumab and is approved for the treatment of colorectal cancer. Ranibizumab has been shown to completely penetrate the retina and enter the subretinal space after intravitreal injection. Co-development of Abgenix with Amgen, panitumumab (rHuMAb-EGFr) targets EGFR. Panitu-mumab is an entirely human monoclonal demonstrating antitumor activity in advanced, refractory colorectal cancer

affinity maturation. In addition, the initial output is intact human mAb including the Fc portion, which allows immediate screening for effector function. Antibodies raised by this technology can be produced either in the same hybridoma cell line generated after immunization or in cell lines such as Chinese hamster ovary. None of the antibodies derived from these mice have yet made it to the market, although 35 have already entered clinical development. Four antibodies anti-EGFR, RANKL, CTLA-4, and CD4 are now in phase 3 development. So far there has been no Anti Antibody Response reported in the clinical trial (Lonberg 2005).

2 Display Technologies

The simplest robust technology for raising mAbs against a given target therapeutic protein is phage display technology (Winter 1994). The libraries encompass a mixture of filamentous bacteriophage each displaying a different antibody fragment and specificity. To build a library, antibodies fragments such as Fab (VH + CH1/VL + CL heterodimers connected via a disulfide bridge) (Griffiths et al. 1994), single chain variable fragment (VH and VL joined by a polypeptide linker of at least

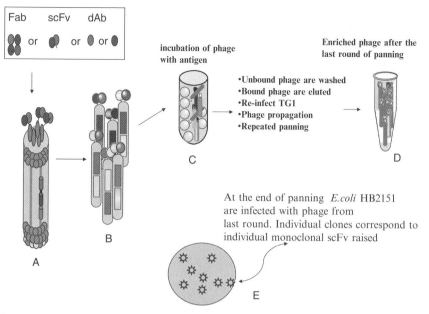

Fig. 2 Principle of phage display. The phage display libraries encompass a mixture of filamentous bacteriophage each displaying a different antibody fragment and specificity. Fab, scFv, or dAb antibody fragments (Fig. 2 inset) are cloned as a fusion with phage coat protein (A, VH in *red*; VL in *orange*; and gIII in *blue*) resulting in libraries of millions or billions of phage each displaying different antibody fragments (Fig. 2A,B). The library is then used to select against an immobilized target protein to capture the phage that bind specifically to the protein (Fig. 2C). Unbound phage are washed while bound phage are eluted and then infect *E. coli* TG-1 bacteria. Phage are propagated and used for further round of selection. At the end of the panning *E. coli* HB2151 are infected and individual bacterial clone producing antibody fragments are screened for binding to the target antigen. For further details see (Harrison et al. 1996)

12 amino acids, (scFv) (Nissim et al. 1994), and single VH or VL domain antibody (dAbs) (Holt et al. 2003) were cloned as a fusion with phage coat protein, resulting in libraries of millions or billions of phage each displaying different antibody fragments (Fig. 2 inset, A and B). The library is then used to select against a target protein to capture the phage that bind specifically to the protein (Fig. 2C–E). The ability to rapidly screen large number of antibodies against the target protein has obvious advantages over the laborious generation of hybridomas. Moreover, the DNA encoding the selected antibody fragment is packaged with the protein (Fig. 2A). This link between phenotype (binding affinity) and genotype (antibody gene segments) allows simultaneous recovery of the gene encoding the selected antibody (Hoogenboom 2005). Libraries were built from immune fragments isolated from immunized animals or infected humans, resulting in biased library toward certain specificities. When an immune library was made from an immunized animal, it basically replaces the hybridoma approach but with the ability to obtain many more antibodies and with rare antibody specificities (McWhirter and Alexion Antibody

Technologies 2006; Throsby 2006). An attractive application of immune libraries is to develop virus or toxins-neutralizing antibody fragments that can replace the current treatment by serum-derived polyclonal antibodies, which suffers from potential drawbacks such as limited production capacity and batch-to-batch variation (de Kruif et al. 2006). Naïve libraries were later on built from a pool of healthy donors followed by a synthetic repertoire rearranged in vitro, which is not biased and therefore can be used for selecting specificities against a wide range of targets (Vaughan 1996; Hoogenboom 2005). Nevertheless, the advantage of the semisynthetic repertoires is the ability to control the type and number of germline gene segments as well as the sequence of the synthetic CDRs (Nissim et al. 1994; de Wildt et al. 2000; Silacci 2005). Large and diverse semisynthetic libraries have been a valuable source of antibodies against a large number of target proteins including self nonimmunogenic as well as antigens that are species-crossreactive. Anti-TNFα antibody, Humira (Adalimumab), derived from phage display is the only human antibody approved by the FDA to treat rheumatoid arthritis. The human mAb Adalimumab appears to be less immunogenic than the chimeric Infliximab. In three randomized trials, the cumulative incidence of anti-Adalimumab antibodies in 1 062 patients with rheumatoid arthritis was 6% (Kress 2002). Concomitant methotrexate therapy was associated with a reduced incidence of antibody development; 12% of patients treated with Adalimumab alone were antibody-positive vs. $<1\%$ of patients treated with Adalimumab and methotrexate (Weinblatt 2003). The question whether fully human mAb are less immunogenic than humanized mAb can not be addressed yet until more human antibodies will be used in clinic. This will come up probably soon as many antibody fragments derived from phage display are now in clinical and preclinical trails (leading candidate listed in Hudson 2005).

A less common route to generate human antibodies includes ribosome display (Hanes and Pluckthun 1997) and yeast display (Boder and Wittrup 1997). The advantage of yeast display is the availability of posttranslational modification in the yeast host but ribosomal display is used more often along side phage display for affinity maturation. In ribosome display, mRNA is transcribed from antibody cDNA libraries, and subsequently translated in vitro to produce complexes where ribosomes are still connected to both mRNA and nascent polypeptide. The ribosome display selection is similar to phage display with antibody–ribosome–mRNA complex being selected by binding to an immobilized target antigen. Selected mRNA is released from the ribosome followed by RT-PCR to generate a population of selected DNA, as the starting point for further rounds of selection. While offering similar benefits as phage display, this technology has the potential ability to generate larger libraries by overcoming the need to transform cells to generate a library. The main advantage, however, is the integral PCR step in the procedure that makes this technology a convenient approach for affinity maturation. An affinity matured ribosomal display antibody was recently developed, CAT-354, which is a human anti-IL-13 monoclonal antibody for potential treatment of severe asthma (Blanchard 2005).

3 Development of Technologies to Tailor the Properties Determining the Clinical Potential of Antibodies

Minimizing immunogenicity in the clinical setting poses considerable challenges but the clinical potential of mAbs does not exclusively depend on that. Other properties such as affinity, effector function, tissue penetration, and pharmacokinetics are also very important. Scientists have gone a long way in the development of technologies to tailor mAb to tune these functions and to make candidate mAbs real drug candidates.

3.1 Affinity

The clinical utility of an antibody depends on its affinity for the target antigen. Improving affinity can improve the potency, pharmacokinetics, and reduce the dosing needed. Nevertheless, increased affinity does not always translate to increased potency and in many cases there is an affinity threshold. This is most common for tumor targeting where higher affinity antibodies do not necessarily have superior tumor targeting as this might diminish penetration or cause binding to normal tissues that have lower expression of the targeted tumor marker. The mAb raised by hybridoma technology either from mice or from transgenic mice usually have high affinity and do not need affinity maturation. The beauty of display technology is the ability to tailor the affinity to the optimal binding affinity and avoid the threshold affinities. In general the initial selected antibody from display libraries often bears lower than the desired affinity. The different approaches to improve antibody affinity can be divided into chain or CDR shuffling. Chain shuffling involves shuffling the VH or VL of a given antibody with a repertoire of the corresponding chain thereby creating a mini-library of the lead antibody. This mini-library is then used for selection for higher affinity binders using stringent selection (Marks 2004). CDR shuffling was developed originally by Barbas et al. (1994) and involved mutation within the CDRs and reselection in stringent conditions (Neri et al. 1997).

3.2 Effector Function

3.2.1 Engineering the Fc

In some cases, binding of mAbs to the target protein and neutralization of its activity is sufficient. For example, two mAbs approved for clinical use, Herceptin (anti-Her2/Neu) and anti-EGFR, provide therapeutic benefit in part by blocking growth signals after binding to their corresponding receptor. More commonly, however, destruction of target cells such as the removal of tumor cells or viral-infected cells is desired. Destruction of target cells is mediated by effector functions and each of these is mediated through interaction of the Fc portion of mAbs with a specific set of Fc receptors. These include antibody-dependent cytotoxicity (ADCC), phagocytosis, and complement-dependent cytotoxicity (CDC). ADCC and phagocytosis are mediated by binding to FcR and CDC by binding to the complement proteins.

The importance of carbohydrate linked to Asn297 of IgG in the interaction with Fc-receptor has long been recognized (Fig. 1). Moreover, the interaction with the Fc is sensitive to changes in the composition of the carbohydrate. Molecular engineering technology has been used to tune the composition of the carbohydrate by mainly reducing the fructose moiety, which was shown to significantly increase binding to FcγR and thus enhance ADCC. ADCC response have also been tuned by engineering the amino acid sequence of the Fc region to improve binding to FcγRs (Shields 2001). More recently, computational design methods have been used to tailor the effector functions of Alemtuzumab and Trastuzumab achieving a more than 100-fold increase in the potency of ADCC, as well as increases in the percentage of tumor cells that are killed (Lazar 2006). In the same manner, detailed mapping of C1q to human IgG1 has been used to improve the CDC of Rituximab (Idusogie 2001).

3.2.2 Arming Mab with Effector Function

Antibody engineering has advanced to the point that other effector functions can be engineered into mAb regardless of the characteristics or presence of the Fc portion. mAb effector functions are increased by arming with either radionuclide drugs (Wu and Senter 2005) or potent toxins (Kreitman 1999; Kreitman et al. 2000) or by engineering recombinant bi-specific antibodies that simultaneously bind the target and activate receptors or immune effector cells such as CD3 and FcR (von Mehren 2003; Baltman Greenberg Science 2004). The FDA has recently approved three mAb conjugates for cancer. Two of these are murine radiolabelled mAbs to treat B cell lymphoma, a CD-20-specific IgG2lk radiolabeled with ^{90}Y (Ibritumomab Tiuxetan) (Wahl 2005) and a CD-20 IgG2al radiolabelled with ^{131}I (Tositumomab) (Borghaei 2004). The third mAb conjugate is a humanized CD-33 specific IgG4k mAb conjugated to a calicheamicin derivative that induces double strand breaks (Gemtuzumab Ozogamicin) for the treatment of leukemia (Linenberger 2005). Gemtuzumab Ozogamicin is actually the only approved mAb-drug conjugate, but many more are in different phases of clinical trials (Wu and Senter 2005). Smaller antibody fragment with shorter half life and rapid blood clearance and therefore with limited unwanted exposure to normal tissues are also been armed with effector function. For example, fragments conjugated to pseudomonase exotoxine QA are been tested (Wu and Senter 2005). An additional approach to increase the effector function of mAb is by antibody-directed enzyme prodrug therapy (ADEPT), which uses mAb to specifically deliver an enzyme that activates a subsequently administered prodrug. Phase 1 trial of ADEPT was reported by Francis et al. (2002) using murine F(ab')2 anti-CEA fragment linked to carboxypeptidase G2 followed by prodrug bis-iodo-phenol mustard (ZD276P) in patients with advanced colorectal carcinoma. The main problem in this trial was, however, the immunogenicity of the murine F(ab')2 and the conjugated enzyme.

3.2.3 Immunocytokines

Fusion of antibody or antibody fragments to cytokines capable of augmenting immune response is an alternative approach to localize therapy (Maas et al. 1993). Such recombinant fusion proteins, called immunocytokines, combine the targeting power of the mAb to direct the cytokine to specific antigens, thus achieving an effective local concentration in the desired microenvironment, without the toxicity associated with systemic cytokine administration. In the past decade, several groups have developed immunocytokines, including those fused to TNFα (Gillies et al. 1991) IL-2, granulocyte/macrophage colony stimulating factor (GM-CSF) (Tao and Levy 1993; Zhao et al. 1999), and IL-12 (Gillies et al. 1998). Indeed, one of the first successful constructions of a fully active immunocytokine was that of a chimeric human/mouse anti-ganglioside GD2 antibody, ch14.18 with IL-2 (Gillies et al. 1992). GD2 is expressed on many tumors of neuroectodermal origin, such as neuroblastoma, melanoma, and certain sarcomas.

4 Pharmacokinetics

The pharmacokinetics of antibodies in blood is an important factor in assessing their clinical potential. Most likely, it is desired to increase the half life of antibody to improve efficacy. Alternatively, it might be advantageous to decrease half life in cases where nonspecific binding is high. Half life of antibody can range from several minutes for antibody fragments such as dAb or scFv up to several weeks for an intact antibody. There are several approaches to improve the pharmacokinetics. In case of intact antibody, it can be tuned by tailoring the interaction between mAb and its salvage receptor, FcRn. This receptor binds and transport IgGs in the circulation, and thus rescues Ab from a default degradation (Ghetie 1997; Ward et al. 2005). Binding to FcRn is pH dependent via His310 and His435 on Fc. IgG can bind FcRn in endosomes under slightly acidic conditions (pH 6.0–6.5) and can recycle to the cell surface, where it is released under almost neutral conditions (pH 7.0–7.4). Fc derivatives that increase binding to FcRn at pH 6.0 are desired to increase half life (Hinton 2004) while Fc mutation attenuating interaction with FcRn are used to reduce half life (Carlos Vaccaro 2005; Kenanova 2005).

Antibody fragment lacking Fc can be engineered to superior molecules with an increased half life (Hudson 2005). The most commonly used format antibody fragment scFv (25kDa) can be engineered to a larger fragment by increasing the number of scFv building block. Depending on the linker length, dimeric diabody of 55 KDa (two scFv), triabody of 80 kDa (three scFv) or tetravalent tetrabodies of 110 kDa (four scFv) were constructed for imaging studies. These fragments are smaller than intact antibody and they can be cleared faster and have improved tumor binding and penetration in comparison with scFv and Fab. It seems that bivalent diabody is advantageous as it has better tumor retention in comparison with scFv but still has more rapid tumor penetration and clearance in comparison with intact antibody (Robinson 2005; Hudson 2005) for review. Minibodies (scFv–CH3 dimer) account for higher tumor uptake but with still better clearance. Both diabody and minibodies augment the avidity alongside increase in size (Fig. 3).

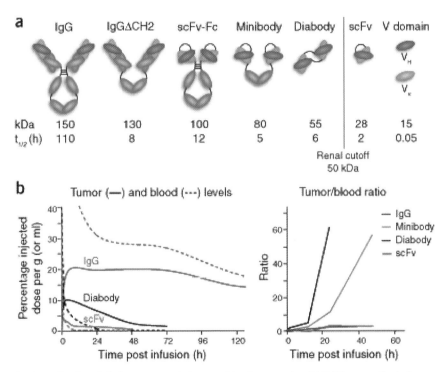

Fig. 3 Antibodies, their fragments, and pharmacokinetic properties: (**a**) Different antibody formats and their respective molecular weights (kDa) and serum half life. VL is indicated in *orange*, VH in *purple*, while C domain in *blue*. (**b**) Biodistribution of different mAb formats in two xenograft models. *Left graph*: tumor (*solid lines*) and blood levels (*dashed lines*) plotted vs. hour after injection (h) for anti-Her2/Neu Mabs IgG 741F8 (*blue*), diabody C6.5 (*black*), and scFv C6.5 (*red*) in severe combined immune deficient (SCID) mice bearing solid subcutaneous SK-OV-3 tumors expressing Her2/Neu. *Right graph*: tumor-to-blood ratios of anti-CEA T84.66 immunoglobulin, minibody, diabody, and scFv in mice with LS174 colon carcinoma xenografts plotted vs. time after infusion. These studies show the superior tumor targeting of diabodies with high tumor uptake and rapid blood clearance when compared with immunoglobulin with higher blood pool and scFv with poor tumor uptake and rapid clearance. The image is reproduced, with permission, from Nature (Hudson 2005)

The half life of antibody fragments can also be modified by conjugation to polyethylene glycol (PEG) (Chapman et al. 1999). At least two PEGylated antibody fragments have progressed to clinical trials, including Certolizumab pegol (Cimzia; UCB; a humanized TNF-specific Fab$'$ conjugated to PEG). Certolizumab pegol has half-life of $\approx$14 days in patients, which is comparable with the parental IgG, and it is well tolerated (Choy 2002). The potential advantages of PEGylated fragments over IgG include the lack of any undesirable Fc-mediated effects (Chapman 2002).

5 Conclusions

Design of a therapeutic antibody involves target selection, antibody generation, and engineering for optimal efficacy. When mAbs were first discovered in the 1980s, the choices of therapeutic application were very limited, but since then tremendous progress has been made. The ability to engineer human like or human antibodies and to improve mAb affinity and effector function of choice has led to a big step in the use of mAbs in clinical settings. The big step was the development of antibody library technology, which already led to one human antibody approved for therapy with many more in clinical and preclinical trials. This technology not only enables the development of intact human antibodies but the development of non-native antibody forms that can be tuned to the desired affinity, pharmacokinetics, and effector function. Since clinical studies are still limited to one approved human mAb developed by these technologies, it remains to be seen if further improvements are needed. For example semisynthetic or synthetic phage or ribosomal display libraries bear nonnative CDR3, which might be immunogenic. Possibly, libraries will need further tuning to generate more human antibody germline-like sequence repertoires for further therapeutic application. So far, apart from the anti-TNFα to treat rheumatoid arthritis, the most promising therapeutic mAbs are the ones developed to kill tumors either by effector function or by delivering death signals. Probably the best approach in the future will be to combine cocktails of anti-tumor mAbs that recognize different tumor epitopes that will be used in combination with chemo- or radiotherapy. It is unlikely that even an optimized mAb will be curative as monotherapy. In contrast to using mAbs to treat cancer, using mAbs as immunomodulatory agonists is much more complicated and many more precautions need to be addressed in regards to structural design of the mAb and clinical trials. This issue has gained urgency after the failure of a clinical trial using an anti-CD28 mAb for treatment of autoimmune diseases. CD-28 normally regulates T cell proliferation and cytokine production and is important in immune system homeostasis (Gardner 2006).

Development of therapeutic mAbs has shifted largely from academia to the industrial sector. This stimulates a lot of competition but due to intellectual property confidentiality less information is available in regards to preclinical trials. Considering the great promise of mAbs in diagnosis and therapy, we hope that the design and conduct of clinical trials will have open access to results and data for the most important reason, the patient.

References

Andrew P, Chapman PA, Spitali M, West S, Stephens S, King DJ (1999) Therapeutic antibody fragments with prolonged in vivo half-lives. Nat Biotechnol 17:780–783

Barbas CF 3rd, Hu D, Dunlop N, Sawyer L, Cababa D, Hendry RM, Nara PL, Burton DR (1994) In vitro evolution of a neutralizing human antibody to human immunodeficiency virus type 1 to enhance affinity and broaden strain cross-reactivity. Proc Natl Acad Sci USA 91:3809–3813

Blanchard C, Mishra A, Saito-Akei H, Monk P, Anderson I, Rothenberg ME (2005) Inhibition of human interleukin-13-induced respiratory and oesophageal inflammation by anti-human-interleukin-13 antibody (CAT-354). Clin Exp Allergy 35:1096–1103

Blattman JN, Greenberg PD (2004) Cancer immunotherapy: a treatment for the masses. Science 305(5681):200–205

Boder ET, Wittrup KD (1997) Yeast surface display for screening combinatorial polypeptide libraries. Nat Biotechnol 15:553–557

Borghaei H, Schilder RJ (2004) Safety and efficacy of radioimmunotherapy with yttrium 90 ibritumomab tiuxetan (Zevalin). Semin Nucl Med 34:4–9

Boulianne GL, Hozumi N, Shulman MJ (1984) Production of functional chimaeric mouse/human antibody. Nature 312:643–646

Cambridge G, Leandro M, Edwards J, Ehrenstein M, Salden M, Bodman-Smith M, Webster A (2003) Serologic changes following B lymphocyte depletion therapy for rheumatoid arthritis. Arthritis Rheum 48:2146–2154

Carlos Vaccaro JZ, Ober RJ, Wardl ES (2005) Engineering the Fc region of immunoglobulin G to modulate in vivo antibody levels. Nat Biotechnol 23:1283–1288

Carter P (2006) Potent antibody therapeutics by design. Nat Rev Immunol 6:343–357

Chapman AP (2002) PEGylated antibodies and antibody fragments for improved therapy: a review. Adv Drug Deliv Rev 54:531–545

Coiffier B, Haioun C, Ketterer N, Engert A, Tilly H, Ma D, Johnson P, Lister A, Feuring-Buske M, Radford JA, Capdeville R, Diehl V, Reyes F (1998) Rituximab (anti-CD20 monoclonal antibody) for the treatment of patients with relapsing or refractory aggressive lymphoma: a multicenter phase II study. Blood 92:1927–1932

Cosimi AB, Burton RC, Colvin RB, Goldstein G, Delmonico FL, LaQuaglia MP, Tolkoff-Rubin N, Rubin RH, Herrin JT, Russell PS (1981) Treatment of acute renal allograft rejection with OKT3 monoclonal antibody. Transplantation 32:535–539

de Kruif J, Baker AB, Marissen WE, Kramer RA, Throsby M, Rupprecht CE, Goudsmit J. Crucell Holland BV, Leiden, (2007) A Human Monoclonal Antibody Cocktail as a Novel Component of Rabies Postexposure Prophylaxis. Annu Rev Med 58:359–368

de Wildt RM, Mundy CR, Gorick BD, Tomlinson IM (2000) Antibody arrays for high-throughput screening of antibody–antigen interactions. Nat Biotechnol 18:989–994

Dyer MJ (1999) The role of CAMPATH-1 antibodies in the treatment of lymphoid malignancies. Semin Oncol 26:52–57

Choy EHS, Smith1 BHM, Moss K, Lisi L, Scott DGI, Patel4 J, Sopwith M, Isenberg DA (2002) Efficacy of a novel PEGylated humanized anti-TNF fragment (CDP870) in patients with rheumatoid arthritis: a phase II double-blinded, randomized, dose-escalating trial. Rheumatology 41:1133–1137

Eiermann W (2001) Trastuzumab combined with chemotherapy for the treatment of HER2-positive metastatic breast cancer: pivotal trial data. Ann Oncol 12(Suppl 1):S57–S62

Elliott MJ, Maini RN, Feldmann M, Long-Fox A, Charles P, Katsikis P, Brennan FM, Walker J, Bijl H, Ghrayeb J et al (1993) Treatment of rheumatoid arthritis with chimeric monoclonal antibodies to tumor necrosis factor alpha. Arthritis Rheum 36:1681–1690

Francis RJ, Sharma SK, Springer C, Green AJ, Hope-Stone LD, Sena L, Martin J, Adamson KL, Robbins A, Gumbrell L, O'Malley D, Tsiompanou E, Shahbakhti H, Webley S, Hochhauser D, Hilson AJ, Blakey D, Begent RH (2002) A phase I trial of antibody directed enzyme prodrug therapy (ADEPT) in patients with advanced colorectal carcinoma or other CEA producing tumours. Br J Cancer 9:600–607

Gardner K (2006) Cytokine storm and an anti-CD28 monoclonal antibody. N Engl J Med 355:2593–2594

Ghetie Vea (1997) Increasing the serum persistence of an IgG fragment by random mutagenesis. Nat Biotechnol 15:637–640

Gillies SD, Lan Y, Wesolowski JS, Qian X, Reisfeld RA, Holden S, Super M, Lo KM (1998) Antibody-IL-12 fusion proteins are effective in SCID mouse models of prostate and colon carcinoma metastases. J Immunol 160:6195–6203

Gillies SD, Reilly EB, Lo KM, Reisfeld RA (1992) Antibody-targeted interleukin 2 stimulates T-cell killing of autologous tumor cells. Proc Natl Acad Sci USA 89:1428–1432

Gillies SD, Young D, Lo KM, Foley SF, Reisfeld RA (1991) Expression of genetically engineered immunoconjugates of lymphotoxin and a chimeric anti-ganglioside GD2 antibody. Hybridoma 10:347–356

Griffiths AD, Williams SC, Hartley O, Tomlinson IM, Waterhouse P, Crosby WL, Kontermann RE, Jones PT, Low NM, Allison TJ et al (1994) Isolation of high affinity human antibodies directly from large synthetic repertoires. Embo J 13:3245–3260

Hanes J, Pluckthun A (1997) In vitro selection and evolution of functional proteins by using ribosome display. Proc Natl Acad Sci USA 94:4937–4942

Hinton PR, Johlfs MG, Xiong JM, Hanestad K, Ong KC, Bullock C, Keller S, Tang MT, Tso JY, Vasquez M, Tsurushita N (2004) Engineered human IgG antibodies with longer serum half-lives in primates. J Biol Chem 279:6213–6216

Harrison JL, Williams SC, Winter G, Nissim A (1996) Screening of phage antibody libraries. Methods Enzymol 267:83–109

Holt LJ, Herring C, Jespers LS, Woolven BP, Tomlinson IM (2003) Domain antibodies: proteins for therapy. Trends Biotechnol 21:484–490

Hoogenboom H (2005) Selecting and screening recombinant antibody libraries. Nat Biotechnol 23:1105–1116

Hudson PHPJ (2005) Engineered antibody fragments and the rise of single domains. Nat Biotechnol 23:1126–1136

Hwang WY, Foote J (2005) Immunogenicity of engineered antibodies. Methods 36:3–10

Idusogie EE, Wong P, Presta LG, Gazzano-Santoro H, Totpal K, Ultsch M, Mulkerrin MG (2001) Engineered antibodies with increased activity to recruit complement. J Immunol 166:2571–2575

Jakobovits A, Moore AL, Green LL, Vergara GJ, Maynard-Currie CE, Austin HA, Klapholz S (1993) Germ-line transmission and expression of a human-derived yeast artificial chromosome. Nature 362:255–258

Jones PT, Dear PH, Foote J, Neuberger MS, Winter G (1986) Replacing the complementarity-determining regions in a human antibody with those from a mouse. Nature 321:522–525

Kenanova V, Olafsen T, Crow DM, Sundaresan G, Subbarayan M, Carter NH, Ikle DN, Yazaki PJ, Chatziioannou AF, Gambhir SS, Williams LE, Shively JE, Colcher D, Raubitschek AA, Wu AM (2005) Tailoring the pharmacokinetics and positron emission tomography imaging properties of anti-carcinoembryonic antigen single-chain Fv-Fc antibody fragments. Cancer Res 65:622–631

Kohler G, Milstein C (1975) Continuous cultures of fused cells secreting antibody of predefined specificity. Nature 256:495–497

Kreitman RJ (1999) Immunotoxins in cancer therapy. Curr Opin Immunol 11:570–578

Kreitman RJ, Wilson WH, White JD, Stetler-Stevenson M, Jaffe ES, Giardina S, Waldmann TA, Pastan I (2000) Phase I trial of recombinant immunotoxin anti-Tac(Fv)-PE38 (LMB-2) in patients with hematologic malignancies. J Clin Oncol 18:1622–1636

Kress A (2002) Adalimumab – for use in the treatment of rheumatoid arthritis: clinical review. Abbott Laboratories Biologic Licensing Application, 1–136. Office of Therapeutics Research and Review; Division of Clinical Trial Design and Analysis; Immunology and Infectious Disease Branch

Lazar GA, Dang W, Karki S, Vafa O, Peng JS, Hyun L, Chan C, Chung HS, Eivazi A, Yoder SC, Vielmetter J, Carmichael DF, Hayes RJ, Dahiyat BI (2006) Engineered antibody Fc variants with enhanced effector function. Proc Natl Acad Sci USA 103:4005–4010

Linenberger ML (2005) CD33-directed therapy with gemtuzumab ozogamicin in acute myeloid leukemia: progress in understanding cytotoxicity and potential mechanisms of drug resistance. Leukemia 19:176–182

Lonberg N (2005) Human antibodies from transgenic animals. Nat Biotechnol 23:1117–1125

Maas RA, Dullens HF, Den Otter W (1993) Interleukin-2 in cancer treatment: disappointing or (still) promising? A review. Cancer Immunol Immunother 36:141–148

Marks J (2004) Antibody affinity maturation by chain shuffling. Methods Mol Biol 248:327–343

Robinson MK, Doss M, Shaller C, Narayanan D, Marks JD, Adler LP, González Trotter DE, Adams GP (2005) Quantitative Immuno-Positron Emission Tomography Imaging of HER2-Positive Tumor Xenografts with an Iodine-124 Labeled Anti-HER2 Diabody. Cancer Res 65:1471–1478

McWhirter JR, K.-R.A., Saven A, Maruyama T, Potter KN, Mockridge CI, Ravey EP, Qin F, Bowdish KS, Alexion Antibody Technologies I (2006) Antibodies selected from combinatorial libraries block a tumor antigen that plays a key role in immunomodulation. Proc Natl Acad Sci USA 1003:1041–1046

Meeker TC, Lowder J, Maloney DG, Miller RA, Thielemans K, Warnke R, Levy R (1985) A clinical trial of anti-idiotype therapy for B cell malignancy. Blood 65:1349–1363

Morris PJ, Russell N (2006) Alemtuzumab (Campath-1H): a systematic review in organ transplantation. Transplantation 81:1361–1367

Neri D, Carnemolla B, Nissim A, Leprini A, Querze G, Balza E, Pini A, Tarli L, Halin C, Neri P, Zardi L, Winter G (1997) Targeting by affinity-matured recombinant antibody fragments of an angiogenesis associated fibronectin isoform. Nat Biotechnol 15:1271–1275

Nissim A, Hoogenboom HR, Tomlinson IM, Flynn G, Midgley C, Lane D, Winter G (1994) Antibody fragments from a 'single pot' phage display library as immunochemical reagents. Embo J 13:692–698

Padlan EA (1991) A possible procedure for reducing the immunogenicity of antibody variable domains while preserving their ligand-binding properties. Mol Immunol 28:489–498

Reichmann L, Clark M, Waldmann H, Winter G (1988) Reshaping human antibodies for therapy. Nature 332(6162):323–327

Shawler DL, Bartholomew RM, Smith LM, Dillman RO (1985) Human immune response to multiple injections of murine monoclonal IgG. J Immunol 135:1530–1535

Shields RL et al. (2001) High resolution mapping of the binding site on human IgG1 for FcγRI, FcγRII, FcγRIII, and FcRn and design of IgG1 variants with improved binding to the FcγR. J Biol Chem 276:6591–6604

Silacci M, Brack S, Schirru G, Marlind J, Ettorre A, Merlo A, Viti F, Neri D (2005) Design, construction, and characterization of a large synthetic human antibody phage display library. Proteomics 5:2340–2350

Tao MH, Levy R (1993) Idiotype/granulocyte-macrophage colony-stimulating factor fusion protein as a vaccine for B-cell lymphoma. Nature 362:755–758

Throsby M, Geuijen C, Goudsmit J, Bakker AQ, Korimbocus J, Kramer RA, Clijsters-van der Horst M, de Jong M, Jongeneelen M, Thijsse S, Smit R, Visser TJ, Bijl N, Marissen WE, Loeb M, Kelvin DJ, Preiser W, ter Meulen J, de Kruif J (2006) Isolation and characterization of human monoclonal antibodies from individuals infected with West Nile Virus. J Virol 80(14):6982–6992

Vaughan TJ, Williams AJ, Pritchard K, Osbourn JK, Pope AR, Earnshaw JC, McCafferty J, Hodits RA, Wilton J, Johnson KS (1996) Human antibodies with sub-nanomolar affinities isolated from a large non-immunized phage display library. Nat Biotechnol 14:309–314

von Mehren M, Adams G, Weiner LM (2003) Monoclonal antibody therapy for cancer. Annu Rev Med 54:343–369

Wahl R (2005) Tositumomab and (131)I therapy in non-Hodgkin's lymphoma. J Nucl Med 46(Suppl 1):128S–140S

Ward S , Mandez C, Vaccaro C, Zhou J, Tang Q, Ober RJ (2005) From sorting endosomes to exo-cytosis: association of Rab4 and Rab11 GTPases with the Fc receptor, FcRn, during recycling. Mol Biol Cell 16:2028–2038

Weinblatt E, Ketystone C, Furst DE et al (2003) Adalimumab, a fully human anti-tumor necro-sis factor α monoclonal antibody, for the treatment of rheumatoid arthritis in patients taking concomitant methotrexate. The ARMADA Trial. Arthritis Rheum 48:35–45

Winter G, G.A., Hawkins RE, Hoogenboom HR (1994) Making antibodies by phage display tech-nology. Annu Rev Immunol 12:433–455

Wu AM, Senter P (2005) Arming antibodies: prospects and challenges for immunoconjugates. Nat Biotechnol 23:1137–1146

Zhang W, Feng J, Li Y, Guo N, Shen B (2005) Humanization of an anti-human TNF-a antibody by variable region resurfacing with the aid of molecular modeling. Mol Immunol 42:1445–1451

Zhao L, Rai SK, Grosmaire LS, Ledbetter JA, Fell HP (1999) Construction, expression, and char-acterization of anticarcinoma sFv fused to IL-2 or GM-CSF. J Hematother Stem Cell Res 8: 393–399

Preclinical Safety Evaluation of Monoclonal Antibodies

C.M. Lynch and I.S. Grewal(⊠)

1   Introduction   20
2   Goals of Preclinical Safety Evaluation   23
    2.1   General Considerations   23
    2.2   Start with the End in Mind.   23
    2.3   Coordinate the Preclinical Safety Program in Step
          with the Phases of Clinical Development   23
    2.4   Plan for Process Development Changes   24
    2.5   Start Assay Development Early   25
3   Critical Issues for Success   26
    3.1   Relevant Species   26
    3.2   Science-Driven Approach   28
    3.3   Exposure   28
4   Preclinical Safety Studies   30
    4.1   Preclinical Safety Studies to Support Phase I   30
    4.2   Preclinical Safety Studies to Support Phase II.   33
    4.3   Preclinical Studies to Support Phase III   34
    4.4   Preclinical Safety Studies to Support Marketing   34
    4.5   Preclinical Studies with Payload Antibodies   38
    4.6   Guidance Documents   40
    4.7   Antibody Toxicities   41
5   Summary   42
References   43

List of abbreviations

ADC, antibody drug conjugates; ADCC, antibody-dependent cellular cytotoxicity; ADCP, antibody-dependent cellular phagocytosis; AUC, area under the serum

I.S. Grewal

Department of Preclinical Therapeutics, Seattle Genetics, Bothell, WA 98021, USA

e-mail: igrewal@seagen.com

Y. Chernajovsky, A. Nissim (eds.) *Therapeutic Antibodies. Handbook of Experimental Pharmacology 181.*
© Springer-Verlag Berlin Heidelberg 2008

concentration–time curve; BLA, Biologics License Application; CDC, complement-dependent cytotoxicity; C_{max}, model-predicted maximum serum concentration; CMC, chemistry manufacturing and controls; C_{min}, model-predicted minimum serum concentration; CNS, central nervous system; CRO, contract research organization; ECL, electrochemiluminescence; ELISA, enzyme-linked immuno sorbent assay; FDA, Food and Drug Administration; GLP, good laboratory practice; HNSTD, highest nonseverely toxic dose; ICH, International Conference on Harmonisation; IND, Investigational New Drug; IV, intra venous; mAb, monoclonal antibody; MS, multiple sclerosis: MTD, maximum tolerated dose; NOAEL, no adverse effect level; OECD, Organisation for Economic Cooperation and Development; PK, pharmacokinetic; PML, progressive multifocal leukoencepphalopathy; PTC, points to consider; TDAR, T cell dependent antibody response; TK, toxicokinetics; VEGF, vascular endothelial cell growth factor.

Abstract Monoclonal antibodies (mAbs) are a well-established product class of biotechnology-derived pharmaceuticals for treating multiple diseases. A growing number of mAbs are being tested in clinical trials worldwide. Many of the second generation mAbs entering the clinic today are highly engineered, produced from recombinant cell lines, and present new safety challenges for regulators and industry scientists responsible for their safety evaluation. The increasing complexity of antibodies and the variety of recombinant production cell systems used for antibody manufacturing require a well thoughtout approach for preclinical safety evaluation of mAbs. The focus of this chapter is to provide the reader with a basic framework for preparing a scientifically sound preclinical package for safety evaluation of therapeutic mAbs. We outline the general considerations for planning a preclinical program and the issues critical for success. We describe the types of preclinical safety studies and the timing for their conduct in relation to clinical trials. We also share some of the lessons learned about toxicity of mAbs from previous antibody development programs. A list of relevant regulatory documents issued by various government agencies and selected references to other useful texts and publications are also provided in the chapter. We believe that applying the principles described in this chapter will improve the quality and relevance of the preclinical safety data generated to support the future development of mAbs therapeutics.

1 Introduction

During the past 20 years, great progress has been made in developing monoclonal antibodies (mAbs) as major biotherapeutics for a wide variety of diseases, including cancers, inflammatory diseases, autoimmune conditions, and infections. There are 19 approved mAbs for therapeutic use in the US today (Table 1) and a growing number of mAbs are being tested in clinical trials worldwide (Reichert et al. 2005; Adams and Weiner 2005; Kim et al. 2005). An ever-increasing number of mAbs for diagnosis and treatment are most likely to fill the pipelines of many companies in

Table 1 Approved antibodies for therapeutic use

Approval date	Antibody	Name	Target	Antibody type	Indication	Company
1986 (US)	Muromonab-CD3	OKT3	CD3	Murine, IgG2a	A & I*	Johnson & Johnson
1984 (US)	Abciximab	ReoPro	PIIb/IIIa	Chimeric, IgG1, Fab	Hemostasis	Centocor
1987 (US) 1988 (EU)	Rituximab	Rituxan	CD20	Chimeric, IgG1	Cancer	Genentech
1997 (US) 1999 (EU)	Daclizumab	Zenapax	CD25	Humanized, IgG1	A & I*	Roche
1998 (US) 1998 (EU)	Basiliximab	Simulect	CD25	Chimeric, IgG1	A & I*	Novartis
1998 (US) 1999 (EU)	Palivizumab	Synagis	RSV	Humanized, IgG1	Infections	MedImmune
1998 (US) 1999 (EU)	Infliximab	Remicade	TNFα	Chimeric, IgG1	A & I*	Centocor
1998 (US) 2000 (EU)	Trastuzumab	Herceptin	HER2	Humanized, IgG1	Cancer	Genentech
2000 (US)	Gemtuzumab ozogamicin	Mylotarg	CD33	Humanized, IgG4, immunotoxin	Cancer	Wyeth
2001 (US) 2001 (EU)	Alemtuzumab	Campath-1H	CD52	Humanized, IgG1	Cancer	Genzyme
2002 (US) 2004 (EU)	Ibritumomab tiuxetan	Zevalin	CD20	Murine, IgG1, radiolabeled (Yttrium 90)	Cancer	Biogen Idec
2002 (US) 2003 (EU)	Adalimumab	Humira	TNFα	Human, IgG1	A & I*	Abbott
2003 (US)	Omalizumab	Xolair	IgE	Humanized, IgG1	A & I*	Genentech
2003 (US)	Tositumomab-I131	Bexxar	CD20	Murine, IgG2a, radiolabeled (Iodine 131)	Cancer	Corixa/GSK
2003 (US) 2004 (EU)	Efalizumab	Raptiva	CD11a	Humanized, IgG1	A & I*	Genentech
2004 (US) 2004 (EU)	Cetuximab	Erbitux	EGFR	Chimeric, IgG1	Cancer	Imclone
2004 (US) 2005 (EU)	Bevacizumab	Avastin	VEGF	Humanized, IgG1	Cancer	Genentech
2004 (US)	Natalizumab	Tysabri	α4-intergrin	Humanized, IgG4	A & I*	Biogen Idec
2006 (US)	Panitumumab	Vectibix	EGFR	Human, IgG2	Cancer	Amgen

*A & I = Autoimmune and inflammatory indications

the near future as a result of breakthroughs in antibody technologies coupled with identification of additional molecular targets of disease. Therefore, it is essential to conduct appropriate preclinical safety studies of mAbs to support more rapid clinical development of antibody therapeutics and ensure patient safety.

The first generations of mAb therapeutics were produced from mouse hybridomas and had limited success in the clinic. This was partially due to their inability to effectively interact with human effector cells and their rapid clearance from the system because of immunogencity (Carter 2006). With the advent of recombinant DNA technology, generation of chimeric and humanized mAbs (by grafting of the Fc portion and variable regions of the mouse antibodies with human counterparts) has alleviated some of these problems (Carter 2006). Many new technologies are now available that allow production of fully human antibodies (Hoogenboom 2005; Lonberg 2005; Carter 2006). Recombinant technology has also allowed further refinements of antibody sequences to alter the binding affinity and Fc effector functions. It is thus possible to customize mAbs for desired effector functions, such as antibody-dependent cellular cytotoxicity (ADCC) and complement-dependent cytotoxicity (CDC). Most of the mAbs in the clinic today are genetically modified to incorporate more human characteristics aimed at reducing immunogenicity and enhancing interaction with human effector cells. The second generation of mAbs that are modified to alter glycosylation, target binding affinity, and half-life are now entering product development in an effort to improve efficacy and to increase the chances for clinical success (Adams and Weiner 2005; Carter 2006).

In parallel with the advances in antibody engineering, there has also been an evolution of the technology for generation of high titer mAb producing cell lines of both mammalian and nonmammalian origins (Carson 2005). A variety of different expression systems and production cell lines are now available for small and large-scale commercial manufacture of mAbs (Birch and Racher et al. 2006). Thus, the increasing complexity of antibody engineering and the variety of recombinant production cell systems available for antibody generation make it more critical than ever that a thorough and thoughtful approach be taken to the preclinical safety evaluation of monoclonal antibodies. In addition to their novel peptide nature, complex structure, unique biologic functions, and longer half-lives, the more routine utilization of engineered antibodies to treat chronic diseases (Kim et al. 2005) also adds to the potential safety concerns for their prolonged clinical use.

In this chapter, we provide a basic framework for preparing a scientifically sound preclinical package for safety evaluation of therapeutic mAbs. We outline the general considerations for planning a preclincal program and the issues critical for success. We describe the types of preclinical safety studies and the timing for their conduct in relation to clinical trials. We also share some of the lessons learned from previous development of antibodies. We identify the relevant regulatory documents along with selected references to other useful texts and publications. The chapter will serve as a roadmap, providing guiding principles and directing the reader to additional sources of information. We hope that application of the principles described in this chapter will improve the quality and relevance of the preclinical safety data generated to support the development of mAbs therapeutics.

2 Goals of Preclinical Safety Evaluation

The three main goals of preclinical safety evaluation of monoclonal antibodies and any biopharmaceutical are:

1. To determine a safe starting dose for the first in human Phase 1 clinical trial and subsequent dose escalation schemes
2. To identify potential target organs of toxicity and to determine whether the toxicity is reversible after a period of time following the end of treatment
3. To identify parameters that can be used to monitor safety in the clinical trials

Meeting these goals is achieved through the conduct of in vitro and in vivo non-clinical studies aimed at defining and understanding the toxicological properties of the antibody. To design an appropriate safety assessment of an antibody, it is best to have first characterized its pharmacological properties such as receptor affinity, receptor occupancy, and biological activity related to its intended therapeutic application. An understanding of the exposure response relationship is an integral part of the preclinical safety evaluation of monoclonal antibodies. Initial estimates of pharmacokinetic (PK) parameters are helpful in designing the duration of the recovery period, for example, in repeated dose-toxicity studies. Since the toxicology package is intended to support the clinical program from Phase I to approval, clearly defined clinical trials are a prerequisite for designing the supporting toxicology program. General considerations for planning a nonclincial safety evaluation program for a monoclonal antibody will be discussed below and the issues that are critical for success will be highlighted.

2.1 General Considerations

2.2 Start with the End in Mind

The most efficient way to plan a nonclincial development strategy is to start with the end in mind and to work backwards. This may seem counter-intuitive, but experience has proven time and time again that it is the most effective approach. A very useful exercise to do at the outset of the program is to write the label for the product in collaboration with clinical, regulatory, and manufacturing. This exercise will help define the key components (e.g., indication, patient population, dosing regimen, duration of treatment, route of administration, formulation, etc.) required for designing the toxicology package.

2.3 Coordinate the Preclinical Safety Program in Step with the Phases of Clinical Development

The next step in the process is to list all of the nonclinical pharmacology and toxicology studies anticipated to be conducted over the entire course of the development of the product from the investigational new drug (IND) phase to postmarketing. Then divide the studies into categories according to when they will be conducted as follows: (1) prior to initiation of Phase I clinical trial, (2) Prior to or concurrently with Phase II, and (3) concurrently with Phase III pivotal trials. Working backwards, this will allow determination of which studies are required for registration of the product i.e., to file the Biologics License Application (BLA), but need not be completed to initiate pivotal Phase III clinical trials. Examples of such studies are chronic toxicity studies and reproductive and developmental toxicology studies. Next identify toxicology studies that are required to be completed to support initiation of Phase III and Phase II trials. Often they are one and the same. Finally, identify which studies are necessary for the IND submission.

The utility of this approach is that it allows coordination of the timing of the conduct of the safety study in step with the phases of drug development. The necessity for safety studies and the timing of their conduct is not solely governed by the clinical trials, but also by the chemistry, manufacturing and controls (CMC) development strategy that will be discussed in the next section. One of the most common occurrences in toxicology programs is need to conduct similar toxicity studies more than once because of lack of coordination with Clinical and CMC. Often the duration of treatment in the Phase I trial is shorter that the intended labeled clinical use of the product. Thus, the duration of treatment is longer in Phase II and beyond. If the IND-enabling studies are designed strictly to support the shorter duration Phase I trial then they will not be adequate to support Phase II and will necessitate the conduct of a second toxicity study of longer duration. The advantage of planning backward is that one can anticipate the need for the longer duration toxicity study beyond the initial IND and elect to conduct the longer duration toxicity study upfront. The longer duration toxicity study will provide toxicology coverage for both Phase I and II, and avoid unnecessary duplication of effort and resources.

2.4 Plan for Process Development Changes

A classic example of a CMC trigger for the need to conduct additional safety evaluations is a process change in the manufacture of the antibody. Changes can consist of upstream changes to the culture conditions of cell lines for recombinant derived mAbs or even a change in the production cell line itself, and downstream purification changes or formulation changes. Efforts will be undertaken to demonstrate comparability of the new product to the old process first using analytical methods. However, if the changes are of a sufficient magnitude that comparability cannot be assured using in vitro analytical methods alone, then a bridging toxicity study or an entirely new toxicity study will be necessary.

2.4.1 Keep Product for Comparability Studies and Bridging Strategies

A bridging toxicity study in which the old and new product is compared in a truncated study design (e.g., a short duration with a subset of endpoints) using at least one dose level of the old product to compare with the new is the most cost effective approach. It is essential that a sufficient supply of the early phase material is retained for a bridging study. It is a widespread practice to continue process development after initiation of the Phase I trial. Therefore, it is prudent to plan for a bridging study and include material for the study in the initial estimates of drug supply needs. If early phase material has not been reserved to conduct a bridging study then it may be necessary to conduct a comprehensive toxicity study de novo with antibody from the new process, essentially repeating what has done already with the early process material.

2.5 Start Assay Development Early

The final general consideration is the need to start assay development early, well in advance of the planning for the toxicity study. The lead time for assay development can be anywhere from nine months to a year. Additional time will be necessary if the assay has to be transferred to a contract research organization (CRO) and validated prior to implementation of testing specimens from the toxicity study. Product specific assays are needed to determine the stability and concentration of the antibody in a number of settings and matrices.

2.5.1 Dose Solution Analysis

It is a Good Laboratory Practice (GLP) requirement that the concentration of the antibody in the solution used for dose administration be verified. The CMC group may have an assay in place for lot release testing of the formulated antibody that can be adapted. Please be aware that the antibody will be diluted to levels considerably lower than that found in the final drug product, so additional assay development will be needed to ensure detection of antibody at low concentrations.

Demonstration of the stability of the dose solution under the conditions of use will also be necessary. Following dilution of the antibody to prepare the dosing solution, it may be held in the viviarium at room temperature for up to 8 h on the day of dose administration. Similarly, stability data are required on the formulated drug product for the duration of the dosing period, i.e., until after the last dose is administered. Quite often the toxicology studies are conducted well in advance of clinical product manufacture and initiation of formal product stability studies. It is wise to alert the CMC group or other group responsible for assay development that an assay to demonstrate antibody product stability will be needed to support the toxicity study in advance of the formal stability program. Stability testing can be conducted concomitantly with the toxicity study.

2.5.2 PK Assay

For the purposes of assessing the PK and toxicokinetics (TK) of the antibody it will be necessary to have an assay to measure the antibody concentration in serum from animals. The assays typically employed for this purpose are enzyme-linked immuno sorbent assay (ELISA) and utilize serum as the matrix rather than plasma. Assay performance in serum from all species employed in the safety evaluation program should be examined. One of the biggest challenges in developing an assay to assess PK is the interference observed in the presence of an immune response against the antibody. It is beyond the scope of this text to discuss the assay development per se; however, it is important to be aware of the assay limitations when examining the PK data and making interpretations about exposure.

2.5.3 Immunogenicity Assay

Many antibodies, whether murine, chimeric, or humanized, are immunogenic in animals. The induction of antibody formation in animals should be included as an endpoint in PK and toxicity studies, particularly if they involve repeated dose administration. Measurement of immunogenicity using ELISA is subject to the same limitations observed with the PK assay because of cross interference between the drug (therapeutic antibody) and antidrug antibodies. The impact of antibody formation on exposure and consequently the evaluation of safety endpoints should be taken into consideration during interpretation of the overall findings of the study. Other assay platforms such as electrochemiluminescence (ECL) can be explored for measurement of immunogenicity. Given the complexities of these assays, the sooner assay development can begin the better.

3 Critical Issues for Success

3.1 Relevant Species

The single most important element in conducting a successful preclinical safety evaluation of a monoclonal antibody is choosing the most relevant animal species for toxicity testing (Chapman et al. 2007). A relevant species is one in which the antibody is pharmacologically active and expression of the target antigen is present and exhibits a similar tissue-cross reactivity profile to humans. Ideally the properties of the antigen in the animal should be comparable with those in humans in biodistribution, function, and structure. This provides the opportunity to evaluate the toxicity arising from binding of the antibody to the target antigen, known as on-target toxicity. Furthermore, the greater the similarities in the tissue distribution of the target antigen in the animal species and in humans the more likely it is that target organs of toxicity identified in animals will be predictive for potential toxicities in humans. An animal species that expresses the target antigen, but has a somewhat different tissue distribution may still be of relevance for evaluating toxicity so long as these differences are taken into consideration for human risk assessment. Absolute equivalence of antigen density or affinity for the mAb is not necessary for an animal model to be useful. The need for a relevant animal model for safety evaluation is so critical to the overall success of the drug development program that species cross-reactivity should be included as part of the selection criteria when screening antibodies during lead selection.

Toxicity studies in nonrelevant species may not simply be uninformative, but may be misleading and are, therefore, discouraged. When no relevant model exists, there are two options, neither of which is entirely satisfactory. The first option is the use of transgenic animals that have been engineered to express the human target antigen. The utility of a transgenic animal for safety evaluation is determined by the extent to which the pharmacodymanics resulting from the antibody antigen interaction are similar to those anticipated in humans. The pharmacokinetic properties of the antibody in the transgenic mouse model are quite likely to be very different than in humans.

The second option is to consider developing a surrogate antibody to the human therapeutic antibody that is cross-reactive with the homologous antigen in animals suitable for toxicity testing. The disadvantage of this approach is that the safety evaluation will not be performed on the antibody that will be administered to humans. It should be noted that no two antibodies are exactly alike and there is inherent risk in this approach. Furthermore, the production process, impurities, pharmacokinetics, binding affinity, and mechanism of action may differ between the surrogate and therapeutic antibodies. In addition, the use of a surrogate antibody adds considerable cost to the product development because of the need to produce two antibodies for the program.

When it is not feasible to use either transgenic animal models or surrogate antibodies, it may still be advisable to conduct an assessment of the off-target toxicities of the antibody focused on evaluation of any functional effects on the major physiological systems (e.g., cardiovascular and respiratory) akin to a safety pharmacology study. Although information may be gained from these studies, the challenge is to know to what extent it is relevant to human risk assessment. The more information available on the pharmacology of the antibody intended for clinical use the better the utility of these alternative approaches can be assessed. Surrogate antibodies have been successfully used to evaluate reproductive and developmental toxicity and support licensure of monoclonal antibody products, e.g., Infliximab (Remicade®) and Efalizumab (Raptiva®).

3.2 Science-Driven Approach

Stating that taking a science-driven approach to design safety studies is the key to success may seem a little bit like stating the obvious. However, many scientists are confronted with the pressure to simply conduct whatever studies are requested of them by a regulatory authority, even if they are not relevant. Taking a "check the box" approach to the safety evaluation of a mAb may ultimately do a disservice to both the mAb product development program and the regulatory agency. First of all, a study critical to elucidating the toxic potential of the antibody may fail to be done during preclinical testing, only to be discovered later in the clinic. Typically, the sponsor will know the properties of the antibody better than the agency. The sponsor can facilitate the review process by furnishing the pharmacology and toxicology reviewer with pertinent information about the mAb so that together they can assure human safety.

3.2.1 Knowledge of the mAb and Target Antigen Biology

Knowledge of the biology of the antibody and its target antigen will allow better design of a toxicity study that will evaluate the safety and potential toxicity of the antibody. In order for mAbs to be clinically effective, a combination of mechanisms of action directed at their desired effects is typically needed. In this regard, mAbs provide multiple effector functions and other properties that make them attractive therapeutics. Some of the most relevant attributes are: (1) mAbs interact with host immune cells to induce ADCC; (2) certain isotypes of mAbs fix complement and thus induce CDC; (3) many mAbs have the potential to alter signal transduction of the target receptors thereby inducing profound changes in the target cell; (4) mAbs can also block interaction of the target antigen with its ligand(s); (5) mAbs also can enhance phagocytic ability of professional phagocytes via antibody-dependent cellular phagocytosis (ADCP); and finally (6) antibodies can also be used for targeted delivery of payloads, including radionuclides, toxins, and cytotoxic drugs.

3.3 Exposure

Antibodies typically have long half-lives compared with small molecule drugs and as a result, the antibodies may be present in the body long-after administration. In addition their pharmacological effects may last for a very long time after mAb administration (Kimby 2005). For this reason, it is important to consider the exposure–response relationship rather than the dose–response relationship during the design and interpretation of results from toxicity studies. For example, to assess if toxicity is reversible a recovery period is typically included in multiple-dose toxicity studies. The recovery period is intended to determine whether toxicity diminishes in the absence of antibody. Although antibody is not administered during the recovery period, it takes 5 half-lives for 97% of the antibody to be eliminated. The duration of the recovery period should take into account the half-life of the antibody and ensure that exposure to the antibody is diminished or absent for a period of time to assess the potential for recovery or reversibility of toxicity.

When there is a difference of greater than tenfold in affinity of the antibody across species, it is helpful to use exposure rather than nominal dose administered to ensure appropriate design of the studies. Specifically, if the affinity of the antibody for the monkey target antigen is tenfold less than for the human target then the dose administered to monkeys should be adjusted upwards to ensure adequate exposure in the toxicity study. Exposure–response relationships are also helpful for interspecies comparisons and determination of the therapeutic index and desired safety margin for the initial starting dose in humans, and subsequent dose-escalation schema. Antibody PK parameters (e.g., clearance) will likely differ across species. Therefore, the dose levels and dose schedule or intervals between doses will need to be adjusted to achieve equivalent exposure levels across species. Failure to adjust dose levels and dose schedules based on the species may result in errors either in direction, i.e. in inadequate dosing in the toxicity studies, or more egregiously in over-dosing in humans in the clinical trials.

Exposure can be estimated by including toxicokinetic assessments in toxicity studies. The ideal approach is to conduct a single-dose PK study where multiple blood samples are collected at numerous time intervals adequate to fully describe the serum concentration–time profile of the antibody. This allows reliable estimates of the PK parameters such as area under the serum concentration–time curve (AUC), clearance, volume of distribution, and half life. If it is not possible to conduct a PK study, then collection of blood samples after the first and in particular the last dose in a multiple-dose toxicity study may provide sufficient serum concentration data to allow estimation of PK parameters. Blood samples can be collected during the recovery period including the recovery necropsy to assist in determination of the terminal elimination half-life. At a minimum it is advisable to collect peak and trough blood samples before and after each dose, respectively. This will at least provide model-predicted maximum serum concentration (C_{max}) and model-predicted minimum serum concentration (C_{min}) values, and an increase in the latter over the time course of the study will indicate dose accumulation. Dose levels in toxicity studies of antibodies usually span 1 to 2 orders of magnitude. It is not uncommon to have disproportionately higher levels of dose accumulation at the top end of the dose range or conversely nonlinear PK at the low dose levels manifest as faster clearance of the antibody and lower exposure. It is important to be aware of these differences in exposure when relating the toxicities observed to the doses administered, especially when defining the highest nonseverely toxic dose (HNSTD) and no adverse effect level (NOAEL) that will be used to determine the starting dose in humans. It is also very helpful to define the multiples of the clinical dose that were evaluated in the toxicity studies when presenting the results to regulatory agencies.

4 Preclinical Safety Studies

The preclinical safety studies described in this section are applicable to monoclonal antibody products that encompass murine, chimeric, humanized or fully human intact immunoglobulins, or any portion of immunoglobulins including fragments, single chain antibodies, and diabodies that can interact with specific target antigens. Antibodies may contain native immunoglobulin sequences or engineered sequences and be produced from hybridomas or recombinant cell lines. Antibody products also include payload antibodies carrying radionuclides, toxins, or cytotoxic drugs, where the antibody is serving as a vector for targeted delivery of the payload. The latter, known as antibody drug conjugates (ADC) or immunoconjugates, are considered as drugs products from a regulatory perspective. Preclinical safety studies that are required for drug products must be conducted in addition to the studies for antibody products to characterize the potential toxicity of the cytotoxic drug. We strongly recommend a Pre-IND meeting with the Food and Drug Administration (FDA) before initiating pivotal preclinical safety studies (Siegel 2004). In the subsections that follow we describe the various types of preclinical safety studies and the timing of their conduct in relation to the phase of clinical development.

4.1 Preclinical Safety Studies to Support Phase I

A typical Phase I IND-enabling safety package for a monoclonal will contain at a minimum: (1) a human tissue cross-reactivity study and (2) a general toxicity study in at least one relevant species. Safety packages should normally include two relevant species; however, it is not uncommon that only one relevant species can be identified, most often a nonhuman primate. All preclinical safety studies intended to support human clinical trials must be conducted in compliance with GLP.

4.1.1 Human Tissue Cross-Reactivity Studies

When the same or related antigenic determinant is expressed on human cells or tissues other than the intended target tissue, binding of the antibody may be observed. Nontarget tissue binding known as tissue cross-reactivity may result in undesired effects that raise a safety concern. Accordingly, the potential for cross-reactivity with nontarget human tissue or cells must be assessed. A panel of 32 tissues from three unrelated human donors should be evaluated by immunohistochemisty with several concentrations of antibody. There are a number of CROs that specialize in cross-reactivity studies. They can furnish the panel of human tissues, generate an appropriate protocol, and conduct any experiments necessary to optimize the conditions for the therapeutic antibody, including labeling with biotin if required, to conduct the IHC study.

4.1.2 General Toxicity Studies

As described earlier in this chapter (Sect. 4.1), the single most important element in conducting a successful preclinical safety evaluation of a monoclonal antibody is choosing the most relevant animal species for toxicity testing. Relevant animal species for testing of monoclonal antibodies are those that express the desired epitope and demonstrate a similar tissue cross-reactivity profile as for human tissues. A variety of techniques, such as immunochemical or functional assays, can be used to identify a relevant species. One of the ways to identify relevant species for toxicity testing is to conduct species cross-reactivity studies. Tissues from a variety of species commonly used for toxicity testing can be surveyed immunohistochemically using commercially available multispecies tissue microarrays. Evaluation of antibody binding to cells from animals by FACS can also be employed and is typically more sensitive than immunohistochemical analysis of tissue sections. Comparison of the DNA and amino acid sequences of the target antigen across species should be performed and the percent homology to the human sequence determined if the sequence of the animal orthologue is available. An understanding of the functional role of the target antigen and whether it is similar across species is another consideration for determining the relevance of a species for preclinical safety evaluation. As described earlier (Sect. 3.2.1) knowledge of the biology of the target antigen, antibody, and it mechanism of action will allow better selection of an appropriate species for toxicity testing. It is customary to include a justification for the relevancy of the species selected for toxicity testing in the IND submission outlining the rationale for the selection. If safety is assessed in only one species, it is wise to provide a summary of experiments conducted that demonstrated the lack of additional relevant species.

Toxicity Study Design

The toxicity study design is determined in a number of ways by the clinical trial duration, size, scope, indication, and phase of development it is intended to support. The duration of the toxicity study should equal or exceed the duration of the clinical trial and use at least the same number or more doses of antibody than will be administered to humans. The route of administration in animals should be the same as for clinical use. Antibodies are most often administered by intravenous infusion to humans. Antibodies can be administered to nonhuman primates as a 1–2 h intravenous infusion and are usually administered to rodents as a slow intravenous (IV) bolus injection rather than an infusion. The dose schedule may be identical to the human dose schedule or the intervals between doses in animals may be decreased compared with the intervals in humans. The shorter intervals may be driven by a need to compensate for faster clearance rates of the antibody in animals or to diminish the impact of immunogenicity on exposure in the study.

A typical toxicity study has three dose levels: low, mid, and high doses of the antibody and includes a control group. The vehicle the antibody is formulated in

Table 2 Typical study design for a toxicity study of a mAb in nonhuman primates

Group	Treatment	Dose Level (mg kg^{-1})	Dose Schedule	Animal Numbers (male/female)	
				Main	Recovery
1	Vehicle control	–	Q1 wk × 4	3M/3F	2M/2F
2	Antibody	Low dose	Q1 wk × 4	3M/3F	2M/2F
3	Antibody	Mid dose	Q1 wk × 4	3M/3F	2M/2F
4	Antibody	High dose	Q1 wk × 4	3M/3F	2M/2F

is traditionally used as the control article. Dose levels should be selected to provide information on the dose–response relationship, including a toxic dose and a NOAEL dose. Toxicity testing should be performed in both male and female animals and results should be segregated according to gender for statistical analysis purposes. Thus, the numbers of animals in toxicity studies are usually quoted as the number per sex per group. An example of a multiple-dose toxicity study design for an antibody in nonhuman primates is presented in Table 2. The number of animals per group may vary depending on the species being tested. The number of animals per group is typically larger for rodents than for nonrodent species, particularly if the nonrodent species is a nonhuman primate. The number of rodents used for general toxicity studies ranges from 10 to 15 per group in the main portion of the study plus an additional 5–10 animals per group in the recovery portion of the study. Much fewer animals per group are used for nonrodent species, ranging from 3 to 4 in the main and 2–3 in the recovery portions of the study, respectively. The number of animals used per dose level determines the probability of detecting a toxic effect and should be adequate to assess potential toxicity. If toxicokinetic analyses are included in the study, additional rodents are typically added to the study for the purpose of blood collection. The number of animals required is dependent on the number of timepoints needed. Normally, sufficient blood samples can be collected from the main and recovery animals in nonrodent species without the need for additional animals dedicated for toxicokinetic analysis.

The standard endpoints assessed in a general toxicity study are listed in Table 3. Clinical signs, body weight, and changes in food consumption can serve as general indicators that the animal is not feeling well and experiencing some type of toxicity. Laboratory measurements of hematology, serum chemistry, and urinalysis parameters, collectively known as clinical pathology, provide information about the functional status of the major organ systems like the liver, kidney, hematopoietic, and immune systems. The frequency of clinical pathology assessments varies depending on the species used for toxicity testing. The blood volumes allowable for sampling for hematology and serum chemistry are greater in larger animals and thus multiple timepoints can be evaluated in life. Anatomic pathology assessments, which include macroscopic and microscopic examination of tissues and organs, allow definitive identification of the target organs of toxicity. For a very comprehensive account of the standard practices for conducting toxicity studies we highly recommend a book chapter by Roy and Andrews (2004). The standard clinical pathology parameters

Table 3 Standard endpoints in a general toxicity study

Endpoint	Frequency of Assessment
Clinical observations (cage side)	Twice daily
Detailed clinical observations	Weekly
Body weight	Weekly
Food consumption	Daily
Ophthalmology	Baseline, once during dosing phase and during recovery if changes observed
Vital signs	Every 30 min for 4 h post dose
ECG	Baseline, once during dosing phase and during recovery if changes observed (nonrodents only)
Hematology (inc. coagulation)	Periodically in-life (nonrodents) and at termination
Serum chemistry	Periodically in-life (nonrodents) and at termination
Urinalysis	Periodically in-life (nonrodents) and at termination
Gross pathology	At termination
Organ weights	At termination
Histopathology	At termination

and anatomic pathology tissues and organs examined in toxicity studies can be obtained from any CRO and are listed in the book chapter by Roy and Andrews recommended earlier.

Single and Multiple-Dose Toxicity Studies

The decision to conduct a single-dose toxicity and/or a multiple-dose toxicity study to support the initial Phase I trial is driven by the patient population, disease indication, intended number of cycles of treatment in humans, and risk benefit relationship. The duration of animal dosing for antibodies has generally been 1–3 months for repeated dose toxicity studies to support Phase I trials. For life-threatening illnesses like cancer, shorter dosing periods or acute single-dose toxicity studies may be adequate to support a short duration Phase I trial.

4.2 Preclinical Safety Studies to Support Phase II

Repeated-dose toxicity studies of longer duration than performed for the IND may be required to support Phase II. The preclinical toxicity study duration generally should meet or exceed the duration of the planned clinical trial. For example, if the Phase I study and supporting toxicity study were 1 month in duration and the proposed Phase II study is for 3 months duration, then a subchronic toxicity study of at least 3 months duration will be required to support the Phase II trial(s). It is not uncommon for a sponsor to want to obtain initial human safety on an antibody product as quickly as possible and to choose to evaluate a shorter dosing period at the early phase of development than required for ultimate licensure and use of the product. If the timeline allows it is obviously a better use of resources (e.g., animals and money) to conduct the 3-month subchronic toxicity study at the outset to support both the 1-month Phase I and 3-month Phase II trials with a single preclinical toxicity study.

4.3 Preclinical Studies to Support Phase III

One-month and 3-month toxicity studies conducted to support the Phase I and II trials may be adequate to support initiation of Phase III trials under certain circumstances. In general, longer duration studies are usually needed owing to the increased number of patients that will be exposed to the antibody. For antibodies intended for chronic administration, studies of 6–9 months duration are required for the Biologics License Application for marketing authorization (Table 4) and may be required to support Phase III depending on the duration of the pivotal Phase III studies.

4.4 Preclinical Safety Studies to Support Marketing

The preclinical safety studies required for the marketing approval of an antibody usually include single and repeated dose toxicity studies, local tolerance studies, reproduction and developmental toxicity studies, and safety pharmacology studies. In addition, antibodies intended for chronic administration require chronic toxicology studies and for nononcology indications may require evaluation of carcinogenic potential for approval. These types of studies and their relation to the conduct of human clinical trials are presented in the International Conference on Harmonisation (ICH) M3 guidance (Table 5). Antibodies whose targets are present on immune cells or can functionally cause immune suppression or stimulation should also be evaluated for immunotoxicity. Genotoxicity studies routinely conducted for small molecule pharmaceuticals are not applicable to antibodies and, therefore, should not be conducted for antibody products.

Table 4 Duration of multiple-dose toxicity studies required for mAb marketing

Duration of Clinical Trial	Duration of Nonclinical Study	
	Rodents	Nonrodents
Up to 2 weeks	1 month	1 month
Up to 1 month	3 months	3 months
Up to 3 months	6 months	3 months
>3 months	6–9 months	6–9 months

Adapted from ICH M3

Table 5 Selected guidance documents for preclinical safety evaluation of mAb

Document	Title	Web site
FDA PTC	Points to Consider in the Manufacture and Testing of Monoclonal Antibody Products for Human Use	http://www.fda.gov/cber/ gdlns/ptc_mab.pdf
ICH S6	Preclinical Safety Evaluation of Biotechnology-Derived Pharmaceuticals	http://www.fda.gov/cder/ Guidance/1859fnl.pdf
ICH M3	Nonclinical Safety Studies for the Conduct of Human Clinical Trials for Pharmaceuticals	www.fda.gov/cder/Guidance/ 1855fnl.pdf
21CFR58	Good Laboratory Practice for Nonclinical Laboratory Studies	http://www.access.gpo.gov/nara/ cfr/waisidx_03/21cfr58_03.html
OECD GLP	Good Laboratory Practice	http://www.oecd.org/department/ 0,2688,en_2649_34381_1_1_1_1, 00.html
ICH S8	Immunotoxicity Studies for Human Pharmaceuticals	http://www.fda.gov/CBER/ gdlns/ichs8immuno.htm

4.4.1 Local Tolerance

Local tolerance at the site of antibody administration should be evaluated. The formulation intended for marketing should be tested. Quite often local tolerance can be evaluated in single or repeated dose toxicity studies, thus obviating the need for separate local tolerance studies.

4.4.2 Reproduction and Developmental Toxicity Studies

The aim of reproduction toxicity studies is to reveal any effect(s) on mammalian reproduction. The combination of studies selected should allow exposure of mature adults and all stages of development from conception to sexual maturity. To allow detection of immediate and latent effects of exposure, observations should be continued through one complete life cycle, i.e., from conception in one generation through conception in the following generation. A combination of studies for effects on (1) fertility and early embryonic development, (2) prenatal and postnatal development, including maternal function, and (3) embryo–fetal development should be conducted. At the earlier phases of clinical development, repeated dose toxicity studies can provide information regarding potential effects on reproduction, particularly male fertility. Evaluation of male fertility, when appropriate, should be completed before Phase III trials.

The need for reproductive and developmental toxicity studies is dependent upon the clinical indication and intended patient population. Studies should be carried out in instances in which the antibody product is intended for repeat or chronic administration to women of childbearing potential. The specific study design and dosing schedule may be modified based on issues related to antibody species specificity, immunogenicity, biological activity, and/or a long elimination half-life. Monoclonal antibodies with prolonged immunological effects may raise specific concerns regarding potential developmental immunotoxicity. These concerns can be addressed in a developmental toxicity study design modified to assess immune function of the neonate. Developmental immunotoxicology studies can be quite challenging depending on the species used for testing and availability or lack thereof of historical data, especially for nonhuman primates. We strongly advise consultation with experts regarding the conduct of developmental immunotoxicology studies.

4.4.3 Safety Pharmacology

Safety pharmacology studies measure functional indices of potential toxicity. The aim of safety pharmacology studies is to reveal any functional effects on the major physiological systems (e.g., cardiovascular, respiratory, renal, and central nervous systems). These functional indices may be investigated in separate studies or incorporated in the design of toxicity studies. Cardiovascular assessments such as electrocardiogram, blood pressure and heart rate, and detailed clinical observations (which may reveal effects on the central nervous system (CNS) and respiratory systems) should be included in the general toxicity studies to support the IND, in particular in nonrodent species. If a safety pharmacology signal is observed in these initial toxicity studies, then specialized studies should be conducted as a follow-up. Data from unanesthetized and unrestrained animals are preferred for in vivo safety pharmacology testing. We recommend the use of telemetry for this purpose. In telemetry studies, a transmitting device implanted into test animals continuously transmits cardiac function data to a remote receiver using radio frequency communications, and allows evaluation of cardiac function in an anesthetized and unrestrained experimental animal. Investigations may also include the use of isolated organs or other test systems not involving intact animals. All of these studies may allow for a physiology-based explanation of specific organ toxicities, which should be considered carefully with respect to human use and indication(s).

4.4.4 Carcinogenicity

Standard carcinogenicity bioassays involving the conduct of long-term carcinogenicity studies in two rodent species, typically the rat and the mouse, are usually inappropriate for antibody products. In general, carcinogenicity has not been evaluated for most of the commercial antibodies on the market today with a couple of exceptions. However, assessment of carcinogenic potential should still be considered depending upon the duration of clinical dosing, patient population, and/or biological activity of the antibody (e.g., antibodies causing immunosuppression). When there is a concern about carcinogenic potential, a variety of approaches may be considered to evaluate risk. Antibody products that have the potential to support or induce proliferation of transformed cells possibly leading to neoplasia should be evaluated for antigen expression in various malignant and normal human cells. The ability of the antibody to stimulate growth of normal or malignant cells expressing the antigen should be determined. When in vitro data give cause for concern about carcinogenic potential, further studies in relevant animal models may be needed. Incorporation of sensitive indices of cellular proliferation in long term repeated dose toxicity studies may provide useful information.

4.4.5 Pharmacokinetics

Pharmacokinetic and toxicokinetic studies are warranted to the extent necessary to understand exposure in the safety studies conducted, to allow cross-species comparisons, and to predict margins of safety for clinical trials based on exposure. The importance of the exposure–response relationship in interpretation of the results from toxicity studies was described earlier in the chapter (Sect. 3.3). Traditional small molecule distribution and excretion studies that attempt to assess mass balance are not relevant for antibodies. However, studies of biodistribution may provide the initial evidence for inappropriate tissue targeting by an mAb or explain toxicities that are observed in animals. Interpretation of the data should consider the antibody species of origin, isotype, binding to serum proteins, route of administration, and level of antigen expression in the recipient. Even if antigen is expressed in an animal model, the mAb may bind the human target antigen and its animal counterpart with different affinities. Antibody half-life may also be affected by glycosylation, susceptibility to proteases, presence of circulating antigen, and host immune response. The presence of antibodies to the therapeutic mAb may alter biodistribution. The expected consequence of metabolism of antibodies is the degradation to individual amino acids. Therefore, classical biotransformation studies as performed for pharmaceuticals are not needed for unconjugated antibodies.

4.4.6 Immunotoxicity Studies

Toxicity to the immune system encompasses a variety of adverse effects. These include suppression or enhancement of the immune response. Suppression of the immune response can lead to decreased host resistance to infectious agents or tumor cells, whereas enhancement of the immune response can stimulate the expansion of autoreactive immune cells and lead to autoimmune disease. Parameters evaluated in standard toxicity studies can indicate signs of immunotoxicity, such as changes in total leukocyte counts (white blood cells) and absolute differential leukocyte counts, gross changes in any lymphoid tissues at necropsy, and histopathological changes of the spleen and thymus. However, with standard toxicity studies, doses near or at the maximum tolerated dose can result in changes to the immune system related to stress. These effects on the immune system are most likely mediated by increased corticosterone or cortisol release. Commonly observed stress-related immune changes include increases in circulating neutrophils, decreases in circulating lymphocytes, decreases in thymus weight, decreases in thymic cortical cellularity and associated histopathologic changes ("starry sky" appearance), and changes in spleen and lymph node cellularity. Increases in adrenal gland weight can also be observed. In situations with clear clinical observations (e.g., decreased body weight gain, decreased activity), some or all of the changes to lymphoid tissue and hematology parameters might be attributable to stress rather than to a direct immunotoxic effect. Caution needs to be exercised when attributing changes in the immune system observed in general toxicity studies to stress rather than to immunotoxicity. The evidence of stress should be compelling.

If immunotoxiciy is suspected then additional endpoints to assess immunotoxicity need to be incorporated in subsequent general toxicity studies or specific immunotoxicity studies need to be conducted. Immunophenotyping is one of the easier endpoints to incorporate into standard toxicity studies. Immunophenotyping is the identification and/or enumeration of leukocyte subsets using antibodies. Immunophenotyping is usually conducted by flow cytometric analysis or by immunohistochemistry. Immunophenotyping is not a functional assay. Studies to assess immune functions such as T cell dependent antibody response (TDAR) have been conducted to assess immunotoxicity of mAb. TDAR plus additional functional assays are described in the ICH S8 draft guidance for immunotoxicity studies for human pharmaceuticals (Table 5). Although the S8 guidance is intended for small molecule drugs and not biologics-like antibodies, it is, nonetheless, informative and relevant portions can be applied to immunotoxicity testing of antibodies.

4.4.7 Additional Comments

We described most of the different types of safety studies earlier that might be conducted for the sake of completeness. Not all of these studies may be required for every antibody product. Indications in life threatening or serious diseases without current effective therapy may warrant a case-by-case approach to the preclinical safety evaluation where particular studies may be abbreviated, deferred, or omitted to expedite development. The studies typically conducted for antibody products based on indications that are life threatening or not, are presented in Table 6

4.5 Preclinical Studies with Payload Antibodies

In addition to the studies outlined earlier for naked or unconjugated monoclonal antibodies, other studies are required for payload antibodies (Table 6). Immunoconjugates should be tested for stability ex vivo in plasma from humans and each of the animal species used for toxicity testing. Immunoconjugate stability should

Table 6 Preclincal Safety Studies of mAbs requited based on disease indication

Study type	Indication	
	Life Threatening	Nonlife Threatening
Tissue cross-reactivity	Yes	Yes
General toxicity	Yes	Yes
Immunotoxicty	Yes	Yes
Safety Pharmacology	Yes	Yes
Chronic toxicity	No	Yes
Reproductive & developmen-tal toxicity	Yes	Yes
Carcinogenicity	No	Yes
Genetic toxicity	No	No
Additional studies for pay-load Abs		
PK/TK: conjugate, Ab & free payload	Yes	NA
Plasma stability	Yes	NA
Metabolism (drug payload)	Yes	NA
Distribution	yes	NA

To date antibodies carrying payloads such as radionuclides, toxin, or cytotoxic drugs have only been developed for life-threatening oncology indications

also be assessed in vivo. Individual components of an immunoconjugate should be measured during pharmacokinetic and tissue distribution studies in animals and compared with the distribution of unconjugated antibody. The target tissues for the various components and the potential toxicities should be established. Immunoconjugates containing radionuclides, toxins, or drugs should undergo animal toxicity testing, even when the target antigen is not present in an animal species, because of possible conjugate degradation and release of the payload or activity in sites that are not the result of mAb targeting. The toxicity studies should contain three dose levels of the immunoconjugate and at least one dose level of the free drug and unconjugated antibody to allow comparisons of toxicities produced by the individual components. For the unconjugated antibody and the free drug, the dose level should be the molar equivalent to the high dose of the immunoconjugate if possible. If the unconjugated free drug at the equivalent high-dose level will not be tolerated then the maximum tolerated dose (MTD) can be used. The toxicity profile of each component should adequately describe the incidence and severity of possible adverse effects. Results should be correlated closely with studies of conjugate stability. Depending upon the nature of the components of the immunoconjugate and the stability of the conjugate itself, separate studies of the components may be warranted. Studies of the immunoconjugate should be performed in a species with the relevant target antigen, whenever available, and generally in rodents if a target antigen-positive species is not available. In cases where the cytotoxic drug in the conjugate is a new chemical entity, toxicity testing in two species, rodent and non-rodent, should be considered. For immunoconjugates containing radionuclides there should be complete accounting of the metabolism of the total dose of administered radioactivity and an adequate number of time points to determine early and late elimination phases in PK and TK assessments.

4.6 Guidance Documents

Table 5 lists the recommended guidance documents that provide useful information that is relevant for planning and executing a preclinical safety evaluation package for a monoclonal antibody product. We recommend starting with the ICH S6 "Preclinical Safety Evaluation of Biotechnology-Derived Pharmaceuticals" document. It is the primary guidance for preclincal safety evaluation of biotechnology-derived products including monoclonal antibodies. It indicates the goals of preclincal studies, outlines principles for study design, and provides an overview of the types of safety studies that are required. The FDA issued a revised version of the "Points to Consider (PTC) in the Manufacturing and Testing of Monoclonal Antibody Products for Human Use" in 1997. The PTC has a broad scope and covers manufacture and testing, and preclinical studies and clinical studies of mAbs. Reading Section III, Preclinical Studies, of the PTC document will provide the necessary information for designing a preclinical safety evaluation program. The information provided is more detailed in some aspects that in the ICH S6 document and is focused on mAbs specifically. There is a thorough description of cross-reactivity studies of mAbs. There is also a section on preclincal studies with immunoconjugates that is helpful. The ICH M3 "Nonclinical Safety Studies for the Conduct of Human Clinical Trials for Pharmaceuticals" guidance is similar in content to S6 with more detailed information on the recommended duration of repeated-dose toxicity studies and types of reproductive toxicity studies required in relation to the phases of clinical development. There are two documents that describe good laboratory practice for the conduct of preclincial safety studies; one issued by the FDA and the second one issued by the Organization for Economic Cooperation and Development (OECD). The FDA document is published in the Code of Federal Regulations, Title 21, Part 58 (21CFR58). It prescribes good laboratory practices that are intended to assure the quality and integrity of the preclinical safety data submitted in support of initiation of clinical trials in humans. Both documents describe the conditions and process by which studies should be performed, monitored, recorded, archived, and reported. The OECD also provides information on the organization and management of multisite studies that is helpful. Finally, the ICH S8 "Immunotoxicity Studies for Human Pharmaceuticals" guideline provides recommendations on nonclinical testing for immunosuppression induced by low molecular weight drugs. Although the S8 guidance is intended for small molecule drugs and not biologics like antibodies, it is, nonetheless, informative and relevant portions can be applied to immunotoxicity testing of antibodies.

4.7 Antibody Toxicities

Toxicity of mAbs can result from their effector functions, the antigen and associated pathways, or mechanism of action and have been encountered in previous development programs of therapeutic antibodies. More recently the potential toxicities associated with the use of super-agonist antibodies have been illustrated. We describe here selected examples of the types of toxicities observed.

A variety of side-effects and toxicities have occurred because of binding of mAbs to antigen on tissues other than the intended target organ or tumor. Binding of Cetuximab (anti-EGFR, Erbitux®) to normal skin due to expression of the target antigen causes significant skin eruptions (Robert et al. 2001; Herbst and Langer 2002). Trials for anti-CD40L antibody were discontinued because of expression of the target on platelets, which resulted in severe thromobolytic events (Sidiropoulos and Boumpas 2004). Toxicity seen with Trastuzumab (anti-Her2, Herceptin®) is the result of binding of this antibody with low levels of target antigen expressed on heart tissue (Slamon et al. 2001). Toxicity can also result from binding to the intended target. Rapid lysis of normal and tumor B cells upon binding of Rituximab (anti-CD20, Rituxan®) results in infusion related toxicity (Byrd et al. 1999). The use of anti-CTLA-4 antibodies in clinical trials demonstrated CTLA-4 pathway related toxicity, which leads to uncontrolled general activation of T cells resulting in autoimmunity (Phan et al. 2003). Treatment of patients with Bevacizumab (anti-VEGF, Avastin®) results in multiple toxicities including hypertension, bleeding, proteinuria, and thrombosis. It is very likely that these toxicities are related to disruption of the normal functions of vascular endothelial cell growth factor (VEGF) (Hurwitz et al. 2004).

Concerns arising from target-biology related toxicities have been most recently illustrated by experiences with two therapeutic mAbs, Natalizumab (α4-intergrin, Tysabri®) and TGN1412 (αCD28) (Suntharalingam et al. 2006). Shortly after accelerated approval of Natalizumab for treatment of multiple sclerosis (MS), it was recalled from the market and clinical trials were suspended because it induced a rare fatal viral demyelinating disease, progressive multifocal leukoencepphalopathy (PML), in two patients (Scott 2005; Berger Koralnik 2005; Berger 2006a). Nataltizumab is an IgG4 mAb, which lacks significant effector function but binds to α4β1-integrin and blocks migration of lymphocytes to the various tissues and organs. Lymphocytes routinely conduct immune surveillance in the body to check for infection emerging from new pathogens or previously dormant viruses. One of the most favored hypotheses is that Natalizumab inhibited the migration and homing of lymphocytes to the CNS, which resulted in the activation of a latent polyomavirus JC in the brain that led to the development of PML (Berger 2006b). The FDA approved return of Natalizumab to the market subject to a special restricted distribution program following a comprehensive review of more than 3 000 patients that revealed a total of five cases of PML.

A second highly publicized case of target-related toxicities with mAbs was the initiation of a Phase I trial with TGN1412, a new super-agonist immune system altering antibody, which targets the CD28 antigen expressed abundantly on T cells.

The first in man administration of this super-agonist mAb in six healthy volunteers led to devastating toxicities because of massive activation of T cells. Minutes after receiving the first dose of the antibody all six healthy volunteers manifested severe systemic inflammatory responses. The response started with a release of pro-inflammatory cytokines, which was manifested clinically as nausea, headaches, diarrhea, hypotension, vasodilatation, and fever. The condition of the subjects became very critical in next 12–16 h and was characterized by pulmonary infiltrates, renal failure, and disseminated intravascular coagulation. Patients also had unexpected depletion of monocytes and marked lymphopenia within 24 h of the initial antibody infusion (Suntharalingam et al. 2006).

It is clear from the above examples that mAbs that are functionally immunomodulatory can alter the immune response in fundamental ways. It is, therefore, recommended that mAbs that work through effector functions such as ADCC, CDC, or ADCP or have the functional ability to induce a robust biologic response should be thoroughly evaluated in relevant in vitro and in vivo models before first in man clinical trials are initiated. Furthermore, it is necessary to understand the biology of the antigen and antibody across species, especially those aspects that cannot be fully evaluated in preclinical animal models, so that human risk assessment is made in light of the limitations of the preclinical models and appropriate starting doses are selected.

5 Summary

Although therapeutic antibody products have been with us for over two decades, the complexity and diversity of antibody products entering clinical development has greatly increased in the past few years. We have a variety of recombinant antibody products (e.g., chimeric and humanized mAb, single chain and dimeric Fvs), fully human antibodies, and a host of methods for their production. Antibodies have been engineered to enhance their effector functions and alter their half lives. It is more important than ever that appropriate preclinical safety evaluations are designed to support clinical development and ensure patient safety. Preclinical testing concerns surrounding mAb products include their effector function(s), tissue cross-reactivity, immunogenicity, and stability. The critical issues for conducting a successful preclinical safety evaluation of a monoclonal antibody product are identifying a relevant species for toxicity testing, using knowledge of the biology of the target antigen and antibody to inform the design of the studies, and interpretating of the results in terms of the exposure–response relationship. Preclinical testing schemes should parallel to the extent feasible those anticipated for clinical use with respect to dose, concentration, schedule, route, and duration. Preclinical safety testing of mAb is designed to identify possible toxicities in humans, to estimate the likelihood and severity of potential adverse events in humans, and to identify a safe starting dose and dose escalation scheme. It is essential that they are designed appropriately to identify key toxicities and parameters for monitoring safety in the clinic. Preclinical studies should be conducted in step with the clinical trials to ensure that appropriate studies for assessing human risk have been conducted prior to each stage of development. It is important to be very familiar with the guidance documents for preclincal safety testing and to be knowledgeable about the biology of antibodies and target antigens through continued review of the literature and interactions with the scientific community. Finally, regular communication with the FDA or other regulatory authorities is essential.

References

Adams GP and Weiner LM (2005) Monoclonal antibody therapy of cancer. Nat Biotechnol 23:1147–1157

Berger JR (2006a) Natalizumab and progressive multifocal leucoencephalopathy. Ann Rheum Dis 65:iii48–iii53

Berger JR (2006b) Natalizumab. Drugs Today 42:639–655

Berger JR and Koralnik IJ (2005) Progressive multifocal leukoencephalopathy and natalizumab–unforeseen consequences. N Engl J Med 353:414–416

Birch JR Racher AJ (2006) Antibody production. Adv Drug Deliv Rev 58:671–85

Byrd JC et al. (1999) Rituximab therapy in hematologic malignancy patients with circulating blood tumor cells: association with increased infusion-related side effects and rapid blood tumor clearance. J Clin Oncol 17: 791–795

Carson KL (2005) Flexibility–the guiding principle for antibody manufacturing. Nat Biotechnol 23:1054–1058

Carter PJ (2006) Potent antibody therapeutics by design. Nat Rev Immunol 6:343–357

Chapman K et al. (2007) Preclinical safety testing of monoclonal antibodies: the significance of species relevance. Nat Rev Drug Discov 6:120–6.

Herbst RS and Langer CJ (2002) Epidermal growth factor receptors as a target for cancer treatment: the emerging role of IMC-C225 in the treatment of lung and head and neck cancers. Semin Oncol 29:27–36

Hurwitz H et al. (2004) Bevacizumab plus irinotecan fluorouracil, and leucovorin for metastatic colorectal cancer. N Engl J Med 350:2335–2342

Hoogenboom HR (2005) Selecting and screening recombinant antibody libraries. Nat Biotechnol 23:1105–1116

Kim SJ et al. (2005) Antibody engineering for the development of therapeutic antibodies. Mol Cells 20:17–29

Kimby E (2005) Tolerability and safety of rituximab (MabThera). Cancer Treat Rev 31:456–73

Lonberg N (2005) Human antibodies from transgenic animals. Nat Biotechnol 23:1117–1125

Phan GQ et al. (2003) Cancer regression and autoimmunity induced by cytotoxic T lymphocyte-associated antigen 4 blockade in patients with metastatic melanoma. Proc Natl Acad Sci USA 100:8372–8377

Reichert JM et al. (2005) Monoclonal antibody successes in the clinic. Nat Biotechnol 23:1073–1078

Robert F et al. (2001) Phase I study of anti-epidermal growth factor receptor antibody cetuximab in combination with radiation therapy in patients with advanced head and neck cancer. J Clin Oncol 19(13):3234–3243

Roy D and Andrews PA (2004) Nonclinical testing from theory to practice. In: Teicher BA and Andrews PA (eds), Anticancer drug development guide, 2nd edn, Humana Press, Totowa, NJ, pp 287–311

Scott CT (2005) The problem with potency. Nat Biotechnol 23:1037–1039

Siegel EB (2004) The Pre-Pre-IND FDA consultation process for preclinical studies: opportunities for launching a rapid drug or biologic development program. Preclinica 2:171

Sidiropoulos PI and Boumpas DT (2004) Lessons learned from anti-CD40L treatment in systemic lupus erythematosus patients. Lupus 13:391–397

Slamon DJ et al. (2001) Use of chemotherapy plus a monoclonal antibody against HER2 for metastatic breast cancer that overexpresses HER2. N Engl J Med 344:783–792

Suntharalingam G et al. (2006) Cytokine storm in a phase 1 trial of the anti-CD28 monoclonal antibody TGN1412. N Engl J Med 355:1018–1028

Part II
Molecular Developments in Antibody Production

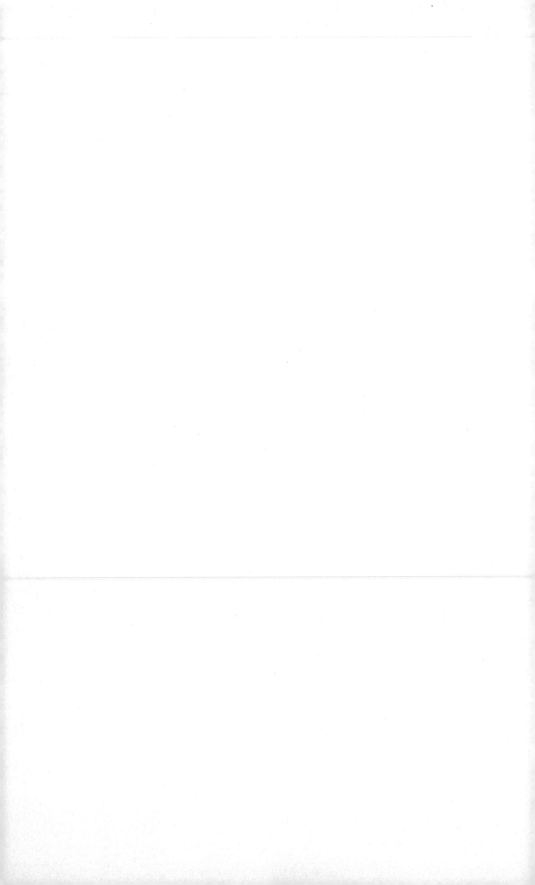

Engineering Antibodies for Stability and Efficient Folding

A. Honegger

1 Introduction 48
2 Antibody Structure 49
3 Antibody Variability 51
4 Variable Domain Stability.. 55
5 Influence of Variable Domain Stability on the Stability of scFv, Fab Fragments,
   and Full-Size Antibodies 56
   5.1   scFv Stability 56
   5.2   Stability of the C_L/C_H1 Heterodimer 57
   5.3   Stability of the Fab Fragment
         and of Full-Size Antibodies... 58
6 Antibody–Antigen Interactions 59
7 Stabilization and Humanization of Antibody Variable
   Domains by Loop Grafts.. 61
   7.1   Selection of a Suitable Acceptor Framework............................ 61
   7.2   Grafting Strategy 62
   7.3   Refinement of the Graft 63
8 Rescuing Problematic Variable Domains
   by Individual Point Mutations 64
9 Concluding Remarks... 66
References 67

Abstract Antibody variable domains vary widely in their intrinsic thermodynamic stability. Despite the mutual stabilization of the domains in the scFv fragment, most scFv derived from monoclonal antibodies without further engineering show poor to moderate stability. The situation gets more complex for Fab fragments and full-sized antibodies: while the disulfide-linked C_L/C_H heterodimer shows very limited thermodynamic stability, its unfolding kinetics are very slow. The same is true for Fab fragments, which, due to this kinetic stabilization, appear to be more stable than

A. Honegger
Biochemisches Institut, Universität Zürich, Winterthurerstrasse 190, CH-8057 Zürich, Switzerland
e-mail: honegger@bioc.uzh.ch

Y. Chernajovsky, A. Nissim (eds.) *Therapeutic Antibodies. Handbook of Experimental Pharmacology 181.*
© Springer-Verlag Berlin Heidelberg 2008

their thermodynamic stability suggests. However, suboptimal variable domains can be engineered for improved stability and folding efficiency while preserving their antigen-binding specificity and affinity, either by a limited number of point mutations or by grafting their antigen specificity to superior variable domain frameworks.

1 Introduction

Today, therapeutic monoclonal antibodies and antibody-derived immunotoxins represent one of the fastest growing areas of pharmacological development. Antibody-based therapeutics make use of the high specificity and selectivity of the antibody–antigen interaction to neutralize venoms, toxins, and pathogenic infections, modulate cell–cell signaling by blocking cell surface receptors and their ligands or by activating cell surface receptors, to direct immune effector functions such as antibody-dependent cellular cytotoxicity and complement-dependent cytotoxicity toward tumor cells expressing particular surface antigens, or to specifically deliver drugs, enzymes, radioisotopes, and toxins to the tumor cells, thus minimizing the systemic toxicity of those drugs.

Many factors influence the clinical potential of an antibody-based therapeutic agent. The clinical efficacy and safety depend first and foremost on the target against which an antibody is directed, and on the epitopes the antibody recognizes within this target. A second factor is the effector functions utilized by the therapeutic agent to elicit the desired response. A third factor is the pharmacokinetics of the antibody-derived construct. Apart from effects mediated by the Fc-part of a full-size antibody, the size of an antibody-derived construct will influence both tissue penetration and clearance rate. A fourth factor is the immunogenicity of the construct, particularly if an antibody-based drug is to be administered repeatedly over a prolonged time span; adverse effects can range from loss of activity and altered pharmacokinetics to life-threatening anaphylactic shock. Although early clinical applications of murine monoclonal antibodies were hampered by the problem of immunogenicity, new technologies have provided solutions to this problem. Because of the modular structure of antibodies, replacement of the murine constant domains by the corresponding human constant domains was relatively simple, giving rise to chimeric antibodies, in which 4 out of 12 domains (two V_L and two V_H domains) retain the murine sequence, and eight domains (C_L, C_H1, C_H2 and C_H3) are derived from a human antibody. This step alone has significantly reduced the fraction of patients that produce human anti-mouse-antibodies. Humanization of the variable domains by CDR graft or resurfacing further reduces the sequence fraction derived from the nonhuman antibody to those residues that in genuine human antibodies show the highest sequence variability.

In addition, the biophysical properties of the therapeutic agent, such as its thermodynamic stability and its aggregation propensity can critically affect the pharmacokinetics of such molecules (Willuda et al. 1999, 2001). Thus the engineering of modern antibody-based therapeutics has gone beyond humanization to address these issues. By combining the knowledge gained from an analysis of the biophysical properties of natural antibody variable domains, the effects of mutations obtained in directed evolution experiments, and the detailed structural comparison of antibodies, it has now become possible to engineer antibodies for higher thermodynamic stability and more efficient folding.

2 Antibody Structure

Figure 1 shows some of the commonly used antibody constructs:

Figure 1A shows a full-length antibody of the IgG class, consisting of two heavy chains (cyan) and two light chains (magenta). Two antigen recognition sites are located at the ends of the two arms. The light chain consists of two domains, the light chain variable domain V_L and the light chain constant domain C_L. In the IgG, the heavy chain consists of four domains: the heavy chain variable domain V_H and three constant domains, C_H1, C_H2, and C_H3. Each domain forms a β-sandwich (immunoglobulin fold) and contains at least one intradomain disulfide bond. Light and heavy chain are linked by a disulfide bond from the C-terminus of the light chain to a cystein within the C_H1 domain or the hinge between C_H1 and C_H2. The two

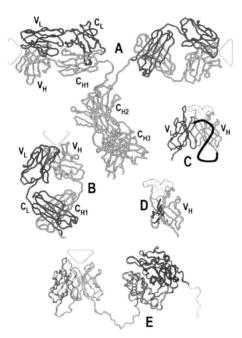

Fig. 1 Structures of various antibody-derived constructs. (**A**) Full-size monoclonal antibody (IgG2a) based on PDB entry 1IGT (Harris et al. 1997). The light chain is shown in *magenta*, the heavy chain in *cyan*. The location of the antigen binding site is indicated by *triangles*. (**B**) Antibody Fab fragment, consisting of the antibody light chain and the first two domains of the heavy chain. (**C**) Antibody single chain Fv fragment, consisting of the variable domains of the light and heavy chain connected by a flexible linker. (**D**) Single domain V_H antibody mimicking the antigen binding mode of camelid heavy chain IgGs. (**E**) Immunotoxin 4D5MocB-ETA, consisting of a scFv recognizing the he epithelial cell adhesion molecule (Ep-CAM) connected by a linker to the to a truncated form of *Pseudomonas aeruginosa* exotoxin A

heavy chains are linked by disulfide bonds between the hinge regions. The antigen recognition sites are formed by the V_L/V_H heterodimer. The C_H2 domains are glycosylated, the sugar residues being located at the interface of the two domains. C_H2 and C_H3 domains of the two heavy chains form the Fc-part of the molecule, which contains the binding sites for complement and Fc-receptor interaction and is thus responsible for harnessing immune effector functions in vivo.

Figure 1B shows a Fab fragment, consisting of a light chain and the Fd-fragment (V_H and C_H1) of the heavy chain. The Fab fragment contains one antigen binding site and is unable to activate immune effector functions. The two chains may or may not be linked by a disulfide bond. If additional hinge region cysteins are retained in the construct, disulfide-linked Fab'_2 can be produced.

Figure 1C shows a single chain fragment (scFv) (Bird et al. 1988; Huston et al. 1988), consisting of a V_L/V_H heterodimer connected by a flexible linker. Depending on the length of this linker, scFv can be monomeric or, if the linker is too short to connect the two domains without strain, form dimers (diabodies), trimers (tribodies), or even tetramers as the V_L domain of one molecule pairs with the V_H domain of a second molecule (Kortt et al. 1997). Since the antigen recognition site of Fab fragments and scFvs is identical to that of a full size antibody, they can be derived from monoclonal antibodies. Alternatively, they can be selected from gene libraries using phage display or ribosome display.

In contrast, single-domain V_H antibodies (Davies and Riechmann 1994; Davies and Riechmann 1995) (Fig. 1D) mimic the antigen recognition sites of a class of antibodies only found in camels, dromedaries, and llama that lack the light chain (Hamers-Casterman et al. 1993). Engineered replacement of hydrophobic residues in the V_L/V_H interface region of the human V_H3 domain give rise to a V_H domain that is stable in the absence of a V_L domain and can be randomized to yield a library that mimics the antigen binding mode of camelid heavy chain IgGs (Tanha et al. 2001).

Since Fabs, scFvs, and single-domain antibodies lack the intrinsic ability of antibodies to activate immune effector functions, they are usually used as building blocks for more complex constructs. Multiple scFv of the same specificity can be combined to obtain constructs with higher avidity, either as diabodies, daisy-chained on the same polypeptide chain, or brought together by multimerization domains (Willuda et al. 2001). The same can be done with scFv of different specificities to yield multispecific constructs, either targeting multiple overexpressed tumor antigens on the same target cell in an attempt to further increase the targeting efficiency or using different specificities to crosslink immune effector cells to the tumor cells. Antibody-derived constructs can be genetically fused to toxins and other biomolecules to give rise to immunotoxins. Peptidic tags can facilitate radiolabeling (Waibel et al. 1999) of such constructs for radioimmunotargeting. ScFv and Fabs can be chemically linked to liposomes to target their load of drugs, DNA, or siRNA to specific cells. (Fig. 1E) shows one example of an immunotoxin currently in Phase II/III clinical trials under the name of Proxinium™ (Viventia Biotech): a humanized scFv derived from a monoclonal antibody against the epithelial cell adhesion molecule (Ep-CAM) genetically fused to a truncated form of *Pseudomonas aeruginosa* exotoxin A (ETA (252-608)KDEL) (Di Paolo et al. 2003).

3 Antibody Variability

The human antibody repertoire comprises five different classes of antibodies, IgA, IgD, IgE, IgG, and IgM, some of which are further subdivided into several subclasses. The different classes differ in their heavy chain constant domains. They fulfill different roles in the natural immune response, as they differ in their ability to interact with the various Fc receptors and their ability to activate complement. Two classes of light chains, lambda and kappa, associate with these heavy chains to form an intact antibody.

Antigen specificity is determined by the variable domains located at the N-terminus of heavy and light chain. Their variability is produced by genetic recombination of gene fragments during the differentiation of a hematopoetic stem cell into a B cell and by somatic hypermutation of the V-domains in the activated B cells. The germline contains a large number of different V genes, and this variety is needed, since antigen binding interactions are not limited to the CDR-3s, which derive their diversity from the genetic recombination of V, J, and D gene segments, but also involve germline-encoded CDR-1s and CDR-2s as well as residues in the outer loop. On the basis of their sequence similarity, human kappa light chains are subdivided into seven distinct germline families (Tomlinson et al. 1995; Lefranc et al. 1999), $V\kappa1$–$V\kappa7$, of which four ($V\kappa1$–$V\kappa4$) are significantly represented in the mature antibody repertoire. Of the 11 lambda light chain families, the first three ($V\lambda1$–$V\lambda3$) are most frequently used in the rearranged repertoire. The different V_L germline families differ not only in their sequence, but also encode CDR-L1 loops of different lengths. Human V_H domains fall into seven sequence families (Tomlinson et al. 1992; Lefranc et al. 1999), which comprise three structural subtypes, characterized by distinct framework conformations and packing of hydrophobic core residues (Honegger and Plückthun 2001). In addition, the different germline families are characterized by different CDR-H1 and CDR-H2 lengths and conformations. Murine antibody sequences are subdivided into 19 $V\kappa$ families and 15 V_H families, representing four distinct structural subtypes. Of three known murine $V\lambda$ germline genes, only one is commonly used in rearranged antibodies. The seven human $V\kappa$ germline family consensus sequences show 43–74% sequence identity, while the murine germline family consensus sequences show 43–78% sequence identity, the genetic distance between any murine germline family consensus sequence and the closest human germline family consensus sequence corresponds to 64–86% sequence identity, using residues L1–L108 for comparison (AHo numbering scheme,[1] L1–L90 according to the Kabat numbering scheme). The seven human V_H germline families share between 36 and 78% sequence identity, comparing

---

[1] The AHo numbering scheme (Honegger and Plückthun 2001). Yet another numbering scheme for immunoglobulin variable domains: an automatic modeling and analysis tool. J Mol Biol 309:657–670.) is used throughout this chapter, since it unambiguously indicates the position of each residues in the 3D-structure of the variable length CDR loops, which is not the case for other numbering schemes used. Figure 2 indicates the correspondence between the residue numbers according to Kabat (Kabat et al. 1991. Sequences of proteins of immunological interest, NIH Publication No. 91-3242) and the AHo numbering scheme.

Light Chain Variable Domain

Heavy Chain Variable Domain

Fig. 2 Alignment of human germline family consensus sequences (chapter 4), and the sequences of the CDR-grafted antibody (chapter 7.3). Color codes in the header summarize conserved structural properties of antibody variable domains. Please refer to the text for details. (**A**) Average solvent accessibility of each residue: yellow, 0–10% accessible, signifies a residue that is fully buried; yellow-green, 10–25%, buried; green, 25–50%; green-blue, 50–75%; semi-buried; blue, 75–100%; dark blue, >100% exposed, signifies a residue is more exposed than it would be in the context of an extended poly-Ala peptide. (**B–D**) Core residues are separated into upper core residues (**C**) and lower core residues (**D**) that are likely to influence antigen affinity, invariant central core residue (**C**) and lower core residues (**D**) that differ according to germline family. (**E–I**) Residues involved in contacts, color coded according to the average relative reduction of solvent accessible surface upon interaction (white, 0% reduction; yellow, 0–20%; yellow-orange, 20–40%; orange, 40–60%; red-orange, 60–80%; red, 80–100%). (**E**) Contacts between variable and constant domains. (**F**) Contacts between light and heavy chain. (**G–I**) Residues involved in hapten binding, binding of linear oligomeric antigens and structural epitopes in proteins. (**J–P**) Human germline family consensus sequences for the four hVκ, three hVλ and seven V_H families represented in the HuCAL library, color-coded according to amino acid properties: Aromatic residues Trp, Tyr, Phe, orange, aliphatic residues Leu, Ile, Val, Pro, Ala as well as Cys and Met, yellow. Gly, yellow-green, uncharged hydrophilic residues Ser, Thr, Asn, Gln, green. Basic His, cyan, Arg, Lys, blue, acidic residues Asp, Glu, red. (**Q, R**) Generic grafting strategy. In the positions highlighted in cyan (**Q**), the sequence of the grafted antibody reflects that of the acceptor framework, and in the positions highlighted in magenta (**R**), it reflects that of the CDR donor. (**S–W**) Loop graft of murine antibody moc31 to the 4D5 framework and refinement of the graft. Sequence positions that are the same in all constructs are colored blue, those that correspond to the sequence of the framework donor are colored cyan, those that correspond to the CDR donor are shown in magenta. Additional positions changed to the sequence of the CDR donor in the actual constructs are highlighted in orange. Variable domain structures extracted from all antibody structures available in the PDB (>500 structures) were superimposed and compared to extract common features. Figure 3 summarizes this information in relation to the sequence positions. For your orientation, residue numbers have been listed both according to the Kabat numbering scheme (Kabat et al. 1991) and the AHo numbering scheme (Honegger and Plückthun 2001), although the sequences have been aligned according to the AHo scheme. Standard header for V_L (top) and V_H (bottom) sequence alignments summarize the consensus structural properties and interaction residues of the domains. White bars indicate CDR boundaries according to the definition of Kabat. Residues highlighted in magenta show where alignment gaps are placed in the Kabat numbering scheme. In contrast, the AHo numbering specifies that alignment gaps are to be centered on the positions highlighted in yellow to reflect the structural equivalence of the positions with the same residue number between antibodies with different CDR lengths. Row A of the header indicates the average relative side chain accessibility in the isolated domain: The solvent accessible surface of each residue was calculated as percentage of the solvent accessible surface the same residue would have in the context of a poly-Ala peptide in extended conformation, using the program NACCESS (Hubbard and Thornton 1993). Comparison of the average solvent accessible surface area of the same residue in the complex and in the free domains yields information on the contribution of each residue to interface formation between variable and constant domains, between light and heavy chain and between antibody and antigen (Rows E-I).

Fig. 2 (continued)

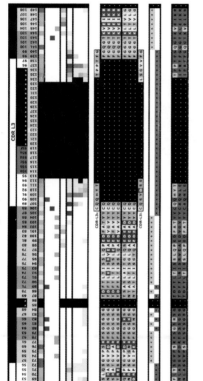

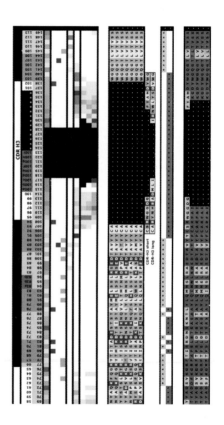

Table 1 Stability of human consensus variable domains against thermal denaturation (Tm) and chemical denaturation by guanidinium chloride

Domain	Tm (°C)	GdmCl$_{50}$ (M)	$\Delta G_{NU}(H_2O)$ (kJ mol^{-1})	m (kJ M^{-1} mol)
HuCAL Vκ1	63.9	2.1	29.0	14.1
HuCAL Vκ2	63.0	1.5	24.8	16.1
HuCAL Vκ3	72.7	2.3	34.5	14.8
HuCAL Vκ4	59.2	1.5	n.d.[2]	n.d.[2]
HuCAL Vλ1	63.8	2.1	23.7	11.1
HuCAL Vλ2	49.9	1.0	16.0	16.2
HuCAL Vλ3	49.0	0.9	15.1	15.9
HuCAL V$_H$1a	n.d.[a]	1.5	13.7	10.1
HuCAL V$_H$1b	n.d.[a]	2.1	26.0	12.7
HuCAL V$_H$2	n.d.[a]	1.4	n.d.[b]	n.d.[2]
HuCAL V$_H$3	n.d.[a]	3.0	52.7	17.6
HuCAL V$_H$4	n.d.[a]	2.3	n.d.[b]	n.d.[b]
HuCAL V$_H$5	n.d.[a]	2.2	16.5	7.0
HuCAL V$_H$6	n.d.[a]	1.2	n.d.[b]	n.d.[2]

[1] No Tm values could be determined for V$_H$ domains, since these domains precipitate upon thermal denaturation

[2] The unfolding curves of hVκ4, hV$_H$2, hV$_H$4, and hV$_H$6 were not compatible with a two-state model

residues H1–H108, the 15 murine V$_H$ domain 31–74%, while any murine germline family consensus sequence shows at least 60% sequence identity to the closest human germline family consensus sequence.

4 Variable Domain Stability

To evaluate the influence of this germline diversity on the biophysical properties of antibody-derived constructs, we have analyzed the human germline family consensus domains on which the Human Combinatorial Antibody Library (HuCAL) is based (Knappik et al. 2000). In Fig. 2, rows J–P, an alignment of these consensus sequences representing the different human germline families is shown, with a header summarizing the location, surface exposure, and likeliness of involvement in antigen binding and other interfaces. Each of these domains was expressed with the CDR-3 sequence appropriate for its type. For isolated V$_H$ domains, the long CDR-H3 sequence was used, as it had a stabilizing effect on the domains and allowed the isolated domain to be expressed in native form, for scFvs, the short CDR-H3 derived from the scFv 4D5 (Eigenbrot et al. 1993) was used. CDR-L3 of the Vκ domains is that of scFv 4D5, for Vλ, a consensus sequence derived from an alignment of rearranged human Vλ sequences was used. The different consensus domains were produced by periplasmic expression in *E. coli*, purified and their thermodynamic stability assessed by thermal and chemical denaturation (Ewert et al. 2003). The results of this analysis are summarized in Table 1.

Generally, thermal unfolding was reversible for the V_L domains, but led to irreversible aggregation and precipitation for the V_H domains. For the V_L domains, the stability against thermal unfolding correlates reasonably well with their thermodynamic stability as assessed by chemical denaturation by guanidinium chloride (Table 1) or urea (data not shown). For $V\kappa4$, V_H2, V_H4, and V_H6, the free energy of unfolding $(\Delta G_{NU}(H_2O))$ could not be quantitated because these domains formed soluble aggregates, which lead to denaturation curves that were not compatible with a two-state model of the unfolding process. The hV_H3 germline family consensus domain was by far the most stable V_H domain. Interestingly, the unpaired V_{HH} domains derived from camelid heavy chain antibodies (Hamers-Casterman et al. 1993; Muyldermans et al. 1994; Ewert et al. 2002) and murine V_H domains selected for their exceptional stabilities (Wörn and Plückthun 1998a) share the structural features that distinguish the human V_H3 domains from V_H domains derived from other germline families. hV_H1 was found to be the next most stable V_H domain, followed by V_H5. In contrast hV_H2, hV_H4, and hV_H6 were found to be barely viable in the absence of a V_L domain, they exhibited low cooperativity during denaturant-induced unfolding, lower production yields, and higher aggregation tendencies. The biophysical properties of V_L domains differed to a lesser extent than those of V_H domains. In general, isolated V_κ domains showed a higher thermodynamic stability and a higher yield of protein expressed in soluble form than isolated V_λ domains. $hV\kappa3$ was found to be the most stable of the kappa domains, $hV_\lambda1$ the most stable of the lambda domains.

5 Influence of Variable Domain Stability on the Stability of scFv, Fab Fragments, and Full-Size Antibodies

5.1 scFv Stability

The interaction between V_L and V_H domain in the scFv leads to a mutual stabilization of the two domains, depending on the intrinsic stability of the two domains and the strength of the interface. (Wörn and Plückthun 1998b; Ewert et al. 2003; Röthlisberger et al. 2005). When two intrinsically weak V-domains interact in a scFv, the resulting construct can be significantly more stable than either of the component domains (Fig. 3A). If one of the domains is significantly more stable than the other, the interface between the two domains stabilizes the weaker domain to some extent, but not sufficiently for the two domains to unfold cooperatively. Depending on the strength of the interaction and the difference in the intrinsic stability of the two domains, an equilibrium unfolding intermediate may be observed in which one of the domain is unfolded, while the other is still native (Fig. 3B,C). If both domains are intrinsically very stable, the interface is not able to stabilize the scFv beyond the stability of the more stable domain. (Fig. 3D).

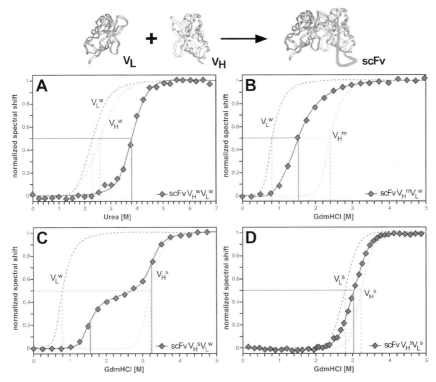

Fig. 3 Influence of domain stability on the stability of the scFv. (**A**) A weak V_L domain (w.t. AB48, Proba et al. 1997) is coupled to a weak V_H domain (ab48 Cys H23 Ala) in V_H-linker-V_L orientation. The resulting scFv shows a cooperative equilibrium unfolding curve with a midpoint at significantly higher denaturant concentration than the midpoints of either of the two constituent domains (indicated by *dashed lines*). (**B**) A weak V_L domain is coupled to a V_H domain of intermediate stability (ab48 Lys H77 Arg, Asn H59 Ser, Tyr H106 Val (Proba, Wörn et al. 1998)). The resulting scFv shows an equilibrium unfolding curve with poor cooperativity and a midpoint denaturant concentration intermediate between those of the two constituent domains. (**C**) A weak V_L domain is coupled to a very strong V_H domain (disulfide-restored ab48 Lys H77 Arg, Asn H59 Ser). The unfolding curve of the scFv shows a clear unfolding intermediate, although the unfolding curve of the V_L domain is shifted to higher denaturant concentrations than that of the free V_L domain, V_L in the scFv fully unfolds at denaturant concentrations at which V_H has not even started to unfold. The unfolding curve of the V_H domain within the scFv is not affected by the presence of the V_L domain. (**D**) A very strong V_L domain (4D5) is coupled to a very strong V_H domain (disulfide-restored ab48 Lys H77 Arg, Asn H59 Ser). The resulting scFv shows an equilibrium unfolding curve with poor cooperativity and a midpoint denaturant concentration intermediate between those of the two constituent domains

5.2 Stability of the C_L/C_H1 Heterodimer

The intrinsic stability of the constant domains was found to be in the same range as that of rather weak variable domains (Röthlisberger et al. 2005). The isolated murine Cκ had a denaturation midpoint of around 1 M GdmCl or 3.2 M Urea. The isolated murine $C_H1\gamma$ domain could not be produced in *E. coli*, neither by periplasmic expression nor as cytoplasmic inclusion bodies, probably due to the rapid degradation of the peptide chain. Despite the large hydrophobic interaction area between the C_H1 and $C\kappa$ domain, unlinked C_H/C_L heterodimers, though produced in soluble form upon periplasmic expression, dissociated upon extraction from the periplasm, leading to the precipitation of the C_H domain. Only the disulfide linked heterodimer could be produced in sufficient amounts to determine its stability. Its equilibrium denaturation midpoint lay at the same denaturant concentration as that of the isolated C_L domain, indicating that the intrinsic stability of the C_H domain cannot be higher than that of the C_L domain, and probably is significantly lower. However, in contrast to the scFv, which unfolds very quickly in the presence of the denaturant, the disulfide-linked C_L/C_H heterodimer equilibrates very slowly, taking up to 2 weeks to reach equilibrium at guanidinium concentrations corresponding to the midpoint of the unfolding curve.

5.3 Stability of the Fab Fragment and of Full-Size Antibodies

In a non-disulfide linked Fab fragment containing both a weak V_L and a weak V_H domain, the Fab fragment showed cooperative unfolding with a midpoint denaturant concentration that was significantly higher than that of either the disulfide-linked C_L/C_H heterodimer or the scFv containing the same variable domains. At the same time, this Fab fragment showed the same very slow unfolding kinetics as the disulfide-linked C_L/C_H heterodimer. In non-disulfide linked Fab fragments containing the more stable variable domains, the constant domains became limiting for the thermodynamic stability, as the unfolding curve revealed a first unfolding transition with very slow equilibration, followed by a second transition at higher denaturant concentration, but with fast equilibration. However, if the interchain disulfide bridge linking the C-termini of the two chains of the Fab was present, the resultant Fab again showed cooperative unfolding, with both the very high unfolding midpoint of the very stable V-domains and the very slow unfolding kinetics of the disulfide-linked C_L/C_H heterodimer (Röthlisberger et al. 2005).

This kinetic barrier to the unfolding of the Fab fragment is not only seen in chemical denaturation, but also in thermal denaturation. Vermeer et al. analyzed the irreversible thermal unfolding of whole IgGs by differential scanning calorimetry (DSC) and circular dichroism spectroscopy. While in the DSC thermogram of a murine IgG1 (murine monoclonal antibody against human chorionic gonadotropin) only a single, though rather broad, endothermic transition was observed (Vermeer, 1998), in a murine IgG2b (murine monoclonal antibody directed against the glycosylated N-terminal region of the β-chain of human hemoglobin A1c), two unfolding peaks were observed, (Vermeer and Norde 2000), which represented the independent unfolding of the Fab and the Fc fragment (Vermeer et al. 2000). The apparent melting temperature (Tm) of the Fab is highly dependent on the heating rate, as is the enthalpy of unfolding. Although the irreversibility of the thermal unfolding and the subsequent aggregation of the denatured protein render the analysis more complex, their results also suggest the presence of a kinetic barrier to the unfolding of the Fab and in addition show that at least in this particular antibody, the FabSS is less stable than the Fc fragment and thus is limiting for the thermal stability of the whole antibody.

6 Antibody–Antigen Interactions

Analysis of the many antibody–antigen complex structures available in the PDB databank (Berman et al. 2000) reveals the diversity of binding modes used in the recognition of different antigens (Fig. 4). The different binding modes correlate with structural features in the antibody, and with the utilization of antibodies derived

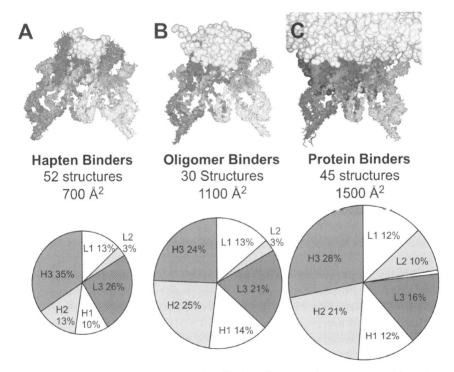

Hapten Binders
52 structures
700 Å²

Oligomer Binders
30 Structures
1100 Å²

Protein Binders
45 structures
1500 Å²

Fig. 4 (**A–C**) Superimposed structures of antibody–antigen complexes were sorted into three classes according to the type of antigen recognized. (**A**) Antibodies recognizing haptens and protruding loops, (**B**) antibodies recognizing peptides and linear epitopes of proteins, and (**C**) antibody recognizing flat structural epitopes in proteins. The antigens are colored yellow, the V_L domains pale pink (framework) and magenta (CDRs), the V_H domains cyan (framework) and blue (CDRs). The solvent accessible surface buried in complex formation was calculated using the program NACCESS (Hubbard and Thornton 1993). Pie charts indicate the average size of the interaction surface and the average contribution of the six CDRs to the interaction surface

from particular germline families. Small antigens (haptens) tend to insert deeply along the axis of the V_L/V_H pseudodimer in antibodies whose CDR-H3 is very short or preferentially assumes an extended conformation. These complexes tend to contain antibodies with a long CDR-L1 and CDR-H2, which help to form a deep binding pocket. The same binding mode is employed by antibodies that bind to highly exposed loops of a protein antigen. In contrast, in antibodies recognizing more or less planar structural epitopes in proteins, a kinked CDR-H3 conformation allows CDR-H3 residues to fill the hapten binding pocket along the pseudo-twofold axis. Short CDR-L1 and CDR-H2 loop contribute to flat shape of the paratope, as CDR-H3 gets buried between antigen and antibody. Linear epitopes in peptides, oligonucleotides, and oligosaccharides also prefer antibodies with an open hapten binding pocket, although they do not insert as deeply. (Fig. 4).

Analysis of the residues involved in antigen contacts shows that residues outside the classical CDR definitions (Chothia and Lesk 1987; Kabat et al. 1981) can be involved in binding interactions. It is thus preferable to refer to these more detailed analyses summarized in Fig. 2, especially if some information on the type of antigen or binding mode of the antibody is available. For protein binders, residues at the N-termini of the domains, the outer half of the CDR-1 loop, and the outer loops may be directly involved in antigen contact, while for hapten and peptide binders, residues usually deeply buried in the V_L/V_H dimer interface and inaccessible to protein antigens are accessible to antigen contact.

The shape of the paratope is not only determined by the residues directly involved in antigen contacts. Residues whose side chains are buried in the domain core may alter the conformation of the CDR loops. Given the large differences of the core packing between V_H domains derived from different germline families, it is at first sight surprising that CDR grafting works as well as it does. This is only possible because a layer of invariant residues (Cys 23, Cys 106, Trp 43, Gln/Glu 6) divides the core of the immunoglobulin variable domain into an upper core, consisting of residues buried directly underneath the CDRs, whose packing can strongly affect antigen affinity and a lower core, whose packing strongly correlates with the framework subtype, but has little or no influence on antigen binding.

Upper core residue 31, which intercalates between the two beta sheets of the immunoglobulin domain and divides the CDR-1 loop into an outer and an inner loop, is probably the prime mediator translating changes of upper core packing into changes of CDR-1 conformation (Honegger and Plückthun 2001). In Vκ, residues L2 and L4 of the N-terminus, residues L25, L29, L31, and L41 of CDR-L1, residues L58 of CDR-L2, residues L80, L82, and L89 of the outer loop, and residues L108 of CDR-L3 pack together to form the upper core of the domain. Some of the positions buried in Vκ are exposed in Vλ, because of the less ordered N-terminus and the different CDR-L1 conformations in lambda light chains. The upper core of the lambda domains is formed by residues L4 of the N-term, residues L25, L31, and L41 of CDR-L1, residue L58 of CDR-L2, residues L80, L82, and L89 of the outer loop, and residues L108 and L138 of CDR-L3. In V_H, residues H2 and H4 of the N-term, residues H25, H29, H31, H39, and H41 of CDR-H1, residues H58 and H60 of CDR-H2, residues H80, H82, and H89 of the outer loop, and residues

H108 and H138 of CDR-H3 pack together to form the upper core of the domain. Although packing interactions in the lower core of the domain could conceivably affect CDR-H2 orientation, and there exists a correlation between germline family, structural subtype, identity of these lower core residues, and CDR-H2 length and conformation in natural antibody domains, deliberate loop grafts to distantly related frameworks (Willuda et al. 1999) showed no loss of binding affinity due to lower core mismatch.

7 Stabilization and Humanization of Antibody Variable Domains by Loop Grafts

7.1 Selection of a Suitable Acceptor Framework

The most frequently used method for the humanization of antibody variable domains is the transfer of the complementary determining regions (CDRs) from their original antibody framework to a human framework (Jones et al. 1986). If this CDR-graft is performed with the primary goal of reducing the immunogenicity of murine antibodies to be used in human in vivo applications, one chooses as graft acceptor the human framework whose sequence most closely matches the original murine sequence. This may be a specific human germline sequence or a germline family consensus sequence. If the closest human germline family consensus sequence is used, the murine CDR donor and the closest human acceptor V-domain typically show between 75% and 85% sequence identity for $V\kappa$ domains and 60–80% sequence identity for V_H domains, excluding CDR 3. However, while a CDR graft to a closely related framework may limit the problems posed by non-CDR residues directly or indirectly affecting the antigen affinity, poor performance of the grafted molecule can result from an insufficiently stable acceptor framework, which is more likely to deform under the strain introduced by the grafted sequences. Although both hV_H3 and hV_H1 offer acceptable biophysical properties, grafts to nonoptimized hV_H2, hV_H4, and hV_H6 frameworks are very likely to yield antibodies with suboptimal properties.

The same technique of CDR grafting can be used to improve the biophysical properties of antibodies by grafting their antigen specificities to a framework with superior biophysical properties (Jung and Plückthun 1997; Jung et al. 1999; Willuda et al. 1999; Wörn et al. 2000). If the most stable human consensus frameworks ($hV\kappa3$ and hV_H3) are chosen as acceptor independent of the sequence of the murine CDR donor, the sequence identity between CDR donor and acceptor framework can be as low as 45%–50% for $V\kappa$ and 35%–40% for V_H, excluding CDR 3. Therefore, particular care has to be taken to transfer not only antigen contact residues, but all residues likely to directly or indirectly influence antigen binding. In addition, care has to be taken to avoid the introduction of destabilizing interactions between CDRs and acceptor framework. In general, simply combining the CDR sequences from one antibody with the framework sequence of a second one is not sufficient to retain antigen recognition.

That grafts to the most distantly related frameworks indeed can succeed is demonstrated by the loop graft from a scFv recognizing the leucine zipper sequence of transcription factor GCN4 (Weber-Bornhauser 1998) (mVλ1 mV$_H$2) to a extremely stable hybrid framework consisting of the hVκ1 domain of antibody 4D5 and the stability-evolved mV$_H$4 domain of ab48 (Proba et al. 1998; Wörn and Plückthun 1998b). The resulting grafted scFv showed significantly enhanced ability to inhibit GCN4-regulated gene expression when expressed as an intrabody in yeast, and served as a starting point for an intrabody library (Wörn et al. 2000; Auf der Maur et al. 2001, 2002). This example involved the transfer of the binding specificity from a murine V$_H$ domain sharing the structural characteristics of the poorly behaved human V$_H$2 and V$_H$4 domains to one sharing the structural characteristics of hV$_H$3 and from a murine Vλ1 domain to hVκ1. The success of this graft depended on the preservation of crucial mVλ1 residues in the V$_L$/V$_H$ interface that make no direct contact to the antigen, but affect the relative orientation of the two domains.

7.2 Grafting Strategy

Rows Q and R in Fig. 2 outline a generic grafting strategy. Residue positions marked in cyan (Row Q) are to be derived from the acceptor framework, residue positions marked in magenta from the CDR donor (Row R). The latter comprise the following:

- *Residues that may contact the antigen.* Unless a structure of the CDR donor in complex with its antigen is available, potential contact residues have to be identified using the information in rows G, H, and I in Fig. 2, which outline the probability of each residue to make contact to the antigen, derived from an analysis of all the antibody–antigen complexes in the PDB.
- *Conformationally critical residues adjacent to the contact residues.* Prolin residues offer less conformational flexibility than other amino acids, while glycines increase the flexibility of the peptide chain. Substitutions involving these residues can result in an altered loop conformation and thus affect the antigen binding affinity.
- *Residues in the upper core of the domain*, indicated in row B. Particularly, positions L80, L82, and L89 in the outer loop of the V$_L$ domain have frequently been implicated in failed grafts, as the side chains of these residues pack against a critical residue in CDR-L1. The side chain of residue L31 intercalates between the two beta sheets of the domain and translates changes in upper core packing to changes in the orientation and conformation of the CDR-L1 double loop. N-terminal residues L2 and L4 pack against the same residue from the other side. The same is true for the corresponding set of upper core residues in V$_H$.
- *Critical residues in the V$_L$/V$_H$ interface* are indicated by red and orange colors in row F. These are usually highly conserved, and a mismatch between CDR donor

and acceptor framework is rare, but any mismatch is quite likely to affect the relative orientation of the two domains.

Application of these rules has been tested in many instances and will usually yield a loop graft that retains most, if not all, of the antigen binding affinity. Rows S, T, and U in Fig. 2 use the graft of the antigen specificity of murine anti-Ep-Cam antibody moc31 (Myklebust et al. 1991) to the hVκ1 and hV$_H$3 framework as a specific example to demonstrate the results obtained with this strategy (Fig. 5).

7.3 Refinement of the Graft

If dealing with a particular antibody rather than a generic assessment, it may be possible to further reduce the number of residues retained from the CDR donor. On the basis of experimental structures or homology models of the CDR donor and the acceptor framework, and a model of the grafted molecule, one may decide to accept some conservative substitutions at the periphery of the putative antigen binding site. In addition, the model of the graft can be analyzed for suboptimal contacts between

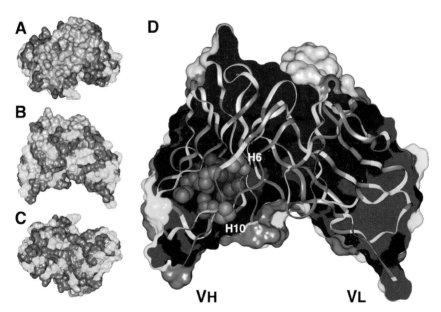

Fig. 5 Structural model of the 4D5mocB loop graft. Sequence postions that are the same in all constructs are colored *blue*, those that correspond to the sequence of the framework donor are colored *cyan*, those that correspond to the CDR donor are shown in *magenta*. Additional positions changed to the sequence of the CDR donor in the actual constructs are highlighted in *orange*. **A**, view onto the putative antigen combining site; **B**, side view; **C**, bottom view; **D**, cross section of the model showing the core residues additionally taken from the sequence of the CDR donor in construct 4D5mocB

residues derived from the two different antibodies that might destabilize the grafted molecule.

In this particular example, the V_H domains of the CDR donor and of the acceptor framework belong to different structural subtypes. The comparison of the structures of V_H domains of the same type as the CDR donor and of V_H domains of the same type as the acceptor framework revealed subtle differences in the takeoff angle of CDR-H2. This could have been either a consequence of the different lower core packing of the two domains or be caused by local sequence details within CDR-H2. A Ser/Gly difference in position H56, affecting the β-bulge in strand c, was corrected toward the sequence of the CDR donor, together with adjacent lower core residue H55, to eliminate this potential cause for the different CDR-H2 takeoff angle, yielding the V_H domain of scFv 4D5mocA (Fig. 2, row V).

To test the alternative hypothesis of the different lower core packing in the two V_H domains affecting CDR-H2, a second construct was designed in which the lower core residues of the CDR donor were retained, yielding the V_H domain of scFv 4D5mocB (Figure 5, row W). As it turned out, both scFv bound the antigen with the same affinity. However, while the CDR donor moc31 was significantly less stable that the 4D5 acceptor framework, scFv 4D5mocB turned out to be more stable than scFv 4D5mocA, despite being closer in sequence to the very unstable moc31 scFv. In the end, this difference in stability had a decisive influence on the biodistribution of the two scFv in a mouse tumor model (Willuda et al. 1999).

8 Rescuing Problematic Variable Domains by Individual Point Mutations

Although CDR grafts to closely related frameworks usually are unproblematic, CDR grafts for stabilization usually require a graft to a hV_H framework of a different subtype, typically hV_H3. As the example of antibody 4D5mocA shows, changing to a different V_H framework subtype may sometimes lead to conflicts between framework and CDRs. On the basis of a compilation of stabilizing mutations reported in the literature, observed in the course of in-vitro evolution of antibody fragments toward increased stability or identified by comparing antibody fragments of different stability, a few rules could be established that allow the identification of problematic residues within an antibody variable domain (discussed in more detail in Ewert et al. 2004).

- An EXCEL worksheet containing the CDR-graft template shown in Fig. 2, the human and murine germline family consensus sequences and a number of EXCEL visual basic macros facilitating the import and analysis of sequences in Microsoft EXCEL is available for download from the AAAAA web site (http://www.bioc.uzh.ch/antibody).
- Align the V_L and V_H sequence of your antibody to the global consensus sequence, the germline family consensus sequences and the header of the alignment

shown in Fig. 2, making sure to center the gaps as specified in (Honegger and Plückthun 2001).

- Any position that would retain the sequence of the CDR donor in a loop graft (as described earlier) should not be changed in this approach. These positions are to be excluded from the subsequent analysis.

- In V_H domains, the subtype-determining residues at position H6, H7, and H10 (Honegger and Plückthun 2001) and the correlated core positions 19, 74, 78, and 93 should match those of the germline family consensus. H6 should either by a Glu or a Gln. If H6 is a Glu, a Pro in H7 will be highly destabilizing, and H10 has to either be a Gly or a Pro. H9 should always be a Gly.

- The more highly conserved a given sequence position is, the more likely a deviation from the consensus will have a negative influence on stability and/or folding.

- Row A in Fig. 2 indicates the average solvent exposure of each position. Hydrophobic framework residues with a relative solvent exposure >75% (indicated in blue) should be replaced by hydrophilic ones, with the exception of Pro residues, which play an important structural role, and Val in positions L3 and H5, where the very high β-sheet propensity of Val outweighs the disadvantage of having a hydrophobic residue on the surface.

- Hydrophilic residues in fully buried positions should be replaced by hydrophobic ones unless the global consensus indicates a highly conserved hydrophilic core residue. If the germline family consensus is hydrophobic, use this residue, otherwise use the hydrophilic residue closest in size to the one found in the germline family consensus. A Lys in position L13 is acceptable and does not need to be replaced, since its side chain amino group can reach the solvent.

- Arg 77 and Asp 100 form a highly conserved, doubly hydrogen bonded buried salt bridge in the lower core of both the V_L and the V_H domains, which should be restored if they are not present in a given V-domain. The absence of this interactions in light chain correlates with fibril formation (Helms and Wetzel 1996). In V_H domains, replacement of Arg H77 by Lys, as found in many murine V_H domains, already leads to a significant loss of stability (Proba, Wörn et al. 1998; Wörn et al. 2000). Replacement by an uncharged residue, as in hV_H5, should have an even stronger effect. Surrounding polar and charged groups form a charge cluster around this central salt bridge and affect the degree of order and definition of the hydrogen bonds connecting the residues contributing to this charge cluster. This is present to the fullest extent only in V_H3 domains (Ewert et al. 2003).

- Gly, because of its exceptionally high flexibility, and Pro, with its very restricted torsional freedom, can have a strong effect both on folding efficiency and on stability. Highly conserved Pro and Gly residues should be conserved, even if the individual sequence and the germline family consensus differ from the global consensus. Non-Gly residues in positions with conserved positive Phi torsion angles should be replaced by Gly.

If possible, analyze the environment of the proposed mutations in a homology model of your antibody (If you are unable to build a homology model, have one built by submitting your sequence to the WAM antibody modeling web site (http://antibody.bath.ac.uk/index.html)), or use the structure of a closely related antibody (http://www.rcsb.org/pdb) or the human consensus Fv model representing the framework combination of your antibody (http://www.bioc.uzh.ch/antibody).

An important point is that it is not necessary to introduce these mutations one-by-one and investigate their contributions and their additivity. This has been done in the past to derive the above mentioned rules. However, for practical applications, we recommend to introduce a set of mutations all at once, making this into a very fast and practicable procedure.

This method was tested successfully with two different scFvs containing the hV_H6 consensus framework (Ewert et al. 2003). Six mutations were proposed, which either improved the expression yield of soluble protein, the thermodynamic stability, or both properties. Combining all six mutations increased the expression yield by a factor 4 to a level similar to that obtained with hV_H3 containing antibodies and increased the thermodynamic stability, measured by denaturant-induced equilibrium unfolding, by 21 kJ mol^{-1}. Five of the six mutations introduced addressed issues common to the three poorly behaved human V_H consensus frameworks, hV_H2, hV_H4, and hV_H6. All six mutations represent mutations toward the global consensus sequence for human V_H domains, which is dominated by the largest human germline family, hV_H3.

In another example, the expression of a very poorly expressed murine antipeptide $mV\kappa1mV_H1$ scFv was dramatically improved by a similar series of nine mutations, improving expression yield and stability sufficiently for us to crystallize the antibody/antigen complex and to determine its structure (Kaufmann et al. 2002). It needs to be stressed again that all mutations were introduced at once, with a rather minimal experimental effort.

9 Concluding Remarks

Both in the process of designing loop grafting and in the process of introducing individual and groups of mutations, the antibody sequence needs to be checked continuously for consistency with structural requirements. This process greatly profits from the availability of tables of preferred and allowed residues at all positions, which are now becoming available (Honegger et al., unpublished). Furthermore, once the rules for the identification of such mutations have been formulated with sufficient precision, the process lends itself to automation.

For the mid-term future, we see three strategies for antibody improvement. First, rule-based engineering, including CDR grafting, can be used, as outlined earlier, to "rescue" antibodies with particularly valuable biological effects or recognition properties. Second, evolutionary approaches (an iteration of randomization and selection) can be used to further refine any antibody, with or without prior rule-based engineering. Third, the sequence changes that reproducibly result in a marked improvement of the biophysical properties of the antibody framework may be introduced into the synthetic frameworks on which combinatorial antibody libraries are based.

References

Auf der Maur A, Escher D, Barberis A (2001) Antigen-independent selection of stable intracellular single-chain antibodies. FEBS Lett 508:407–412

Auf der Maur A, Zahnd C, Fischer F et al. (2002) Direct in vivo screening of intrabody libraries constructed on a highly stable single-chain framework. J Biol Chem 277:45075–45085

Berman HM, Westbrook J, Feng Z et al. (2000) The Protein Data Bank. Nucl Acids Res 28:235–242

Bird RE, Hardman KD, Jacobson JW et al. (1988) Single-chain antigen-binding proteins. Science 242:423–426

Chothia C, Lesk AM (1987) Canonical structures for the hypervariable regions of immunoglobulins. J Mol Biol 196:901–917

Davies J, Riechmann L (1994) 'Camelising' human antibody fragments: NMR studies on V_H domains. FEBS Lett 339:285–290

Davies J, Riechmann L (1995) Antibody V_H domains as small recognition units. Bio-Technology 13:475–479

Di Paolo C, Willuda J, Kubetzko S et al. (2003) A recombinant immunotoxin derived from a humanized epithelial cell adhesion molecule-specific single-chain antibody fragment has potent and selective antitumor activity. Clin Cancer Res 9:2837–2848

Eigenbrot C, Randal M, Presta L et al. (1993) X-ray structures of the antigen-binding domains from three variants of humanized anti-p185HER2 antibody 4D5 and comparison with molecular modeling. J Mol Biol 229: 969–995

Ewert S, Honegger A, Plückthun A (2003) Structure-based improvement of the biophysical properties of immunoglobulin V_H domains with a generalizable approach. Biochemistry 42:1517–1528

Ewert S, Cambillau C, Conrath K et al. (2002) Biophysical properties of camelid V_{HH} domains compared to those of human V_H3 domains. Biochemistry 41:3628–3636

Ewert S, Huber T, Honegger A et al. (2003) Biophysical properties of human antibody variable domains. J Mol Biol 325:531–553

Hamers-Casterman C, Atarhouch T, Muyldermans S et al. (1993) Naturally occurring antibodies devoid of light chains. Nature 363:446–448

Harris LJ, Larson SB, Hasel KW et al. (1997) Refined structure of an intact IgG2a monoclonal antibody. Biochemistry 36:1581–1597

Helms LR, Wetzel R (1996) Specificity of abnormal assembly in immunoglobulin light chain deposition disease and amyloidosis. J Mol Biol 257:77–86

Honegger A, Plückthun A (2001) The Influence of the buried glutamine or glutamate residue in position 6 on the structure of immunoglobulin variable domains. J Mol Biol 309:687–699

Honegger A, Plückthun A (2001) Yet another numbering scheme for immunoglobulin variable domains: an automatic modeling and analysis tool. J Mol Biol 309:657–670

Hubbard SJ, Thornton JM (1993) NACCESS. computer program

Huston JS, Levinson D, Mudgett-Hunter M et al. (1988) Protein engineering of antibody binding sites: recovery of specific activity in an anti-digoxin single-chain Fv analogue produced in *Escherichia coli*. Proc Natl Acad Sci USA 85:5879–5883

Jones PT, Dear PH, Foote J et al. (1986) Replacing the complementarity-determining regions in a human antibody with those from a mouse. Nature 321:522–525

Jung S, Plückthun A (1997) Improving in vivo folding and stability of a single-chain Fv antibody fragment by loop grafting. Prot Eng 10:959–966

Jung S, Honegger A, Plückthun A (1999) Selection for improved protein stability by phage display. J Mol Biol 294:163–180

Kabat EA, Wu TT, Terry H et al. (1991) Sequences of proteins of immunological interest, NIH Publication No. 91–3242

Kaufmann M, Lindner P, Honegger A et al. (2002) Crystal Structure of the Anti-His Tag Antibody 3D5 Single-chain Fragment Complexed to its Antigen. J Mol Biol 318:135–147

Knappik A, Ge L, Honegger A et al. (2000) Fully synthetic human combinatorial antibody libraries (HuCAL) based on modular consensus frameworks and CDRs randomized with trinucleotides. J Mol Biol 296:57–86

Kortt AA, Lah M, Oddie GW et al. (1997) Single-chain Fv fragments of anti-neuraminidase antibody NC10 containing five- and ten-residue linkers form dimers and with zero-residue linker a trimer. Prot Eng 10:423–433

Lefranc MP, Giudicelli V, Ginestoux C et al. (1999) IMGT, the international ImMunoGeneTics database. Nucl Acids Res 27:209–212

Muyldermans S, Atarhouch T, Saldanha J et al. (1994) Sequence and structure of VH domain from naturally occurring camel heavy chain immunoglobulins lacking light chains. Prot Eng 7:1129–1135

Myklebust AT, Beiske K, Pharo A et al. (1991) Selection of anti-SCLC antibodies for diagnosis of bone marrow metastasis. Brit J Cancer Suppl 14:49–53

Proba K, Honegger A, Plückthun A (1997) A natural antibody missing a cysteine in V_H: consequences for thermodynamic stability and folding. J Mol Biol 265:161–172

Proba K, Wörn A, Honegger A et al. (1998) Antibody scFv fragments without disulfide bonds made by molecular evolution. J Mol Biol 275:245–253

Röthlisberger D, Honegger A, Plückthun A (2005) Domain interactions in the Fab fragment: a comparative evaluation of the single-chain Fv and Fab format engineered with variable domains of different stability. J Mol Biol 347:773–789

Tanha J, Xu P, Chen Z et al. (2001) Optimal design features of camelized human single-domain antibody libraries. J Biol Chem 276:24774–24780

Tomlinson IM, Walter G, Marks JD et al. (1992) The repertoire of human germline V_H sequences reveals about fifty groups of V_H segments with different hypervariable loops. J Mol Biol 227:776–798

Tomlinson IM, Cox JP, Gherardi E et al. (1995) The structural repertoire of the human V kappa domain. EMBO J 14:4628–4638

Vermeer AWP, Norde W (2000) The thermal stability of immunoglobulin: Unfolding and aggregation of a multi-domain protein. Biophys J 78: 394–404

Vermeer AWP, Norde W, van Amerongen A (2000) The unfolding/ denaturation of immunogammaglobulin of isotype 2b and its F-ab and F-c fragments. Biophys J 79:2150–2154

Waibel R, Alberto R, Willuda J et al. (1999) Stable one-step technetium-99m labeling of His-tagged recombinant proteins with a novel Tc(I)-carbonyl complex. Nat Biotech 17:897–901

Weber-Bornhauser S, Eggenberger J, Jelesarov I et al. (1998) Thermodynamics and kinetics of the reaction of a single-chain antibody fragment (scFv) with the leucine zipper domain of transcription factor GCN4. Biochemistry 37:13011–13020

Willuda J, Kubetzko S, Waibel R et al. (2001) Tumor targeting of mono-, di-, and tetravalent anti-p185(HER-2) miniantibodies multimerized by self-associating peptides. J Biol Chem 276:14385–14392

Willuda J, Honegger A, Waibel R et al. (1999) High thermal stability is essential for tumor targeting of antibody fragments: engineering of a humanized anti-epithelial glycoprotein-2 (epithelial cell adhesion molecule) single-chain Fv fragment. Cancer Res 59:5758–5767

Wörn A, Plückthun A (1998a) Mutual stabilization of V_L and V_H in single-chain antibody fragments, investigated with mutants engineered for stability. Biochemistry 37:13120–13127

Wörn A, Plückthun A (1998b) An intrinsically stable antibody scFv fragment can tolerate the loss of both disulfide bonds and fold correctly. FEBS Lett 427:357–361

Wörn A, Auf der Maur A, Escher D et al. (2000) Correlation between in vitro stability and in vivo performance of anti-GCN4 intrabodies as cytoplasmic inhibitors. J Biol Chem 275:2795–2803

Human Monoclonal Antibodies from Transgenic Mice

N. Lonberg

1   Immunogenicity of Therapeutic Antibodies: Problem and Solutions 70
2   Development of Techniques for Manipulation
     of the Mouse Genome 72
    2.1   Pronuclear Microinjection 72
    2.2   Embryonic Stem Cells 72
3   Transgenic Mice with Human Immunoglobulin Genes 74
    3.1   Expression of Human Antibody Repertoires 74
    3.2   Transgenic Mouse Platforms for Therapeutic MAb Drug Discovery 75
4   Transgenic Mouse-Derived Human MAbs 78
5   Transgenic Mouse-Derived Human MAbs in the Clinic 79
    5.1   Panitumumab and Zalutumumab 79
    5.2   MAbs in Phase 3 Clinical Testing 81
    5.3   MAbs in Phase 1 and 2 Clinical Testing 88
6   Conclusions 89
References 89

Abstract Since the 1986 regulatory approval of muromonomab-CD3, a mouse monoclonal antibody (MAb) directed against the T cell CD3ε antigen, MAbs have become an increasingly important class of therapeutic compounds in a variety of disease areas ranging from cancer and autoimmune indications to infectious and cardiac diseases. However, the pathway to the present acceptance of therapeutic MAbs within the pharmaceutical industry has not been smooth. A major hurdle for antibody therapeutics has been the inherent immunogenicity of the most readily available MAbs, those derived from rodents. A variety of technologies have been successfully employed to engineer MAbs with reduced immunogenicity. Implementation of these antibody engineering technologies involves in vitro optimization of lead molecules to generate a clinical candidate. An alternative technology, involving

N. Lonberg
Medarex, 521 Cottonwood Drive, Milpitas, CA 95035, USA
e-mail: nlonberg@medarex.com

Y. Chernajovsky, A. Nissim (eds.) *Therapeutic Antibodies. Handbook of Experimental Pharmacology 181.*

the engineering of strains of mice to produce human instead of mouse antibodies, has been emerging and evolving for the past two decades. Now, with the 2006 US regulatory approval of panitumumab, a fully human antibody directed against the epidermal growth factor receptor, transgenic mice expressing human antibody repertoires join chimerization, CDR grafting, and phage display technologies, as a commercially validated antibody drug discovery platform. With dozens of additional transgenic mouse-derived human MAbs now in clinical development, this new drug discovery platform appears to be firmly established within the pharmaceutical industry.

1 Immunogenicity of Therapeutic Antibodies: Problem and Solutions

The discovery of hybridoma methods in 1975 for isolating high specificity and high affinity rodent monoclonal antibodies (MAbs) opened the door to a new class of therapeutic compounds with potential applicability across a wide range of disease indications (Kohler and Milstein 1975). This promise appeared to be fulfilled with the 1986 US regulatory approval of muromonab-CD3 for the treatment of kidney transplant rejection (Goldstein et al. 1985). However, despite the fact that muromonomab-CD3 acts as a potent immunosuppressive drug, it turned out to be an intrinsically immunogenic molecule. Because rodent antibodies are foreign proteins, the human immune system mounts its own antibody response to them, leading to rapid clearance, reduced efficacy (Goldstein et al. 1985; Pendley et al. 2003; Kuus-Reichel et al. 1994), and an increased risk of infusion reactions (Baert et al. 2003). A potential solution to the problem of immunogenicity, fully human MAbs, did not at the time appear to be practical because of the limited availability of target specific human antibodies (Larrick and Bourla 1986; James and Bell 1987; Houghton 1983; Olsson et al. 1984). Although very large panels of rodent MAbs could be easily assembled and screened for optimal binding to the intended target and low cross-reactivity to related molecules, analogous technologies for generating and isolating human MAbs with the full range of specificities and affinities afforded by rodent hybridoma methods did not exist. The smaller pools of available reactive human antibodies might have been a factor in the selection of early human MAb clinical candidates such as HA-1A, which entered clinical testing for treatment of sepsis in the late 1980s and gained European regulatory approval in 1991 (Brun-Buisson 1994). This polyreactive authentic human MAb bound to its intended target, lipid A, through relatively nonspecific hydrophobic interactions of heavy chain V region framework residues (Helmhorst et al. 1998; Bieber et al. 1995). The 1992 clinical, and US regulatory, failure of HA-1A (Spalding 1992; Edgington 1992; McCloskey et al. 1994), together with the observed immunogenicity of muromonomab-CD3, contributed to a considerable cooling of enthusiasm for antibody-based drugs within the pharmaceutical industry. However, 8 years after the approval of muromonomab-CD3, a second MAb-based drug, the engineered chimeric antibody fragment abciximab (Simoons et al. 1994), gained approval. This was followed by the approval of 18 additional MAb-based drugs in the last 10 years. As a class of drug compounds, MAbs appear to have been rescued by the use of technologies for reengineering rodent antibodies in vitro to replace framework amino acid residues with corresponding human sequences (Morrison et al. 1984; Jones et al. 1986). Additional technologies were also developed to directly isolate synthetic MAbs from libraries of human and synthetic immunoglobulin sequences (McCafferty 1990). Although these existing antibody engineering technologies appear to have been very successful in generating therapeutic products with acceptable safety and efficacy, there may still be room for improvement. Although some of the products generated by antibody engineering have not elicited patient immune responses, most of the approved MAb products, including examples from chimerization, CDR grafting and phage display, have been found to be immunogenic (Pendley et al. 2003).

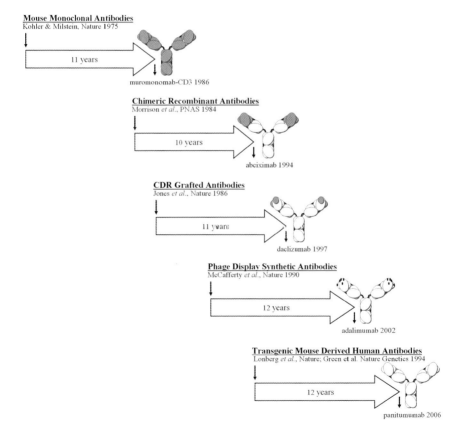

Fig. 1 Evolution of therapeutic antibody technology and progress to the clinic. FDA-approved MAbs have emerged between 10 and 12 years after the date that the new technologies on which they were based were reported in the scientific literature (Morrison et al. 1984; Jones et al. 1986; McCafferty et al. 1990; Kohler and Milstein 1975; Lonberg et al. 1994; Green et al. 1994)

Transgenic mouse strains comprising human immunoglobulin repertoires represent an alternative platform technology for discovering low immunogenicity therapeutic MAbs (Fig. 1). In contrast to antibody engineering technologies, which involve the downstream modification and optimization of individual protein molecules, transgenic technology is used for the upstream genetic engineering of strains of mice that are then used as drug discovery tools to directly generate human sequence antibodies that can be moved into the clinic without further optimization. Twelve years after their appearance in the scientific literature (Lonberg et al. 1994, Green et al. 1994), immunoglobulin transgenic mice have now been validated as drug discovery platforms by the regulatory approval of their first product, panitumumab (Gibson et al. 2006). In this review, I discuss the development of the technology and drugs derived from it.

2 Development of Techniques for Manipulation of the Mouse Genome

2.1 Pronuclear Microinjection

Fundamental basic research in mouse embryology and molecular biology by a large number of laboratories (Nagy et al. 2003) led to the development, in the early 1980s, of a set of tools for the manipulation of the mouse genome (Fig. 2). The generation of genetically engineered mice by direct microinjection of cloned DNA sequences into the pronuclei of single-cell half-day embryos was reported by several groups in 1981 (Gordon and Ruddle 1981; Costantini and Lacy 1981; Brinster et al. 1981; Harbers et al. 1981; Wagner et al. 1981a, 1981b). The microinjected DNA constructs, which are inserted into mouse chromosomes and are propagated through the germline, could include transcriptional regulatory sequences to direct expression to restricted differentiated cell types, including B cell expression of antibody genes (Brinster et al. 1983). This first report of an expressed immunoglobulin gene in transgenic mice involved a very small transgene; however, despite the fact that very fine glass needles are employed for pronuclear microinjection, the sheer forces experienced by the injected DNA do not prevent the use of this technique for introducing much larger (>100 kb) transgenes into the mouse germline. (Costantini and Lacy 1981; Taylor et al. 1992; Schedl et al. 1993; Lonberg and Huszar 1995; Fishwild et al. 1996).

2.2 Embryonic Stem Cells

Because microinjected transgenes integrate relatively randomly over a large number of potential sites within the mouse genome, it does not provide for easy manipulation of specific endogenous mouse genes. Microinjection could generate mice

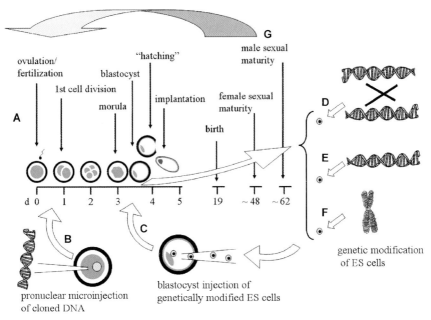

Fig. 2 Techniques developed for the manipulation of mouse embryos provide access for the modification of the germline. (**A**) Overview of mouse development. (**B**) Direct introduction of cloned DNA sequences inserted randomly into mouse chromosomes through pronuclear microinjection of half day embryos. (**C**) Embryonic Stem (ES) cells derived from 3.5-day blastocyst stage embryos can be grown in culture, genetically modified, and then reintroduced into developing blastocysts by insertion of a glass pipet into the blastocoel cavity. (**D**) Site-specific modifications of ES cell genomes can be engineered through homologous recombination followed by selection and screening for specific recombinants in culture. (**E**) Large DNA fragments can be inserted into ES cell chromosomes by transfection or yeast/bacterial cell fusion. (**F**) Entire chromosomes or chromosome fragments, which replicate without integration into endogenous mouse chromosomes, can be introduced into ES cells by microcell-mediated chromosome transfer (MMCT). (**G**) The very short (ca. 2–3 months) generation time of the mouse allows for rapid crossbreeding to combine multiple independent genetic modifications into a single animal

that expressed human genes, but the mouse ortholog was typically still active. This technical hurdle was overcome with the development of positive–negative selection vectors that allowed for the selection and screening of specifically targeted homologous recombination events in cultured cells, and with the parallel development of embryonic stem (ES) cell lines that could be cultured and manipulated in vitro and reintroduced into 3.5-day old blastocyst stage embryos to populate the germline of the resulting chimeric mice. The combination of these two technologies led to the generation of strains of engineered mice comprising specifically targeted modifications of their germlines (Mansour et al. 1988; Zijlstra et al. 1989; Schwartzberg et al. 1989). The most commonly introduced specific modification leads to the inactivation of an endogenous gene and the creation of what are commonly referred to as gene knockout mouse strains. Gene knockout technology has proved to be of enormous value for basic research, and applied to the endogenous mouse immunoglobulin loci, important for the development of transgenic mouse platforms for human antibody drug discovery.

In addition to applications for modifying endogenous mouse genes, ES cells have also proved useful as an alternative to pronuclear microinjection for the introduction of large DNA clones such as YAC clones (Strauss et al. 1993; Choi et al. 1993; Jakobovits et al. 1993; Davies et al. 1993). Very large human chromosome fragments have also been introduced into the mouse germline using ES cell technology. In this approach, called microcell-mediated chromosome transfer (MMCT), human fibroblast-derived microcells are fused with mouse ES cells resulting in pluripotent cell lines having a single human chromosome or chromosome fragment – including a centromere and both telomeres – that replicates and assorts during cell division without insertion into an endogenous mouse chromosome (Tomizuka et al. 1997).

3 Transgenic Mice with Human Immunoglobulin Genes

3.1 Expression of Human Antibody Repertoires

It was quickly recognized that the new tools developed for manipulating the mouse germline might be practically applied toward the generation of human immunoglobulin expressing transgenic mice. In 1985, Alt et al. (1985) suggested that transgenic technology could be useful for generating new human sequence MAbs starting from unrearranged, germline-configuration transgenes. The authors concluded that although this was "conceptually outlandish," it might "be realized in the not-too-distant future." A year later, Yamamura et al. (1986) reported the cell type specific expression of a human immunoglobulin gamma heavy chain transgene. This was followed by reports of expression and rearrangement of germline configuration (unrearranged) chicken and rabbit light chain transgenes in transgenic mice (Bucchini et al. 1987, Goodhardt et al. 1987), a milestone that was recognized at the time as contributing toward the development of a transgenic platform for discovering human MAbs. Buttin (1987) commented that "recent progress in this field invites us to believe that the creation of transgenic mice with B cells secreting a wide spectrum of [human] antibodies is no longer out of reach." In 1989, Bruggemann et al. (1989) reported the expression of a repertoire of human IgM heavy chains and the generation of a transgene-encoded immune response in mice. Three years later, Taylor et al. (1992) reported mice comprising germline configuration human heavy- and κ light-chain transgenes that produced a repertoire of human IgM and IgG antibodies. This group showed in a later paper (Taylor et al. 1994) that the IgG antibodies were a product of class switching, and that they comprised somatic mutations consistent with functional affinity maturation. These reports, and many others from a number of different laboratories, demonstrated that human gene sequences could direct cell type specific expression of human immunoglobulins in mice, and that those exogenous gene sequences could undergo the normal rearrangements and modifications required for generating primary and secondary antibody repertoires. However, human immunoglobulin transgenic mice with intact functional endogenous immunoglobulin loci also express mouse antibodies and chimeric mouse–human antibodies. Creation of a more useful platform for human antibody drug discovery, a mouse with disrupted endogenous immunoglobulin loci, requires combining methods for introducing human immunoglobulin transgenes with the methods described earlier for generating gene knockout mice.

3.2 Transgenic Mouse Platforms for Therapeutic MAb Drug Discovery

In 1994, two articles, one from my laboratory (Lonberg et al. 1994) and the other from Green et al. (1994), reported the generation of mice with four different germline modifications: two targeted disruptions (the endogenous mouse heavy- and κ light-chain genes) and two introduced human transgenes (encoding the heavy chain and κ light chain). Although both articles report the use of homologous recombination in mouse ES cells to engineer similar disruptions of the endogenous mouse loci, different technologies were used to construct and deliver the human sequence transgenes. Lonberg et al. (1994) used pronuclear microinjection to introduce reconstructed minilocus transgenes – the heavy chain containing 3 heavy-chain variable (V_H), 16 diversity (D), and all 6 heavy-chain joining (J_H) regions together with μ and γ1 constant-region gene segments. In the transgenic strains, this construct underwent VDJ joining, together with somatic mutation and correlated class switching (Taylor et al. 1994). The light-chain transgene included four Vκ, all five Jκ and the κ constant region (Cκ). In contrast, Green et al. (1994) used fusion of yeast protoplasts to deliver yeast artificial chromosome (YAC)-based minilocus transgenes. In this case, the heavy chain included $5 V_H$, all 25 D and all 6 J_H gene segments together with μ and δ constant-region gene segments. This construct underwent VDJ joining and expressed both IgM and IgD. The light-chain YAC construct included two functional Vκ and all five Jκ segments, together with Cκ. Neither group inactivated the endogenous λ-light-chain locus, which in typical laboratory mouse strains contributes to only ∼5% of the B cell repertoire. Functional λ-light-chain expression leads to a subpopulation of B cells producing hybrid B cell receptors and secreted antibodies that have human heavy- and mouse λ-light chains. However, the presence of this subpopulation did not prevent the isolation of hybridoma cell lines secreting fully human monoclonal IgM (Green et al. 1994) and IgG (Lonberg et al. 1994) MAbs recognizing the target antigens against which the mice had been immunized.

The ability of these engineered mouse strains, each comprising only a fraction of the natural human primary V gene segment repertoire, to generate antibodies to a variety of targets may reflect the relative importance of combinatorial diversity (encoded in the germline library of V, D, and J gene segments) and junctional and somatic diversity (a product of the assembly and maturation of antibody genes).

Although naive B cell CDR1 and CDR2 sequences are completely encoded by the germ line, junctional diversity, which is intact in minilocus transgenes, creates much of the heavy-chain CDR3 repertoire. CDR3 sequences appear to be critical for antigen recognition by unmutated B cell receptors and may be largely responsible for the primary repertoire (Ignatovitch et al. 1997; Davis 2004; Tomlinson et al. 1996). Primary repertoire B cells having low affinity for the immunogen can then enter into the T cell-mediated process of affinity maturation, which has been shown to generate high-affinity antibodies from a very limited V-gene repertoire. An extreme example of this is offered by a report of an engineered mouse strain having only a single functional human V_H gene and three mouse $V\lambda$ genes (Xu and Davis 2000). These animals demonstrated a specific antibody responses to a variety of T-dependent antigens. High affinity, somatically mutated MAbs were characterized, including a very high, 25 pM, affinity MAb against hen egg-white lysozyme. However, the minimal V-repertoire mice did not respond to the T-independent antigen, dextran B512, and the authors suggested that responses to carbohydrate antigens might drive evolutionary selection for large primary repertoires. Germline-encoded recognition of such antigens may be important for developing a rapid primary protective response to pathogens, a feature that would be selected for in the wild, but less important for isolating high-affinity antibodies from laboratory mice using hyperimmunization protocols that trigger T cell-dependent affinity maturation.

In addition to affecting the response to T-independent antigens and the kinetics of overall immune reactions, repertoire size may have an impact on B cell development and the size of different B cell compartments. Fishwild et al. (1996) compared mice having different numbers of light-chain V gene segments and found that the introduction of larger repertoires encoded by a κ light-chain YAC clone comprising approximately half the Vκ repertoire led to increased population of the peripheral and bone marrow B cell compartments relative to transgenic strains comprising only four Vκ genes. The relative number of mature and immature B cells in these compartments also appeared more normal in mice with larger V gene repertoires. Mendez et al. (1997) generated transgenic mice having nearly complete heavy-chain V repertoires and approximately half the κ-light-chain V repertoire, and compared them with the minilocus mice of Green et al. (1994). This paper, and a later analysis of the same mouse strains by Green and Jakobovits (1998), showed that V-region repertoire size had a profound effect on multiple checkpoints in B cell development, with larger repertoires capable of restoring B cell compartments to near normal levels. Despite the fact that human immunoglobulin transgenic mice express B cell receptors that are essentially hybrids of mouse and human components (e.g., human immunoglobulin, mouse Igα, Igβ, and other signaling molecules), their B cells develop and mature into what appear to be all of the normal B cell subtypes. Furthermore, the immunoglobulin transgenes undergo V(D)J joining, random nucleotide (N-region) addition, class switching, and somatic mutation to generate high-affinity MAbs to a variety of different antigens. The process of affinity maturation in these animals even recapitulates the normal pattern of somatic mutation hotspots observed in authentic human secondary repertoire antibodies (Harding and Lonberg 1995).

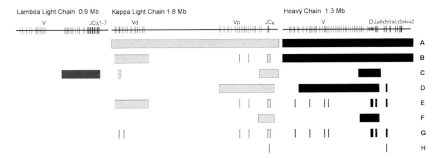

Fig. 3 Human immunoglobulin sequences introduced in the germ line of mice comprising endogenous Ig heavy-chain and κ-light-chain gene inactivations. The germline configuration of the human immunoglobulin λ-light chain, κ-light chain and heavy chain is depicted above *bars* representing those sequences used to assemble transgenes introduced into strains of mice used for generation and isolation of human sequence MAbs. **A** (Tomizuka et al. 2000), **B** (Ishida et al. 2002), **C** (Nicholson et al. 1999), **D** (Mendez et al. 1997), **E** (Fishwild et al. 1996), **F** (Green et al. 1994), **G** (Lonberg et al. 1994), **H** (Zou et al. 1994)

There have now been multiple reports in the literature of transgenic mice having immunoglobulin repertoires comprising human heavy- and light-chain sequences in the background of disrupted endogenous heavy- and κ-light-chain loci (Fig. 3). Several different technologies – including pronuclear microinjection and yeast protoplast fusion with ES cells – have been employed for engineering these mouse strains. The introduction of the largest fraction of the human germline repertoire has been facilitated by microcell-mediated chromosome transfer. Using this technique, Tomizuka et al. (1997) generated ES cell lines and chimeric mice containing fragments of human chromosomes 2 and 14, including the human κ-light-chain and heavy-chain loci, respectively. In addition, they generated chimeric mice that incorporated an apparently intact human chromosome 22, comprising the λ light chain locus. Germline transmission was obtained with the human κ-light-chain ES cell lines. In a subsequent report, germline transmission was obtained with a human heavy-chain ES cell line, and mice were created that expressed complete human heavy- and light-chain repertoires in a genetic background that included disruptions of the mouse heavy- and κ-light-chain loci (Tomizuka et al. 2000). Completely human, high-affinity (<nanomolar) MAbs were isolated from the animals. Although both chromosome fragments could be transmitted through the germ line, the κ-light chain-containing chromosome-2 fragment was found to be less mitotically stable. The observed stability of the heavy chain-containing fragment may derive from the fortuitous location of the immunoglobulin heavy-chain locus (IgH) at the very telomere of the long arm of human chromosome 14. Because of the structure of chromosome 14, a random deletion between IgH and the centromere removed most of the nonimmunoglobulin genes leaving IgH, the centromere and both telomeres functionally intact. The resulting 10- to 20-Mb fragment minimizes cross-species trisomy, which would presumably be selected against during cell division.

The observed stability of this fragment has now been exploited to create artificially constructed human chromosome fragments that include the entire human heavy-chain locus together with the entire human λ-light-chain locus (Kuroiwa et al. 2000). Bruggemann and colleagues (Popov et al. 1999) have also generated human λ-light-chain locus transgenes, using them to create transgenic mice that express partial repertoires of all three human immunoglobulin loci in the background of disrupted endogenous κ-light-chain and heavy-chain loci (Nicholson et al. 1999).

Another transgenic mouse platform, which generates chimeric antibodies rather than fully human sequence antibodies, was developed by Rajewsky and colleagues in 1994 (Zou et al. 1994). These mice comprise relatively precise replacements of the mouse κ and γ1 constant-region gene segments with the corresponding human gene sequences. The κ constant-region gene segment was replaced using homologous recombination in mouse ES cells. For the γ1 gene, only the secreted exons were replaced, and the engineering was accomplished in two steps using the Cre-*loxP* recombination system, also in mouse ES cells.

4 Transgenic Mouse-Derived Human MAbs

The scientific literature includes a large number of reports describing the characteristics of human MAbs derived from transgenic mouse platforms, and a review of this literature provides an assessment of the functionality of these platforms (Lonberg 2005). A very diverse set of antigens have been successfully targeted with transgenic derived MAbs. These include small molecules (Ball et al. 1999; Farr et al. 2002), pathogen-encoded proteins (Tzipori et al. 2004; Mukherjee et al. 2002; Mukherjee et al. 2002b; He et al. 2002; Greenough et al. 2005; Sheoran et al. 2005; Babcock et al. 2006; Coughlin et al. 2006; Vitale et al. 2006), polysaccharide antigens (Chang et al. 2002; Maitta 2004), human-secreted proteins (Mendez et al. 1997; Ishida et al. 2002; Villadsen et al. 2003; Bekker et al. 2004; Yang et al. 1999b; Huang et al. 2002; Mian et al. 2003; Ostendorf et al. 2003; Suarez et al. 2004; Parry et al. 2005; Rathanaswami et al. 2005; Burgess et al. 2006; Melnikova and Bar-Eli 2006), cell-surface proteins (Fishwild et al. 1996; Mendez et al. 1997; Fishwild et al. 1999; Yang et al. 1999, 2001; Holmes 2001; Borchmann et al. 2003; Skov et al. 2003; Teeling et al. 2004; Schuler et al. 2004; Rowinski et al. 2004; Heuck et al. 2004; Ramakrishna et al. 2004; Keler et al. 2003; Bleeker et al. 2004; Suzuki et al. 2004; Imakiire et al. 2004; Mori et al. 2004; Garambois et al. 2004; Trikha et al. 2004; Tai et al. 2005; Boll et al. 2005; Cohen et al. 2005; Kuroki et al. 2005; Sanderson et al. 2005; Tse et al. 2006; van Royen-Kerkhoff et al. 2005; Wang et al. 2005; Ma et al. 2006; Melnikova and Bar-Eli 2006; Teeling et al. 2006; Wu et al. 2006; Villadsen et al. 2007), and human tumor-associated glycosylation variants (Nozawa et al. 2004).

Most of the transgenic mouse-derived MAbs have binding affinities in the 0.1–10 nM range, the same affinity range typically seen for MAbs derived from wild-type mice (Ball et al. 1999; Yang et al. 1999, 1999b; Keler et al. 2003; Cohen et al. 2005; Burgess et al. 2006). This range is probably a function of the natural constraints on affinity maturation operating in vivo (Foote and Eisen 1995; Roost et al. 1995). However, there are also examples of transgenic-derived human MAbs with pico-molar and even subpicomolar affinities. Villadsen et al. (2003) described a 10 pM affinity antibody to IL-15, Wang et al. (2005) described a 4 pM affinity MAb to the insulin-like growth factor receptor, and Rathanaswami et al. (2005) reported several anti-IL-8 MAbs in the 1–10 pM range, with one MAb having a measured affinity in the 0.5–1 pM range.

5 Transgenic Mouse-Derived Human MAbs in the Clinic

5.1 Panitumumab and Zalutumumab

The 2006 regulatory approval in the US for panitumumab was a significant milestone for transgenic mouse-derived MAbs, and marked the first commercial validation of immunoglobulin transgenic mouse drug discovery platforms. Panitumumab binds to the epidermal growth factor receptor (EGFR) with very high affinity ($K_d = 5 \times 10^{-11} M^{-1}$) and blocks ligand binding (Rowinski et al. 2004; Yang et al. 1999, 2001; Foon et al. 2004). In preclinical mouse xenograft models, it was found to be more potent than the lower affinity mouse antibody m225 (Yang et al. 1999), the parent of the already marketed mouse/human IgG1 chimeric anti-EGFR antibody, cetuximab (Cunningham et al. 2004).

There has been no direct comparison of the safety and efficacy of cetuximab and panitumumab in a side-by-side clinical study. In addition, the fact that ce-tuximab is an IgG1 antibody and panitumumab an IgG2 antibody further com-plicates any attempt to compare the two drugs. However, an initial survey of the available literature suggests that the fact that panitumumab is a fully human anti-body derived from a transgenic mouse may differentiate it from the chimeric ce-tuximab (Cohenuram and Saif 2007). In early phase I and II trials, panitumumab was associated with a higher frequency of skin rashes than cetuximab; however, skin rashes (which are related to the mechanism of action of EGFR-targeted drugs, including small molecules, and in this case are not a product of drug immuno-genicity) have been positively correlated with activity for cetuximab (Calvo and Rowinsky 2005), and in a renal cell carcinoma trial, involving a relatively small number of patients, skin rashes correlated with longer cancer progression–free sur-vival for panitumumab (Rowinski et al. 2004). Later trials appear to indicate that the two molecules have similar clinical activity. In a randomized, 2-arm (231 pa-tients in the treatment arm) phase III trial in 2nd line, chemotherapy refractory, $EGFR^+$, metastatic colorectal carcinoma patients (Gibson et al. 2006), there was an 8% objective response rate, with 28% of the patients having stable disease (com-pared with a 0% response rate and 10% stable disease in the control cohort). This compares to the clinical responses seen for cetuximab monotherapy in a 346 patient phase II trial in a similar set of refractory, EGFR$^+$, metastatic colorectal carcinoma patients (Lenz et al. 2006). Approximately, 12% of the cetuximab-treated patients were classified as objective responders, and 32% as stable disease. Panitumumab was dosed at $6\,mg\,kg^{-1}$ every 2 weeks while the chimeric cetuximab was first given at a (roughly) 50% higher loading dose ($400\,mg\,m^{-2}$), followed by a similar weekly dose of $250\,mg\,m^{-2}$. The lower dosing schedule selected for panitumumab was a reflection of the longer clearance time for the fully human antibody; however, the terminal half life (7.5 days) is still shorter than is typically found for IgG molecules. This is presumably due to the large antigen sink provided by normal tissue expression of EGFR. Gibson et al. (2006) reported that no patients had detectable levels of anti-panitumumab antibodies after treatment, and that while 5% of the patients had low-grade infusion reactions, none had grade 3 or 4 reactions. In contrast, 7.5% of the cetuximab patients experienced hypersensitivity reactions with 1.7% having grade 3 or 4 reactions, despite the fact that most of those patients had been pretreated with antihistamines to prevent infusion reactions. Lenz et al. (2006) also reported that over 4% of the cetuximab-treated patients developed human antichimeric antibodies.

Because panitumumab is a human IgG2 antibody and, because IgG2 antibodies are poor mediators of Fc dependent cell killing, the activity of the drug may be a function of non-Fc mediated mechanisms. These could involve blockade of ligand-induced receptor signaling and/or altered signaling directed by MAb binding. This is consistent with the observation that the MAb is active in mouse xenograft models while a sibling human IgG2 antibody that does not block ligand binding has no activity (Yang et al. 2001). However, although IgG2 molecules do not show significant binding to human FcγRIII (CD16), they do bind to the common H131 variant of FcγRIIa (CD32A, Parren et al. 1992). This variant is also associated with clinical responses to rituximab (Weng and Levy 2003). It is, therefore, a formal possibility that in human patients some of the activity of the panitumumab is mediated through FcγRIIa in H131 individuals. Gibson et al. (2006) did not report any data on the FcγRIIa allotype of the patients that responded to panitumumab; however, if a positive correlation between the H131 allotype and clinical responses were found it might indicate that some of the activity of the MAb is Fc mediated. Because IgG1 is a more potent mediator of Fc-dependent activity, it might then follow that a human IgG1 variant of panitumumab could have improved activity. This theory could be tested in the near future as clinical data becomes available for a second EGFR binding MAb, zalutumumab, derived from transgenic mice (Bleeker et al. 2004; Lammerts et al. 2006). Zalutumumab is now in phase 3 testing for treatment of EGFR-positive squamous cell cancer of the head and neck. Preclinical studies of 2F8 show that like panitumumab, it is also more potent than m225 in mouse xenograft models (Bleeker et al. 2004). However, unlike panitumumab it is an IgG1 antibody and may function by eliciting Fc-mediated effector cell activity in addition to blocking ligand binding and normal receptor functioning. A comparison of the clinical activity of these two molecules may provide some insight into the role of Fc-receptor interaction on the efficacy and safety of these drugs.

5.2 MAbs in Phase 3 Clinical Testing

There are at least eight transgenic mouse-derived human MAbs in Phase 3 clinical trials (Table 1). These include zalutumumab, the EGFR binding MAb discussed earlier, two different antibodies directed against CTLA-4, and one each directed against CD20 and CD4 for treatment of cancer, two neutralizing MAbs directed against TNFα and the common subunit of IL-12 and IL-23 for inflammatory indications, and an antibody directed against RANKL for bone loss.

5.2.1 Denosomab

Denosomab is an antibody directed against RANKL, a TNF family member that stimulates the maturation and activation of osteoclasts, which mediate bone resorption. The drug is now in phase 3 clinical trials for treatment of bone loss in postmenopausal women and in cancer patients with treatment induced bone loss or skeletal disease caused by bone metastases. A single subcutaneous dose escalation, phase 1 study in osteoporotic patients showed dose-dependent and sustained activity (up to 6 months) in blocking bone resorption, with no reported serious drug-related adverse events (Bekker et al. 2004). Denosomab was found to have dose-dependent pharmacokinetics (PK), with a terminal half life of 32 days at the highest $3\,mg\,kg^{-1}$ dose. A second single dose trial in patients with multiple myeloma or bone metastases from breast cancer showed decreased bone metabolism that persisted for the 84-day study follow-up period, and a mean half life of 46 days after a single $3\,mg\,kg^{-1}$ dose (Body et al. 2006). These studies measured bone metabolism using urine concentrations of peptide products of collagen catabolism as an indirect measure. Another trial, in postmenopausal women, looked at 3-month and 6-month repeat dosing, and also directly measured bone density (McClung et al. 2006). Consistent with the reduction in bone metabolism seen in the single dose studies, bone density was found to be increased for the 12 months of the study, even for patients given only 60 mg of drug every 6 months. The adverse event profile for the treatment group was not significantly different from that of the placebo group, and only 2 of the 314 treated patients showed transient levels of anti-denosomab antibodies in single blood samples, which were not confirmed in later blood samples. The low incidence of measurable antidrug antibodies, the safety profile, and the very long half-life and sustained drug activity are all consistent with an antibody that is relatively nonimmunogenic. Because infrequent dosing may be very important for patient compliance for a parenterally delivered protein-based therapeutic that is directed at chronic indications such as osteoporosis, low immunogenicity could be a critical feature for the success of this product.

Table 1 Disclosed targets for transgenic mouse derived antibody drugs tested in human subjects

Target	Drug	Indication	Company (developer)	Company (technology)	Highest Development Stage
EGFR	panitumumab	Colorectal cancer and non-small cell lung cancer, renal cell carcinoma	Amgen	Abgenix	Launched
CD20	ofatumumab	Non-Hodgkin lymphoma	Genmab	Medarex	Phase 3
CD4	zanolimumab	Lymphoma	Genmab	Medarex	Phase 3
CTLA-4	ipilimumab	Melanoma and various other cancers	Medarex	Medarex	Phase 3
CTLA-4	CP-675206	Melanoma	Pfizer	Abgenix	Phase 3
EGFR	zalutumumab	Head and neck cancer	Genmab	Medarex	Phase 3
IL-12/IL-23 p40	CNTO 1275	Psoriasis and multiple sclerosis	Johnson & Johnson	Medarex	Phase 3
RANKL	denosomab	Osteoporosis and treatment-induced bone loss	Amgen	Abgenix	Phase 3
TNFα	golimumab	Inflammatory disease	Johnson & Johnson	Medarex	Phase 3
CD30	MDX-060	Lymphoma	Medarex	Medarex	Phase 2
Clostridium difficile toxins A and B	MDX-066/ MDX-1388[a]	Hospital acquired C. difficile associated diarrhea	MBL/Medarex	Medarex	Phase 2
IGF-1R	CP-751,871	Cancer	Pfizer	Abgenix	Phase 2
IL-15	AMG 714	Rheumatoid arthritis	Amgen/Genmab	Medarex	Phase 2
IGF-1R	CP-751,871	Cancer	Pfizer	Abgenix	Phase 2
IL-15	AMG 714	Rheumatoid arthritis	Amgen/Genmab	Medarex	Phase 2
PSMA	MDX-070	Prostate cancer	Medarex	Medarex	Phase 2

Target	Antibody	Indication			Phase
αv Integrins	CNTO 95	Solid tumors	Johnson & Johnson	Medarex	Phase 2
CTGF	FG-3019	Diabetic nephropathy and pulmonary fibrosis	Fibrogen	Medarex	Phase 1b
PDGF-D	CR002	Inflammatory kidney disease	Curagen	Abgenix	Phase 1b
CD89	MDX – 214[b]	Solid tumors	Medarex	Medarex	Phase 1/2
Alpha Interferons	MDX-1103/MEDI-545	Lupus	Medimmune/Medarex	Medarex	Phase 1
Anthrax protective antigen	MDX-1303	B. Anthracis infection	Pharmathene/Medarex	Medarex	Phase 1
CCR5	CCR5 mAb	HIV Infection	Human Genome Sciences	Abgenix	Phase 1
CD30	MDX – 1401[c]	Lymphoma	Medarex	Medarex	Phase 1
CD3ε	NI-0401	Autoimmune disease	NovImmune	Medarex	Phase 1
CD40	CP-870,893	Cancer	Pfizer	Abgenix	Phase 1
CD40	CHIR-12.12	Chronic lymphocytic leukemia	Novartis/Xoma	Abgenix	Phase 1
CDw137	BMS-66513	Cancer	Bristol-Myers Squibb	Medarex	Phase 1
CXCL10	MDX-1100	Ulcerative colitis	Medarex	Medarex	Phase 1
Dendritic cell mannose receptor	MDX – 1307[d]	Human gonadotropin–positive cancers	Celldex	Medarex	Phase 1
HGF/SF	AMG 102	Solid Tumors	Amgen	Abgenix	Phase 1
IL-8	ABX-IL8	Psoriasis	Abgenix	Abgenix	Phase 1
Melanoma antigen glyco-protein NMB	CR011 – vcMMAE[e]	Melanoma	Curagen	Abgenix	Phase 1

Table 1 (continued)

Target	Drug	Indication	Company (developer)	Company (technology)	Highest Development Stage
Muc18	ABX-MA1	Melanoma	Abgenix	Abgenix	Phase 1
Parathyroid hormone	ABX-PTH	Hyperparathyroidism	Amgen	Abgenix	Phase 1
PD-1	MDX-1106/ ONO-4538	Cancer	Ono Pharmaceuticals/ Medarex	Medarex	Phase 1
PDGFRα	IMC-3G3	Cancer	ImClone	Medarex	Phase 1
PSCA	AGS-PSCA/ MK-4721	Prostate cancer	Agensys/Merck	Abgenix	Phase 1
TRAIL-R2	HGS-TR2J	Solid tumors	Human Genome Sciences	Kirin	Phase 1

[a] Combination of two different monoclonal antibodies directed against each of the two toxins
[b] Human antigen-binding fragment (Fab) fused to epidermal growth factor
[c] Nonfucosylated Fc variant of MDX-060
[d] Human Fab fused to βhCG
[e] Antibody-drug conjugate with the small molecule microtubule inhibitor MMAE

5.2.2 Ipilimumab and CP-675206

The two transgenic mouse-derived human antibodies directed against CTLA-4, ipilimumab, and CP-675206, also do not appear to elicit strong patient antidrug antibody responses, despite the fact that the mechanism of action for these drugs results in a very potent up-modulation of patient immune responses. CTLA-4 is a negative T cell signaling molecule that binds to the two ligands CD80 and CD86, both of which are also recognized by the positive T cell signaling molecule CD28 (Korman et al. 2006). Ipilimumab (Keler et al. 2003) is a human IgG1 antibody, while CP-675206 (Ribas et al. 2005) is an IgG2 antibody. Both molecules bind to human CTLA-4 so as to block ligand binding and antagonize CTLA-4 signaling, resulting in the activation of certain T cell responses. Experiments with hamster MAbs that block mouse CTLA-4 show that the resulting enhanced immune responses can mediate tumor rejection in syngeneic mouse tumor models (Leach et al. 1996). Preclinical experiments in cynomolgus monkey models demonstrated that ipilimumab could stimulate humoral immune responses to coadministered vaccines (Keler et al. 2003). Clinical data in cancer patients has been reported for both ipilimumab (Phan et al. 2003; Hodi et al. 2003; Ribas et al. 2004; Attia et al. 2005; Blansfield et al. 2005; Maker et al. 2005, 2005b, 2006 Sanderson et al. 2005; Beck et al. 2006; Thompson et al. 2006) and CP-675206 (Ribas et al. 2004, 2005, Reuben et al. 2006). Objective and durable antitumor responses were observed for both drugs. Rosenberg and colleagues conducted a trial in patients with metastatic melanoma who were treated with ipilimumab at $3\,\mathrm{mg\,kg}^{-1}$ every 3 weeks for up to six cycles or were given a loading dose of ipilimumab at $3\,\mathrm{mg\,kg}^{-1}$ followed by $1\,\mathrm{mg\,kg}^{-1}$ every 3 weeks for up to six cycles. All patients were administered a subcutaneous gp100 peptide vaccine (Attia et al. 2005). The overall objective response rate for the 56 patients in the combined cohorts was 13%, with ongoing complete and partial responses reported at 25, 26, 30, 31, and 34 months. A follow-up paper by this group included additional metastatic melanoma patients treated with and without the vaccine, some receiving ipilimumab doses as high as $9\,\mathrm{mg\,kg}^{-1}$, together with 61 renal cell carcinoma patients treated with ipilimumab at up to $3\,\mathrm{mg\,kg}^{-1}$ (Beck et al. 2006). The overall objective response rate for the 198 patients in this report was 14%. This group also combined ipilimumab and high dose IL-2 in metastatic melanoma patients and reported a 22% objective response rate in patients administered ipilimumab at $3\,\mathrm{mg\,kg}^{-1}$. In a phase 1 single dose, monotherapy, dose escalation trial of CP-675206 in metastatic melanoma, with patients receiving doses as high as $15\,\mathrm{mg\,kg}^{-1}$, the authors reported a 10% objective response rate (Ribas et al. 2005), although one of the four responders had also received ipilimumab (Ribas et al. 2004). The serious adverse events reported for both ipilimumab and CP-675206 comprise a spectrum of immune-related inflammatory responses including rash, enterocolitis, and hypophysitis (Jaber et al. 2006; Blansfield et al. 2005; Ribas et al. 2005; Beck et al. 2006). However, because the mechanism of action of CTLA-4 blocking MAbs involves the activation of immune responses, these have been considered as target-related toxicities, and have in fact correlated with clinical responses (Beck et al. 2006, Reuben et al. 2006). Beck et al.

(2006) reported 36% and 35% objective response rates for melanoma and renal cell cancer patients having enterocolitis, with response rates of only 11% and 2% for patients without enterocolitis. The inflammatory adverse events have been reported to respond to medical management, which may include corticosteroids. Interestingly, corticosteroid treatment does not appear to abrogate objective tumor responses (Attia et al. 2005; Beck et al. 2006). Despite the observed up-regulation of immune responses in patients treated with these two MAbs, the drugs themselves do not appear to be readily recognized and cleared by the human immune system. A terminal half-life of 22 days was reported for CP-675206 (Ribas 2005), and 1-month post-dosing serum trough levels of $10\,\mu g\,ml^{-1}$ ipilimumab were reported after 5 months of repeated monthly dosing at $3\,mg\,kg^{-1}$ (Sanderson et al. 2005). Sanderson et al. (2005) also reported that these repeatedly dosed patients did not develop a measurable antibody response to ipilimumab. These data are consistent with the data from preclinical studies that showed no evidence of monkey anti-human antibody formation in cynomolgus macaques dosed five times over 140 days (Keler et al. 2003), despite the fact that the MAb upregulated the monkey humoral immune responses to coadministered vaccines. There was no sign of immune clearance by monkey anti-human antibodies, with drug titers never falling below $20\,\mu g\,ml^{-1}$ over the course of the 5-month study.

5.2.3 CNTO 1275 and Golimumab

Another transgenic-derived human MAb in phase 3 development is CNTO 1275, which is directed against the common p40 subunit shared by IL-12 and IL-23. Results have been reported from a phase 1 trial in multiple sclerosis (Kasper et al. 2006) and from phase 1 and 2 trials in psoriasis (Kauffman et al. 2004, Toichi et al. 2006, Krueger et al. 2007). In the phase 1 psoriasis trial, the drug showed sustained activity over 16 weeks of follow-up with a single i.v. administration, with 67% of the patients achieving at least a 75% improvement (assessed by the Psoriasis Area and Severity Index). There were no treatment-related serious adverse events, and no infusion reactions. Antidrug antibodies were detected in 1 of 18 patients; however, presence of drug in the serum because of the very long terminal half life, 19–27 days, precluded accurate assessment in most of the patients. A similar 20–31 day terminal half-life was observed in the multiple sclerosis trial where the drug was given by subcutaneous administration. One of the 16 treated patients developed a detectable antidrug response; however, as with the psoriasis trial, the persistence of the drug in the serum made it difficult to accurately measure antidrug antibodies. In the phase 2 psoriasis trial, 237 patients received the drug for up to four weekly 90 mg subcutaneous doses. Antidrug antibodies were detected once or more in the 52 weeks of monitoring in 12 (4%) of the treated patients. However, the measured antibody response did not correlate with injection site reactions, which occurred at the same 2% frequency in both placebo and drug-treated cohorts. Patients given only a single subcutaneous dose, at either 45 or 90 mg, showed sustained disease-modifying responses for over 6 months following treatment. Together with the observed sustained clinical benefit, the approximately 20–30 day terminal half-life of CNTO 1275 appears to indicate that it does not elicit a strong drug-clearing antibody response. As further clinical data are reported, it will be interesting to compare the immunogenicity, PK, safety, and efficacy of the transgenic mouse-derived CNTO 1275 to the phage display derived ABT-874, which is also directed against the common p40 subunit of IL12 and IL-23 (Mannon et al. 2004, Fuss et al. 2006). The phage display antibody also showed some signs of immunogenicity, with antidrug antibodies detectable in 3 of 63 patients, and 2 of those patients showing evidence of early clearance of the drug from the serum (Mannon et al. 2004); however, because patients received up to 7 weekly doses of the drug, it is difficult to compare the data to that reported for CNTO 1275. The terminal half life of ABT-874 was not reported.

Data should also soon be available to compare a second pair of antibodies directed against a shared target but derived from the competing transgenic mouse and phage display technology platforms. Both golimumab, a human sequence antibody from transgenic mice is now in phase 3 clinical testing in rheumatoid arthritis, and adalimumab, a phage display derived antibody currently approved for the same indication, are high affinity TNFα blocking MAbs (Weinblatt et al. 2003). Both are also IgG1 molecules formulated for subcutaneous administration. This comparison may be of particular interest because adalimumab has been reported to elicit antidrug antibodies at a high frequency, despite the fact that it was genetically engineered from a lead molecule originally isolated from a phage display library constructed from human immunoglobulin sequences. The formation of these antidrug antibodies correlated with adverse events and reduced efficacy in a study of 15 rheumatoid arthritis patients (Bender et al. 2007). Another approved TNFα blocking antibody, infliximab, is a chimeric mouse–human antibody that also elicits a strong antidrug antibody response, which correlates with infusion reactions and reduced efficacy (Baert et al. 2003). Data from a third MAb derived from an alternative technology may provide some insight into the relative importance of factors such as drug target, patient population, and intrinsic immunogenicity on the efficacy and safety of antibody-based therapeutics.

5.2.4 Zanolimumab

Zanolimumab is a transgenic mouse-derived human antibody directed against the T cell antigen CD4 (Fishwild et al. 1999). Results from an 85 patient, placebo-controlled, phase 2 trial in psoriasis have been reported (Skov et al. 2003), and the drug is now in phase 3 clinical testing in cutaneous T cell lymphoma. In the published psoriasis study, there was an observed dose-dependent decrease in circulating CD4$^+$ cells, particularly in the CD45RO$^+$ memory T cell population. This may translate to efficacy in the cancer setting where the drug is currently being developed (Villadsen et al. 2007). The drug was well tolerated with one likely drug-related serious adverse event, a rash appearing after the second dose at 160 mg. No patients developed antidrug antibodies. In the published preclinical study (Fishwild et al. 1999), the antibody was found to be nonimmunogenic in chimpanzees; however,

it did induce a blocking antibody response in a majority of the dosed cynomolgus monkeys (demonstrating that primate models may, in some cases, overestimate
immunogenicity).

5.2.5 Ofatumumab

Ofatumumab (Teeling et al. 2004), a transgenic mouse-derived antibody directed at
the B cell surface antigen CD20, is also in phase 3 clinical development. Although
this antibody shares the same target as the mouse–human chimeric MAb rituximab,
which is currently approved for treatment of non-Hodgkin's lymphoma (NHL) and
rheumatoid arthritis (Coiffier et al. 1998, Cohen et al. 2006), it recognizes a distinct
epitope and may, as a result, have a different mechanism of action (Teeling et al.
2006). Rituximab appears to recognize only one of the two extracellular loops of
CD20, while the ofatumumab epitope comprises residues from both loops and the
antibody is a more potent mediator of complement-dependent cytotoxicity in vitro
than rituximab. This difference in potency is more pronounced at lower antigen
density, and may translate into greater activity in low CD20 expressing lymphomas
such as chronic lymphocytic leukemia (CLL), where the drug is currently being
tested in phase 3 clinical trials. Because of the potential difference in mechanism
of action and activity between ofatumumab and rituximab, a comparison of their
relative safety and efficacy profiles may not be as useful for evaluating the potential
of human vs. chimeric antibodies; however, the process for selecting ofatumumab
as the lead clinical candidate (Teeling et al. 2004, Teeling et al. 2006) does highlight
an important advantage of the transgenic mouse platform over other antibody drug
discovery platforms. Unlike antibody engineering technologies for making low immunogenicity MAbs, where an early lead candidate is then modified or optimized
in vitro to reduce immunogenicity, with the transgenic mouse platforms, the process of lead optimization is bypassed, making it possible to test each potential lead
candidate in a series of increasingly sophisticated in vitro and in vivo assays in
essentially the same molecular form as it will eventually be used in humans. Resources that would otherwise be devoted to optimization of a small number of lead
hits can be devoted to better characterization of a larger number of lead candidates
comprising a wider variety of functional properties.

5.3 MAbs in Phase 1 and 2 Clinical Testing

The available published scientific literature does not include the same level of detailed data on drug tolerability, PK, and efficacy for molecules that have not yet
entered phase 3 clinical testing; however, published abstracts from scientific meet-
ings and discussions in review articles does provide some information. A transgenic
mouse-derived anti-CD30 MAb, MDX-060 (Borchmann et al. 2003; Heuck et al.
2004; Boll et al. 2005), has been tested in Hodgkin's lymphoma and anaplastic

large cell lymphoma patients (Borchmann et al. 2004; Borchmann et al. 2005; Klimm et al. 2005). Fifty-six patients were reported to have been treated with up to 15 mg kg^{-1} every week for 4 weeks without significant infusion reactions. The preliminary results were interpreted to indicate that the drug was well tolerated and had clinical activity. Preclinical results have also been published for additional transgenic-derived MAbs now in clinical testing. These include antibodies directed against IL-15 (Villadsen et al. 2003), PSMA (Holmes 2001), *Clostridium difficile* toxins A and B (Babcock et al. 2006), CD40 (Tai et al. 2005), anthrax protective antigen (Vitale et al. 2006), hepatocyte growth factor (Burgess et al. 2006), melanoma antigen glycoprotein NMB (Tse et al. 2006), insulin-like growth factor receptor (Cohen et al. 2005), and αv integrins (Trikha et al. 2004; Martin et al. 2005).

6 Conclusions

Transgenic mice that express human antibody repertoires have proven to be useful for generating high-affinity human sequence MAbs against a wide variety of potential drug targets. The clinical experience with a variety of transgenic mouse derived fully human antibodies in human patients shows promising efficacy and safety profiles for several of these molecules. Furthermore, the overall experience to date is that the technology has succeeded in delivering human MAbs that demonstrate relatively low immunogenicity and have relatively long in vivo half lives. Twelve years after the first publications describing transgenic mice having disrupted endogenous immunoglobulin loci and expressing human heavy and light chain repertoires, the US regulatory approval of panitumumab provides commercial validation for this drug discovery platform. In addition, the variety and very large number of different clinical and preclinical programs involving human MAbs from transgenic mice suggest that the technology will continue to contribute new therapeutic drugs.

Acknowledgements I thank Michelle Temple for assistance with the manuscript.

References

Alt FW, Blackwell TK, Yancopoulos GD (1985) Immunoglobulin genes in transgenic mice. Trends Genet 1:231–236

Attia P, Phan GQ, Maker AV et al. (2005) Autoimmunity correlates with tumor regression in patients with metastatic melanoma treated with anti-cytotoxic T-lymphocyte antigen-4. J Clin Oncol 23:6043–6053

Babcock GJ, Broering TJ, Hernandez HJ et al. (2006) Human monoclonal antibodies directed against toxins A and B prevent Clostridium difficile-induced mortality in hamsters. Infect Immun 74:6339–6347

Baert F, Noman M, Vermeire S et al. (2003) Influence of immunogenicity on the long-term efficacy of imfliximab in Crohn's disease. N Engl J Med 348:601–608

Ball WJ, Kasturi R, Dey P et al. (1999) Isolation and characterization of human monoclonal antibodies to digoxin. J Immunol 163:2291–2298

Beck KE, Blansfield JA, Tran KQ et al. (2006) Enterocolitis in patients with cancer after antibody blockade of cytotoxic T-lymphocyte-associated antigen 4. J Clin Oncol 24:2283–2289

Bekker PJ, Holloway D, Rasmussen S et al. (2004) A single-dose placebo-controlled study of AMG 162, a fully human monoclonal antibody to RANKL, in postmenopausal women. J Bone Miner Res 19:1059–1066

Bender NK, Heilig CE, Dröll B et al. (2007) Immunogenicity, efficacy and adverse events of adalimumab in RA patients. Rheumatol Int 27:269–274

Bieber MM, Bhat NM, Teng NN (1995) Anti-endotoxin human monoclonal antibody A6H4C5 (HA-1A) utilizes the VH4.21 gene. Clin Infect Dis 21(Suppl 2):S186–S189

Blansfield JA, Beck KE, Tran K et al. (2005) Cytotoxic T-lymphocyte-associated antigen-4 blockage can induce autoimmune hypophysitis in patients with metastatic melanoma and renal cancer. J Immunother 28:593–598

Bleeker WK, Lammerts van Bueren JJ, van Ojik HH et al. (2004) Dual mode of action of a human anti-epidermal growth factor receptor monoclonal antibody for cancer therapy. J Immunol 173:4699–4707

Body JJ, Facon T, Coleman RE et al. (2006) A study of the biological receptor activator of nuclear factor-kappaB ligand inhibitor, denosumab, in patients with multiple myeloma or bone metastases from breast cancer. Clin Cancer Res 12:1221–1228

Boll B, Hansen H, Heuck F et al. (2005) The fully human anti-CD30 antibody 5F11 activates NF-{kappa}B and sensitizes lymphoma cells to bortezomib-induced apoptosis. Blood 106:1839–1842

Borchmann P, Treml JF, Hansen H et al. (2003) The human anti-CD30 antibody 5F11 shows in vitro and in vivo activity against malignant lymphoma. Blood 102:3737–3742

Borchmann P, Schnell R, Schulz H et al. (2004) Monoclonal antibody-based immunotherapy of Hodgkin's lymphoma. Curr Opin Investig Drugs 5:1262–1267

Borchmann P, Schnell R, Engert A (2005) Immunotherapy of Hodgkin's lymphoma. Eur J Haematol 75(Suppl 66):159–165

Brinster RL, Chen HY, Trumbauer M et al. (1981) Somatic expression of herpes thymidine kinase in mice following injection of a fusion gene into eggs. Cell 27:223–231

Brinster RL, Ritchie KA, Hammer RE et al. (1983) Expression of a microinjected immunoglobulin gene in the spleen of transgenic mice. Nature 306:332–336

Bruggemann M, Caskey HM, Teale C et al. (1989) A repertoire of monoclonal antibodies with human heavy chains from transgenic mice. Proc Natl Acad Sci USA 86:6709–6713

Brun-Buisson C (1994) The HA-1A saga: the scientific and ethical dilemma of innovative and costly therapies. Intensive Care Med 20:314–316

Bucchini D, Reynaud CA, Ripoche MA et al. (1987) Rearrangement of a chicken immunoglobulin gene occurs in the lymphoid lineage of transgenic mice. Nature 326:409–411

Burgess T, Coxon A, Meyer S et al. (2006) Fully human monoclonal antibodies to hepatocyte growth factor with therapeutic potential against hepatocyte growth factor/c-Met-dependent human tumors. Cancer Res 66:1721–1729

Buttin G (1987) Exogenous Ig gene rearrangement in transgenic mice: a new strategy for human monoclonal antibody production? Trends Genet 3:205–206

Calvo E, Rowinsky EK (2005) Clinical experience with monoclonal antibodies to epidermal growth factor receptor. Curr Oncol Rep 7:96–103

Chang Q, Zhong Z, Lees A et al. (2002) Structure-function relationships for human antibodies to pneumococcal capsular polysaccharide from transgenic mice with human immunoglobulin Loci. Infect Immun 70:4977–4986

Choi TK, Hollenbach PW, Pearson BE et al. (1993) Transgenic mice containing a human heavy chain immunoglobulin gene fragment cloned in a yeast artificial chromosome. Nat Genet 4:117–123

Cohen BD, Baker DA, Soderstrom C et al. (2005) Combination therapy enhances the inhibition of tumor growth with the fully human anti-type 1 insulin-like growth factor receptor monoclonal antibody CP-751,871. Clin Cancer Res 11:2063–2073

Cohen SB, Emery P, Greenwald MW et al. (2006) Rituximab for rheumatoid arthritis refractory to anti-tumor necrosis factor therapy: Results of a multicenter, randomized, double-blind, placebo-controlled, phase III trial evaluating primary efficacy and safety at twenty-four weeks. Arthritis Rheum 54:2793–806

Cohenuram M, Saif MW (2007) Panitumumab the first fully human monoclonal antibody: from the bench to the clinic. Anticancer Drugs 18:7–15

Coiffier B, Haioun C, Ketterer N et al. (1998) Rituximab (anti-CD20 monoclonal antibody) for the treatment of patients with relapsing or refractory aggressive lymphoma: a multicenter phase II study. Blood 92:1927–32

Costantini F, Lacy E (1981) Introduction of a rabbit beta-globin gene into the mouse germ line. Nature 294:92–94

Coughlin M, Lou G, Martinez O et al. (2006) Generation and characterization of human monoclonal neutralizing antibodies with distinct binding and sequence features against SARS coronavirus using XenoMouse((R)). Virology 361:93–102

Cunningham D, Humblet Y, Siena S et al. (2004) Cetuximab monotherapy and cetuximab plus irinotecan in irinotecan-refractory metastatic colorectal cancer. N Engl J Med 351:337–345

Davies NP, Rosewell IR, Richardson JC et al. (1993) Creation of mice expressing human antibody light chains by introduction of a yeast artificial chromosome containing the core region of the human immunoglobulin kappa locus. Nat Bio 11:911–914

Davis MM (2004) The evolutionary and structural 'logic' of antigen receptor diversity. Semin Immunol 16:239–243

Edgington SM (1992) What went wrong with Centoxin? Nat Bio 10:617–619

Farr CD, Tabet MR, Ball WJ et al. (2002) Three-dimensional quantitative structure-activity relationship analysis of ligand binding to human sequence antidigoxin monoclonal antibodies using comparative molecular field analysis. J Med Chem 45:3257–3270

Fishwild D, O'Donnell SL, Bengoechea T et al. (1996) High-avidity human IgG kappa monoclonal antibodies from a novel strain of minilocus transgenic mice. Nat Bio 14:845–851

Fishwild D, Hudson DV, Deshpande U et al. (1999) Differential effects of administration of a human anti-CD4 monoclonal antibody, HM6G, in nonhuman primates. Clin Immunol 92:138–152

Foon KA, Yang XD, Weiner LM et al. (2004) Preclinical and clinical evaluations of ABX-EGF, a fully human anti-epidermal growth factor receptor antibody. Int J Radiat Oncol Biol Phys 58:984–990

Foote J, Eisen H (1995) Kinetic and affinity limits on antibodies produced during immune responses. Proc Natl Acad Sci USA 92:1254–1256

Fuss IJ, Becker C, Yang Z et al. (2006) Both IL-12p70 and IL-23 are synthesizedduring active Crohn's disease and are down-regulated by treatment with anti-IL-12 p40 monoclonal antibody. Inflamm Bowel Dis 12:9–15

Garambois V, Glaussel F, Foulquier E et al. (2004) Fully human IgG and IgM antibodies directed against the carcinoembryonic antigen (CEA) Gold 4 epitope and designed for radioimmunotherapy (RIT) of colorectal cancers. BMC Cancer 4:75

Gibson TB, Ranganathan A, Grothey A (2006) Randomized phase III trial results of panitumumab, a fully human anti-epidermal growth factor receptor monoclonal antibody, in metastatic colorectal cancer. Clin Colorectal Cancer 6:29–31

Goldstein G et al. (1985) A randomized clinical trial of OKT3 monoclonal antibody for acute rejection of cadaveric renal transplants. Ortho Multicenter Transplant Study Group. N Engl J Med 6:337–342

Goodhardt M, Cavelier P, Akimenko MA et al. (1987) Rearrangement and expression of rabbit immunoglobulin kappa light chain gene in transgenic mice. Proc Natl Acad Sci USA 84:4229–4233

Gordon JW, Ruddle FH (1981) Integration and stable germ line transmission of genes injected into mouse pronuclei. Science 214:1244–1246

Green LL, Jakobovits A (1998) Regulation of B cell development by variable gene complexity in mice reconstituted with human immunoglobulin yeast artificial chromosomes. J Exp Med 188:483–495

Green LL, Hardy MC, Maynard-Currie CE et al. (1994) Antigen-specific human monoclonal antibodies from mice engineered with human Ig heavy and light chain YACs. Nat Genet 7:13–21

Greenough TC, Babcock GJ, Roberts A et al. (2005) Development and characterization of a severe acute respiratory syndrome-associated coronavirus-neutralizing human monoclonal antibody that provides effective immunoprophylaxis in mice. J Infect Dis 191:507–514

Harbers K, Jahner D, Jaenisch R (1981) Microinjection of cloned retroviral genomes into mouse zygotes: integration and expression in the animal. Nature 293:540–542

Harding FA, Lonberg N (1995) Class switching in human immunoglobulin transgenic mice. Ann NY Acad Sci 764:536–546

He Y, Honnen WJ, Krachmarov CP et al. (2002) Efficient isolation of novel human monoclonal antibodies with neutralizing activity against HIV-1 from transgenic mice expressing human Ig loci. J Immunol 169:595–605

Helmerhorst EJ, Maaskant JJ, Appelmelk MJ (1998) Anti-lipid A monoclonal antibody centoxin (HA-1A) binds to a wide variety of hydrophobic ligands. Infect Immun 66:870–873

Heuck F, Ellermann J, Borchmann P et al. (2004) Combination of the human anti-CD30 antibody 5F11 with cytostatic drugs enhances its antitumor activity against Hodgkin and anaplastic large cell lymphoma cell lines. J Immunother 27:347–353

Hodi FS, Mihm MC, Soiffer RJ et al. (2003) Biologic activity of cytotoxic T lymphocyte-associated antigen 4 antibody blockade in previously vaccinated metastatic melanoma and ovarian carcinoma patients. Proc Natl Acad Sci USA 100:4712–4717

Holmes EH (2001) PSMA specific antibodies and their diagnostic and therapeutic use. Expert Opin Investig Drugs 10:511–519

Houghton AN, Brooks H, Cote RJ et al. (1983) Detection of cell surface and intracellular antigens by human monoclonal antibodies. Hybrid cell lines derived from lymphocytes of patients with malignant melanoma. J Exp Med 158:53–65

Huang S, Mills L, Mian B et al. (2002) Fully humanized neutralizing antibodies to interleukin-8 (ABX-IL8) inhibit angiogenesis, tumor growth, and metastasis of human melanoma. Am J Pathol 161:125–134

Ignatovitch O, Tomlinson IM, Jones PT et al. (1997) The creation of diversity in the human immunoglobulin V(lambda) repertoire. J Mol Biol 268:69–77

Imakiire T, Kuroki M, Shibaguchi H et al. (2004) Generation, immunologic characterization and antitumor effects of human monoclonal antibodies for carcinoembryonic antigen. Int J Cancer 108:564–570

Ishida I, Tomizuka K, Yoshida H et al. (2002) Production of human monoclonal and polyclonal antibodies in TransChromo animals. Cloning Stem Cells 4:91–102

Jaber SH, Cowen EW, Haworth LR et al. (2006) Skin Reactions in a Subset of Patients With Stage IV Melanoma Treated With Anti–Cytotoxic T-Lymphocyte Antigen 4 Monoclonal Antibody as a Single Agent. Arch Dermatol 142:166–172

Jakobovits A, Moore AL, Green LL et al. (1993) Germ-line transmission and expression of a human-derived yeast artificial chromosome. Nature 362:255–258

James K, Bell GT (1987) Human monoclonal antibody production. Current status and future prospects. J Immunol Methods 100:5–40

Jones PT, Dear PH, Foote J et al. (1986) Replacing the complementarity-determining regions in a human antibody with those from a mouse. Nature 321:522–525

Kauffman CL, Araia N, Toichi E et al. (2004) A phase I study evaluating the safety, pharmacokinetics, and clinical response of a human IL-12 p40 antibody in subjects with plaque psoriasis. J Invest Dermatol 123:1037–1044

Kasper LH, Everitt D, Leist TP (2006) A phase I trial of an interleukin-12/23 monoclonal antibody in relapsing multiple sclerosis. Curr Med Res Opin 22:1671–1678

Keler T, Halk E, Vitale L et al. (2003) Activity and safety of CTLA-4 blockade combined with vaccines in cynomolgus macaques. J Immunol 171:6251–6259

Klimm B, Schnell R, Diehl V et al. (2005) Current treatment and immunotherapy of Hodgkin's lymphoma. Haematologica 90:1680–1692

Kohler G, Milstein C (1975) Continuous cultures of fused cells secreting antibody of predefined specificity. Nature 256:495–497

Korman AJ, Peggs KS, Allison JP (2006) Checkpoint blockade in cancer immunotherapy. Adv Immunol 90:297–339

Krueger GG, Langley RG, Leonardi C et al. (2007) A human interleukin-12/23 monoclonal antibody for the treatment of psoriasis. N Engl J Med 356:580–592

Kuroiwa Y, Tomizuka K, Shinohara T et al. (2000) Manipulation of human minichromosomes to carry greater than megabase-sized chromosome inserts. Nat Biotechnol 18:1086–1090

Kuroki M, Yamada H, Shibaguchi H et al. (2005) Preparation of human IgG and IgM monoclonal antibodies for MK-1/Ep-CAM by using human immunoglobulin gene-transferred mouse and gene cloning of their variable regions. Anticancer Res 25:3733–3739

Kuus-Reichel K, Grauer LS, Karavodin LM et al. (1994) Will immunogenicity limit the use, efficacy, and future development of therapeutic monoclonal antibodies? Clin Diagn Lab Immunol 1:365–372

Lammerts van Bueren JJ, Bleeker WK, Bogh HO et al. (2006) Effect of target dynamics on pharmacokinetics of a novel therapeutic antibody against the epidermal growth factor receptor: implications for the mechanisms of action. Cancer Res 66:7630–7638

Larrick JW, Bourla JM (1986) Prospects for the therapeutic use of human monoclonal antibodies. J Biol Response Mod 5:379–393

Leach DR, Krummel, MF, Allison JP (1996) Enhancement of antitumor immunity by CTLA-4 blockade. Science 271:1734–1736

Lenz H-J, Van Cutsem E, Khambata-Ford S et al. (2006) Multicenter phase II and translational study of cetuximab in metastatic colorectal carcinoma refractory to irenotecan, oxaloplatin, and fluoropyrimidines. J Clin Onc 24:4914–4921

Lonberg N (2005) Human antibodies from transgenic animals. Nat Biotechnol 23:1117–1125

Lonberg N, Huszar D (1995) Human antibodies from transgenic mice. Int Rev Immunol 13:65–93

Lonberg N, Taylor LD, Harding FA et al. (1994) Antigen-specific human antibodies from mice comprising four distinct genetic modifications. Nature 368:856–859

Ma D, Hopf CE, Malewicz, AD et al. (2006) Potent antitumor activity of an auristatin-conjugated, fully human monoclonal antibody to prostate-specific membrane antigen. Clin Cancer Res 12:2591–2596

Maitta RW (2004) Protective and nonprotective human immunoglobulin M monoclonal antibodies to Cryptococcus neoformans glucuronoxylomannan manifest different specificities and gene use profiles. Infect Immun 72:4810–4818

Maker AV, Phan GQ, Attia P et al. (2005) Tumor regression and autoimmunity in patients treated with cytotoxic T lymphocyte-associated antigen 4 blockade and interleukin 2: a phase I/II study. Ann Surg Oncol 12:1005–1016

Maker AV, Attia P, Rosenberg SA (2005b) Analysis of the cellular mechanism of antitumor responses and autoimmunity in patients treated with CTLA-4 blockade. J Immunol 175: 7746–7754

Maker AV, Yang JC, Sherry RM et al. (2006) Intrapatient dose escalation of anti-CTLA-4 antibody in patients with metastatic melanoma. J Immunother 29:455–463

Mannon PJ, Fuss IJ, Mayer L et al. (2004) Anti-interleukin-12 antibody for active Crohn's disease. N Engl J Med 351:2069–2079

Mansour SL, Thomas KR, Capecchi MR (1988) Disruption of the proto-oncogene int-2 in mouse embryo-derived stem cells: a general strategy for targeting mutations to non-selectable genes. Nature 336:348–352

Martin PL, Jiao Q, Cornacoff J, Hall W et al. (2005) Absence of adverse effects in cynomolgus macaques treated with CNTO 95, a fully human anti-alphav integrin monoclonal antibody, despite widespread tissue binding. Clin Cancer Res 11:6959–6965

McCafferty J, Griffiths AD, Winter G et al. (1990) Phage antibodies: filamentous phage displaying antibody variable domains. Nature 348:552–554

McCloskey RV, Straube RC, Sanders et al. (1994) Treatment of septic shock with human monoclonal antibody HA-1A. A randomized, double-blind, placebo-controlled trial. CHESS Trial Study Group. Ann Intern Med 121:1–5

McClung MR, Lewiecki EM, Cohen SB et al. (2006) Denosumab in postmenopausal women with low bone mineral density. N Engl J Med 354:821–31

Melnikova VO, Bar-Eli M (2006) Bioimmunotherapy for melanoma using fully human antibodies targeting MCAM/MUC18 and IL-8. Pigment Cell Res 19:395–405

Mendez MJ, Green LL, Corvalan JRF et al. (1997) Functional transplant of megabase human immunoglobulin loci recapitulates human antibody response in mice. Nat Genet 15:146–156

Mian BM, Dinney CPN, Bermejo CE et al. (2003) Fully human anti-interleukin 8 antibody inhibits tumor growth in orthotopic bladder cancer xenografts via down-regulation of matrix metalloproteases and nuclear factor-kappaB. Clin Cancer Res 9:3167–3175

Mori E, Thomas M, Motoki K et al. (2004) Human normal hepatocytes are susceptible to apoptosis signal mediated by both TRAIL-R1 and TRAIL-R2. Cell Death Differ 11:203–207

Morrison SL, Johnson MJ, Herzenberg LA et al. (1984) Chimeric human antibody molecules: mouse antigen-binding domains with human constant region domains. Proc Natl Acad Sci USA 81:6851–6855

Mukherjee J, Chios K, Fishwild D et al. (2002) Human Stx2-specific monoclonal antibodies prevent systemic complications of Escherichia coli O157:H7 infection. Infect Immun 70:612–619

Mukherjee J, Chios K, Fishwild D et al. (2002b) Production and characterization of protective human antibodies against Shiga toxin 1. Infect Immun 70:5896–5899

Nagy A, Gerstenstein M, Vinterstein K et al. (2003) Manipulating the Mouse Embryo, A Laboratory Manual, 3rd edn. Cold Spring Harbor Laboratory Press, Cold Spring Harbor, NY

Nicholson IC, Zou X, Popov AV et al. (1999) Antibody repertoires of four- and five-feature translocus mice carrying human immunoglobulin heavy chain and kappa and lambda light chain yeast artificial chromosomes. J Immunol 163:6898–6906

Nozawa S, Aoki D, Tsukazaki K et al. (2004) HMMC-1: a humanized monoclonal antibody with therapeutic potential against Mullerian duct-related carcinomas. Clin Cancer Res 10:7071–7078

Olsson L, Andreasen RB, Ost A et al. (1984) Antibody producing human-human hybridomas. II. Derivation and characterization of an antibody specific for human leukemia cells. J Exp Med 159:537–550

Ostendorf T, van Roeyen CRC, Peterson JD et al. (2003) A fully human monoclonal antibody (CR002) identifies PDGF-D as a novel mediator of mesangioproliferative glomerulonephritis. J Am Soc Nephrol 14:2237–2247

Parren PW, Warmerdam PA, Boeije LC et al. (1992) On the interaction of IgG subclasses with the low affinity Fc gamma RIIa (CD32) on human monocytes, neutrophils, and platelets. Analysis of a functional polymorphism to human IgG2. J Clin Invest 90:1537–1546

Parry R, Schneider D Hudson D et al. (2005) Identification of a novel prostate tumor target, mindin/RG-1, for antibody-based radiotherapy of prostate cancer. Cancer Res 65:8397–8405

Pendley C, Schantz A, Wagner C (2003) Immunogenicity of therapeutic monoclonal antibodies. Curr Opin Mol Ther 5:172–179

Phan GQ, Yang JC, Sherry RM et al. (2003) Cancer regression and autoimmunity induced by cytotoxic T lymphocyte-associated antigen 4 blockade in patients with metastatic melanoma. Proc Natl Acad Sci USA 100:8372–8377

Popov AV, Zou X, Xian J et al. (1999) A human immunoglobulin lambda locus is similarly well expressed in mice and humans. J Exp Med 189:1611–1620

Ramakrishna V, Treml JF, Vitale L et al. (2004) Mannose receptor targeting of tumor antigen pmel17 to human dendritic cells directs anti-melanoma T cell responses via multiple HLA molecules. J Immunol 172:2845–2852

Rathanaswami P, Roalstad S, Roskos L et al. (2005) Demonstration of an in vivo generated subpicomolar affinity fully human monoclonal antibody to interleukin-8. Biochem Biophys Res Commun 334:1004–1013

Reuben JM, Lee BN, Li C et al. (2006) Biologic and immunomodulatory events after CTLA-4 blockade with ticilimumab in patients with advanced malignant elanoma. Cancer 106: 2437–2444

Ribas A, Camacho LH, Lopez-Berestein G et al. (2005) Antitumor activity in melanoma and anti-self responses in a phase I trial with the anti-cytotoxic T lymphocyte-associated antigen 4 monoclonal antibody CP-675206. J Clin Oncol 23:8968–8977

Ribas A, Glaspy JA, Lee Y et al. (2004) Role of dendritic cell phenotype, determinant spreading, and negative costimulatory blockade in dendritic cell-based melanoma immunotherapy. J Immunother 27:354–367

Roost HP, Bachmann MF, Haag A et al. (1995) Early high-affinity neutralizing anti-viral IgG responses without further overall improvements of affinity. Proc Natl Acad Sci USA 92: 1257–1261

Rowinski EK, Schwartz GH, Gollob JA et al. (2004) Safety, pharmacokinetics, and activity of ABX-EGF, a fully human anti-epidermal growth factor receptor monoclonal antibody in patients with metastatic renal cell cancer. J Clin Oncol 22:3003–3015

Sanderson K, Scotland R, Lee P et al. (2005) Autoimmunity in a phase I trial of a fully human anti-cytotoxic T-lymphocyte antigen-4 monoclonal antibody with multiple melanoma peptides and Montanide ISA 51 for patients with resected stages III and IV melanoma. J Clin Oncol 23:741–750

Schedl A, Larin Z, Montoliu L et al. (1993) A method for the generation of YAC transgenic mice by pronuclear microinjection. Nucleic Acids Res 21:4783–4787

Schuler W, Bigaud M, Brinkmann V et al. (2004) Efficacy and safety of ABI793, a novel human anti-human CD154 monoclonal antibody, in cynomolgus monkey renal allotransplantation. Transplantation 77:717–726

Schwartzberg PL, Goff SP, Robertson EJ (1989) Germ-line transmission of a c-abl mutation produced by targeted gene disruption in ES cells. Science 246:799–803

Sheoran AS, Chapman-Bonofiglio S, Harvey BR et al. (2005) Human antibody against shiga toxin 2 administered to piglets after the onset of diarrhea due to Escherichia coli O157:H7 prevents fatal systemic complications. Infect Immun 73:4607–4613

Simoons ML, de Boer MJ, van den Brand MJ et al. (1994) Randomized trial of a GPIIb/IIIa platelet receptor blocker in refractory unstable angina. European Cooperative Study Group. Circulation 89:596–603

Skov L, Kragbelle K, Zachariae C et al. (2003) HuMax-CD4: a fully human monoclonal anti-CD4 antibody for the treatment of psoriasis vulgaris. Arch Dermatol 139:1433–1439

Spalding BJ (1992) FDA setback flattens Centocor. Nat Bio 10:616

Strauss WM, Dausman J, Beard C et al. (1993) Germ line transmission of a yeast artificial chromosome spanning the murine alpha 1(I) collagen locus. Science 259:1904–1907

Suarez E, Yáñez R, Barrios Y, Díaz-Espada F (2004) Human monoclonal antibodies produced in transgenic BABkappa,lambda mice recognising idiotypic immunoglobulins of human lymphoma cells. Mol Immunol 41:519–526

Suzuki N, Aoki D, Tamada Y et al. (2004) HMOCC-1, a human monoclonal antibody that inhibits adhesion of ovarian cancer cells to human mesothelial cells. Gynecol Oncol 95:290–298

Tai YT, Li X, Tong X et al. (2005) Human anti-CD40 antagonist antibody triggers significant antitumor activity against human multiple myeloma. Cancer Res 65:5898–5906

Taylor LD, Carmack CE, Schramm SR et al. (1992) A transgenic mouse that expresses a diversity of human sequence heavy and light chain immunoglobulins. Nucleic Acids Res 20:6287–6295

Taylor LD, Carmack CE, Huszar D et al. (1994) Human immunoglobulin transgenes undergo rearrangement, somatic mutation and class switching in mice that lack endogenous IgM. Int Immunol 6:579–591

Teeling JL, French RR, Cragg MS et al. (2004) Characterization of new human CD20 monoclonal antibodies with potent cytolytic activity against non-Hodgkin lymphomas. Blood 104: 1793–1800

Teeling JL, Mackus WJ, Wiegman LJJM et al. (2006) The biological activity of human CD20 monoclonal antibodies is linked to unique epitopes on CD20. J Immunol 177:362–371

Thompson RH, Allison JP, Kwon ED (2006) Anti-cytotoxic T lymphocyte antigen-4 (CTLA-4) immunotherapy for the treatment of prostate cancer. Urol Oncol 24:442–447

Toichi E, Torres G, McCormick TS (2006) An anti-IL-12p40 antibody down-regulates type 1 cytokines, chemokines, and IL-12/IL-23 in psoriasis. J Immunol 177:4917–4926

Tomizuka K, Yoshida H, Uejima H et al. (1997) Functional expression and germline transmission of a human chromosome fragment in chimaeric mice. Nat Genet 16:133–143

Tomizuka K, Shinohara T, Yoshida H et al. (2000) Double trans-chromosomic mice: maintenance of two individual human chromosome fragments containing Ig heavy and kappa loci and expression of fully human antibodies. Proc Natl Acad Sci USA 97:722–727

Tomlinson IM, Walterb G, Jonesc PT et al. (1996) The imprint of somatic hypermutation on the repertoire of human germline V genes. J Mol Biol 256:813–817

Trikha M, Zhou Z, Nemeth JA et al. (2004) CNTO 95, a fully human monoclonal antibody that inhibits alpha v integrins, has antitumor and antiangiogenic activity in vivo. Int J Cancer 110:326–335

Tse KF, Jeffers M, Pollack VA et al. (2006) CR011, a fully human monoclonal antibody-auristatin E conjugate, for the treatment of melanoma. Clin Cancer Res 12:1373–1382

Tzipori S, Sheoran A, Akiyoshi D et al. (2004) Antibody therapy in the management of shiga toxin-induced hemolytic uremic syndrome. Clin Microbiol Rev 17:926–941

van Royen-Kerkhof A, Sanders EA, Walraven V et al. (2005) A novel human CD32 mAb blocks experimental immune haemolytic anaemia in FcgammaRIIA transgenic mice. Br J Haematol 130:130–137

Villadsen LS, Schuurman J, Beurskens F et al. (2003) Resolution of psoriasis upon blockade of IL-15 biological activity in a xenograft mouse model. J Clin Invest 112:1571–1580

Villadsen LS, Skov L, Dam TN et al. (2007) In situ depletion of $CD4^+$ T cells in human skin by Zanolimumab. Arch Dermatol Res 298:449–455

Vitale L, Blanset D, Lowy I et al. (2006) Prophylaxis and therapy of inhalational anthrax by a novel monoclonal antibody to protective antigen that mimics vaccine-induced immunity. Infect Immun 74:5840–5847

Wagner EF, Stewart TA, Mintz B (1981a) The human beta-globin gene and a functional viral thymidine kinase gene in developing mice. Proc Natl Acad Sci USA 78:5016–5020

Wagner TE, Hoppe PC, Jollick JD et al. (1981b) Microinjection of a rabbit beta-globin gene into zygotes and its subsequent expression in adult mice and their offspring. Proc Natl Acad Sci USA 78:6376–6380

Wang Y, Hailey J, Williams D et al. (2005) Inhibition of insulin-like growth factor-I receptor (IGF-IR) signaling and tumor cell growth by a fully human neutralizing anti-IGF-IR antibody. Mol Cancer Ther 4:1214–1221

Weinblatt ME, Keystone EC, Furst DE et al. (2003) Adalimumab, a fully human anti-tumor necrosis factor alpha monoclonal antibody, for the treatment of rheumatoid arthritis in patients taking concomitant methotrexate: the ARMADA trial. Arthritis Rheum 48:35–45

Weng WK, Levy R (2003) Two immunoglobulin G fragment C receptor polymorphisms independently predict response to rituximab in patients with follicular lymphoma. J Clin Oncol 21:3940–3947

Wu Y, Zhong Z, Huber J et al. (2006) Anti-vascular endothelial growth factor receptor-1 antagonist antibody as a therapeutic agent for cancer. Clin Cancer Res 12:6573–6584

Xu JL, Davis, MM (2000) Diversity in the CDR3 region of V(H) is sufficient for most antibody specificities. Immunity 13:37–45

Yamamura K-I, Kudo A, Ebihara T et al. (1986) Cell-type-specific and regulated expression of a rearranged human gamma1 heavy-chain immunoglobulin gene in transgenic mice. Proc Natl Acad Sci USA 83:2152–2156

Yang X-D, Jia X-C, Corvalan JR et al. (1999) Eradication of established tumors by a fully human monoclonal antibody to the epidermal growth factor receptor without concomitant chemotherapy. Cancer Res 59:1236–1243

Yang X-D, Corvalen JR, Wang P et al. (1999b) Fully human anti-interleukin-8 monoclonal antibodies: potential therapeutics for the treatment of inflammatory disease states. J Leukoc Biol 66:401–410

Yang X-D, Jia X-C, Corvalan JR et al. (2001) Development of ABX-EGF, a fully human anti-EGF receptor monoclonal antibody, for cancer therapy. Crit Rev Oncol Hematol 38:17–23

Zijlstra M, Li E, Sajjadi F et al. (1989) Germ-line transmission of a disrupted beta 2-microglobulin gene produced by homologous recombination in embryonic stem cells. Nature 342:435–438

Zou YR, Muller W, Gu H et al. (1994) Cre-loxP-mediated gene replacement: a mouse strain producing humanized antibodies. Curr Biol 4:1099–1103

Part III
Antibodies to Cytokines

Anti-TNF Antibodies: Lessons from the Past, Roadmap for the Future

D.J. Shealy and S. Visvanathan(✉)

1	Introduction	102
2	Lessons from TNF Characterization and Receptor Activation	103
3	Lessons from In Vitro Studies	105
4	Lessons from Animal Models	106
	4.1 TNF-Deficient Mice	106
	4.2 Tumorigenesis..	107
	4.3 Sepsis...	107
	4.4 Arthritis	108
	4.5 Inflammatory Bowel Disease...	108
	4.6 Psoriasis..	109
5	Development of TNF-Specific Antibodies for Clinical Use	109
	5.1 Infliximab	110
	5.2 Adalimumab	110
	5.3 Certolizumab Pegol	111
6	Pharmacokinetics of Anti-TNF Antibody Therapeutics	111
	6.1 Infliximab	111
	6.2 Adalimumab	112
	6.3 Certolizumab Pegol	113
7	Pharmacodynamics of Anti-TNF Antibody Therapeutics	113
	7.1 Infliximab	114
	7.2 Adalimumab	118
	7.3 Certolizumab Pegol	118
8	The Road Ahead for Anti-TNF Antibody Therapeutics	119
References		120

D.J. Shealy,

Centocor Research and Development, Inc., 145 King of Prussia Road, Radnor, PA 19087

e-mail: dshealy@cntus.jnj.com

S. Visvanathan

Centocor Research and Development, Inc., 145 King of Prussia Road, Radnor, PA 19087

e-mail: svisvana@cntus.jnj.com

Y. Chernajovsky, A. Nissim (eds.) *Therapeutic Antibodies. Handbook of Experimental Pharmacology 181.*
© Springer-Verlag Berlin Heidelberg 2008

Abstract Tumor necrosis factor alpha (TNF) is an important cell-signaling component of the immune system. Since its discovery over 20 years ago, much has been learned about its functions under normal and disease conditions. Nonclinical studies suggested a role for TNF in chronic immune-mediated inflammatory diseases, such as rheumatoid arthritis, Crohn's disease, and psoriasis, and therefore neutralizing monoclonal antibodies specific to human TNF were developed for clinical evaluation. Treatment with anti-TNF monoclonal antibodies (infliximab, adalimumab, and certolizumab pegol) has been shown to provide substantial benefit to patients through reductions in both localized and systemic expression of markers associated with inflammation. In addition, there are beneficial effects of anti-TNF treatment on markers of bone and cartilage turnover. Further exploration of changes in these markers and their correlation with clinical measures of efficacy will be required to allow accurate prediction of those patients most in need of these treatments. Both the clinical and commercial experience with these anti-TNF antibodies provide a wealth of information regarding their pharmacological effects in humans.

1 Introduction

Tumor necrosis factor-alpha (TNF) is a proinflammatory cytokine, and is a known mediator of chronic immune-mediated inflammatory diseases, such as rheumatoid arthritis (RA), Crohn's disease (CD), and psoriasis. TNF is expressed as a transmembrane precursor that undergoes proteolytic processing to form a soluble trimer. The binding of both the membrane-bound and soluble forms of TNF to its receptors, TNFR1 and TNFR2, initiates the expression of several other proinflammatory cytokines (eg., interleukin [IL]-1, IL-6, and interferon [IFN]-γ), cell adhesion molecules (eg., intracellular adhesion molecule [ICAM]-1), and general inflammatory markers. Several animal and disease models have provided the foundation for the development of anti-TNF antibodies as treatments for chronic inflammatory diseases.

Two TNF-specific monoclonal antibodies, infliximab (Remicade®) and adalimumab (Humira®), have been approved for patient use (Table 1). In addition, the TNF-specific, pegylated Fab' antibody fragment certolizumab pegol (Cimzia®) has reached the final phase of clinical development (Table 1), and other TNF antagonist therapies are also approved or under development. The goal of therapy with anti-TNF antibodies is to reduce the levels of TNF in the circulation to ameliorate the clinical signs of disease, without causing systemic immunosuppression in the patient.

Here, we will discuss the role of TNF (and its receptors) in chronic inflammatory diseases, including the results of several animal and disease models. In addition, we describe the development of three anti-TNF antibodies (infliximab, adalimumab, and certolizumab pegol), and their pharmacokinetic and pharmacodynamic properties.

Table 1 Anti-TNF monoclonal antibodies

	Infliximab (Remicade®, Centocor)	Adalimumab (Humira®, Abbott)	Certolizumab-pegol (CDP-870/Cimzia®, UCB)
Description	Human/mouse chimeric IgG1, kappa	Human IgG1, kappa	Human Fab′ fragment pegylated
Cell line for manufacture	Mouse myeloma	Chinese hamster ovary	*Escherichia coli*
Route of administration	Intravenous	Subcutaneous	Subcutaneous
Half-life (days)	7.7–9.5	10–20	14
Current/approved dosing	$3–10 \, \text{mg kg}^{-1}$ at 0, 2, and 6 weeks and then every 8 weeks	40 mg weekly or every other week	400 mg every 4 weeks
Indications	Approved for: CD, RA, AS, PsA, UC, Ps	Approved for: CD, RA, AS, PsA	In Phase III studies for: CD, RA
Changes in biomarkers	CRP, inflammatory cytokines, anti-CCP, RF, MMPs, bone and cartilage markers, regulatory T cells	CRP, inflammatory cytokines, anti-CCP, RF, MMPs	CRP

CD, Crohn's disease; RA, rheumatoid arthritis; AS, ankylosing spondylitis; PsA, psoriatic arthritis; UC, ulcerative colitis; Ps, psoriasis; CRP, C-reactive protein; CCP, cyclic citrullinated peptide; RF, rheumatoid factor; MMPs, matrix metalloproteinases

Another anti-TNF biologic therapy, etanercept (Enbrel®), is a fusion protein of two TNFR2 receptor extracellular domains and the Fc portion of human IgG, and this agent has also been approved for the treatment of several immune-mediated inflammatory diseases. However, because this product is not an anti-TNF monoclonal antibody, it is not discussed in this review.

2 Lessons from TNF Characterization and Receptor Activation

An endotoxin-induced serum factor originally described by Old and colleagues (Carswell et al. 1975) demonstrated a remarkable ability to lyse specific murine tumor cells, and this biologic activity is reflected in the name for this protein–tumor necrosis factor, or TNF. When TNF was purified to homogeneity (Aggarwal et al. 1985), and the gene encoding TNF was cloned (Pennica et al. 1984), it was soon recognized to be identical to cachectin, a protein that suppressed anabolic enzymes in adipocytes (Beutler et al. 1985a). Two specific receptors were also identified: TNFR1 (also known as p55 or CD120a) and TNFR2 (also known as p75 or CD120b). TNF and its receptors became the prototypes for the TNF ligand superfamily and the corresponding TNF receptor superfamily (Aggarwal 2003), whose members are integral to the control of cell differentiation, proliferation, and apoptosis necessary for mammalian development, in particular immune function and hematopoiesis. In contrast, uncontrolled excessive production of TNF can lead

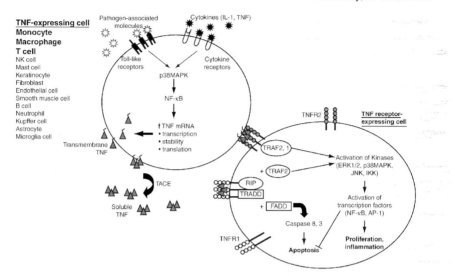

Fig. 1 Mechanisms for TNF expression and signaling. TNF, tumor necrosis factor; IL-1, interleukin-1; NF-κB, nuclear factor kappa B; TACE, TNF-alpha converting enzyme; TNFR1, TNF receptor 1; TNFR2, TNF receptor 2; TRADD, TNF receptor-associated death domain; TRAF2, TNF receptor-associated factor 2; RIP, receptor-interacting protein; FADD, Fas-associated death domain; AP-1, activator protein-1; ERK1/2, extracellular signal-related kinase 1/2; p38 MAPK, p38 mitogen-activated protein kinase; JNK, c-Jun N-terminal kinase; IKK, I kappaB kinase

to the chronic inflammation (Feldmann et al. 2004) that is the hallmark of diseases such as RA, CD, and psoriasis.

TNF is secreted primarily by activated monocytes, macrophages, and T cells, although a number of other cell sources have also been described (Fig. 1). Activation of Toll-like receptors by a variety of pathogen-associated molecules, or the activation of cytokine receptors such as IL-1, stimulates nuclear factor kappa B (NF-κB) transcription factors that increase TNF gene transcription, as well as genes encoding trans-acting factors that significantly increase TNF mRNA stability (Seko et al. 2006), and rapidly increase TNF protein secretion. TNF is expressed as a 26 kDa type II membrane-bound protein that self-associates into the bioactive homotrimer (Black et al. 1997; Moss et al. 1997), and is rapidly released by the protease TNF-alpha converting enzyme (TACE, also known as ADAM17). Both the transmembrane (Smith and Baglioni 1987) and soluble trimeric forms of TNF (Perez et al. 1990) can activate the TNF receptors. The extracellular domains of TNFR1 and TNFR2 bind to the cleft between TNF subunits, which causes the clustering of the receptor cytoplasmic domains and initiates signaling (Bazzoni and Beutler 1996).

The existence of two receptors contributes to the diversity of processes involving TNF. TNFR1 is constitutively expressed on virtually all nucleated cells, while expression of TNFR2 is limited to immune cells and endothelial cells (Aggarwal 2003). In addition to tissue distribution, there are clear differences in the signaling pathways activated by these two receptors. Activation of TNFR1 can have several outcomes, depending upon the expression of various accessory proteins present in the specific cell types. The cytoplasmic domain of TNFR1 includes a death do-main motif that can form signaling complexes that directly activate caspase-3 and caspase-8 and initiate apoptosis (Ashkenazi and Dixit 1998). After TNF binding, the death domain recruits accessory proteins such as TNF receptor-associated death domain (TRADD), receptor-interacting protein (RIP), and TNF receptor-associated factor 2 (TRAF2). At this point, the presence of other accessory proteins in the cell determines whether signaling will initiate or inhibit apoptosis. Further recruitment of the Fas-associated death domain (FADD) leads to the binding and activation of procaspase-8, which in turn activates caspase-3 and induces apoptosis.

Alternatively, TRAF2 can recruit cellular inhibitors of apoptosis (cIAP-1 and cIAP-2) and activate signaling pathways leading to nuclear translocation of the antiapoptotic transcription factors NF-κB and activator protein-1 (AP-1), which reg-ulate the expression of genes necessary to block apoptosis and to increase cell prolif-eration and proinflammatory proteins (Baud and Karin 2001). The NF-κB pathway alone activates over 200 proinflammatory genes (Kumar et al. 2004). The control of the molecular switch that determines whether the cell will undergo apoptosis or pro-liferation is not well understood. Several reports suggest that internalization of the TNF/TNFR1 signaling complex is necessary for activation of apoptosis (Micheau and Tschopp 2003; Schutze et al. 1999), while the clustering of the TNF/TNFR1 signaling complex in lipid rafts leads to activation of the NF-κB and AP-1 path-ways (Legler et al. 2003). Additional studies will be necessary to understand these important mechanistic features of the TNF/TNFR1 signaling complex.

TNFR2 does appear to have specific signaling functions in T cells that lack the TNFR1 receptor (Grell et al. 1998). Through interactions with TRAF2 (Rothe et al. 1994), TNF binding to TNFR2 can also activate the NF-κB and AP-1 pathways. Although TNFR2 lacks the death domain motif found on TNFR1, it can mediate apoptosis through a currently unknown pathway (Haridas et al. 1998). TNFR2 pref-erentially binds to the transmembrane form of TNF (Grell et al. 1995); this binding, therefore, requires cell cell contact, which may provide greater control over the ac-tivation of TNFR2.

3 Lessons from In Vitro Studies

The availability of purified TNF, and antibodies to TNF, led to an escalation in stud-ies using various cell lines. The effect of TNF on cell survival was evaluated with a variety of tumor and normal cell lines (Sugarman et al. 1985). Although TNF did kill some tumor cell lines, it behaved as a growth factor for the majority of cell lines, as well as for diploid human fibroblasts. Normal fibroblasts expressed IL-1 and IL-6 following exposure to TNF (Zhang et al. 1990), and synovial fibro-blasts from patients with RA produced a wide variety of cytokines, chemokines, and growth factors (Koch et al. 1995). The addition of anti-TNF antibody to the cultured synovial fibroblasts specifically reduced the expression of IL-1, IL-6, IL-8, and granulocyte-macrophage colony stimulating factor (GM-CSF), and provided the first clue that TNF might be a primary regulator of proinflammatory cytokines

(Feldmann and Maini 2001). The addition of TNF to cultured human endothelial cells induced the expression of adhesion proteins and a procoagulant factor identified later as tissue factor (Bevilacqua and Gimbrone 1987). An antibody specific for TNF was shown to reduce the expression of E-selectin, ICAM-1, and vascular cell adhesion molecule (VCAM)-1 by endothelial cells, even when added 4–10 h after the TNF challenge (Nakada et al. 1998). Changes in human epithelial cells treated with TNF include reduced transepithelial resistance and increased permeability of the epithelial barrier. The effects were concentration-dependent, reversible, and inhibited by anti-TNF antibody (Mullin and Snock 1990). TNF has been shown to enhance antigen-stimulated human B cell proliferation and differentiation in the presence of IL-2, independent of similar activities mediated by IL-1 (Jelinek and Lipsky 1987). Primary activation of T cells by TNF induced expression of TNF receptors. The addition of TNF to activated T cells also increased the expression of HLA-DR antigens and high affinity IL-2 receptors, and was effective as a costimulator of IL-2-dependent IFN-γ production (Scheurich et al. 1987).

The addition of anti-TNF antibody to murine calvarial cells suppresses secretion of IL-6 and differentiation into bone-resorbing osteoclasts. IL-6 production in response to exogenous IL-6 or parathyroid hormone was also blocked by anti-TNF antibody (Passeri et al. 1994). The role of TNF in the maturation of osteoclast progenitor cells has recently been reviewed (Boyce et al. 2006). Cultured human chondrocytes treated with TNF show increased levels of caseinase activity and prostaglandin E2, as well as increased resorption of human articular cartilage (Bunning and Russell 1989).

It is clear from these examples that TNF is capable of modulating the survival and activity of many different cell types. As discussed later in this chapter, these in vitro effects of TNF are reflected in the systemic pharmacodynamic changes seen in both animal models and in patients, and this underscores the value of these types of studies in developing a clear understanding of the biological disease processes.

4 Lessons from Animal Models

4.1 TNF-Deficient Mice

Several laboratories have generated TNF-deficient mouse strains and reported on the phenotype of these animals (Korner et al. 1997; Marino et al. 1997; Pasparakis et al. 1996). Although these mice are viable, fertile, and have no gross structural or morphological defects, they do exhibit altered cellular organization in lymph nodes and Peyer's patches following challenge with antigen or pathogens. Specifically, primary B cell follicles are absent from the spleen, no organized follicular dendritic cell networks or germinal centers can be found, and there is a lack of granuloma formation. Phagocytic and T cell responses appear normal while humoral responses to T cell-dependent antigens are reduced. Compared with wild-type mice, the TNF-deficient mice are resistant to lipopolysaccharide challenge following D-galactosamine treatment, but are more susceptible to infectious agents such as *Listeria monocytogenes*, *Candida albicans*, and *Cryptosporidum parvum*. A similar increased susceptibility to infection with *Mycobacterium tuberculosis* has been reported in anti-TNF treated mice (Flynn et al. 1995).

4.2 Tumorigenesis

Despite its name, TNF does not induce cell death in the majority of evaluated tumor cell lines (Sugarman et al. 1985). Nonetheless, treatment with TNF has been studied in a number of tumor models and in patients (Burke 1999). Systemic toxicity (hypertension and organ failure) has limited its clinical use to isolated limb perfusion for regionally advanced melanomas and soft tissue sarcomas of the limbs, in combination with an effective chemotherapeutic compound, such as the alkylating agent melphalan (Lejeune et al. 2006). Conversely, several authors have recently presented convincing arguments that TNF behaves as a tumor promoter within the context of the tumor microenvironment (Karin and Greten 2005; Szlosarek et al. 2006). The induction of nitric oxide and angiogenic factors, induction of matrix metalloproteinases (MMPs), enhancement of tumor cell motility, as well as a role as an autocrine survival and growth factor, are all tumor-promoting properties described for TNF. Overexpression of TNF by a Chinese hamster ovary cell line conferred invasive properties on tumor xenografts, while treatment with neutralizing anti-TNF antibodies blocked metastasis (Malik et al. 1990). In TNF-deficient mice (Moore et al. 1999) or wild-type mice treated with anti-TNF antibodies (Scott et al. 2003), significant reductions in carcinogen-induced skin tumors were observed compared with control animals.

NF-κB has also been described as a key link between inflammation and cancer. The spontaneous development of cholestatic hepatitis followed by hepatocellular carcinoma in Mdr2-deficient mice was accompanied by chronic expression of TNF in adjacent inflammatory and endothelial cells, and persistent activation of NF-κB. Late stage tumor development was significantly reduced by switching off the NF-κB signaling pathway or blocking TNF with neutralizing antibodies (Pikarsky et al. 2004).

4.3 Sepsis

Administration of TNF to rats resulted in hypotension, metabolic acidosis, acute pulmonary inflammation, and death within hours, similar to symptoms caused by bacterial endotoxin (Tracey et al. 1986). Treatment with a polyclonal antibody specific for TNF protected mice from a subsequent lethal challenge of endotoxin (Beutler et al. 1985b). The protective effect of TNF-neutralizing antibodies has been seen in a variety of sepsis animal models, including nonhuman primates (Bodmer et al. 1993). However, clinical trials with anti-TNF monoclonal antibodies were uniformly disappointing (Freeman and Natanson 2000) and are no longer being actively pursued.

4.4 Arthritis

Cartilage explants treated with recombinant human TNF show evidence of tissue destruction as indicated by enhanced resorption and inhibition of proteoglycan synthesis (Saklatvala 1986). Further data demonstrating the direct role of TNF in inflammatory arthritis came from the laboratory of George Kollias, which developed genetically engineered mice that constitutively express human TNF (Keffer et al. 1991). These mice developed clinical and histological changes characteristic of RA, and prophylactic treatment with anti-TNF antibody significantly inhibited disease activity. Interestingly, arthritic disease was also seen in mice that overexpressed a modified *TNF* gene that lacked the protease cleavage site, and therefore only expressed the transmembrane form of TNF. This result suggests that production of transmembrane TNF alone, which presumably would be restricted to local tissues and signaling by cell–cell contact, was sufficient for development and progression of arthritis in this model (Georgopoulos et al. 1996). Additional studies in the human TNF transgenic mouse model demonstrated that the features and symptoms of existing arthritic disease were reversed by anti-TNF antibody treatment. Amelioration of disease was associated with reduced arthritic scores and reversal of existing structural damage, including synovitis and periosteal bone erosions evident on histology. Repair of cartilage was age-dependent, as reversal of proteoglycan degradation was observed only in younger mice (Shealy et al. 2002).

Three laboratories corroborated these observations by showing that anti-TNF antibodies could reduce disease activity in the standard collagen-induced arthritis model (Piguet et al. 1992; Thorbecke et al. 1992; Williams et al. 1992). Anti-TNF treatment was effective when administered both prior to disease onset, and after significant disease was evident (Williams et al. 1992). Together, these studies provided a strong rationale for the initiation of clinical trials with anti-TNF monoclonal antibodies in patients with RA.

4.5 Inflammatory Bowel Disease

A wide variety of animal models that mimic inflammatory bowel disease in humans have been developed, including spontaneous or chemically-induced disease in normal mice, immune-mediated models, and disease in genetically-modified mice (Pizarro et al. 2003). The cotton top tamarin develops a spontaneous colitis with attributes that parallel ulcerative colitis in humans. When treated with an anti-TNF antibody, these animals showed a rapid improvement in body weight, fecal matter consistency, and rectal biopsy pathology (Watkins et al. 1997). Treatment with anti-TNF antibodies was also effective in a mouse model of chronic colitis induced by 2,4,6-trinitrobenzene sulfonic acid (TNBS) (Neurath et al. 1997). Macrophage-enriched lamina propria cells isolated from anti-TNF-treated mice produced considerably less IL-1 and IL-6 in culture. TNF-deficient mice challenged with TNBS did not develop disease, while introduction of a mouse TNF transgene in these mice was sufficient to render them sensitive to TNBS-induced colitis.

Mice deficient in IL-10 develop a chronic colitis of the colon with transmural involvement. When anti-TNF treatment was initiated in 4-week-old mice, disease activity was significantly suppressed compared with untreated animals, as indicated by reduced disease scores, histological analysis of the gut, and reduced levels of soluble TNFR2 and IL-1β in stool samples (Scheinin et al. 2003). Adoptive transfer of the CD45RBhi subset of CD4+ cells into immune-deficient mice has also been shown to result in intestinal inflammation. Anti-TNF treatment during the first 4 weeks following cell transfer had little effect, but continued treatment reduced the severity of colitis compared with untreated control animals (Powrie et al. 1994).

A recently described mouse strain derived from the SAMP1/Yit mouse has been shown to develop chronic ileitis, similar to CD, with perianal fistulas. A single injection of anti-TNF antibody rapidly suppressed the degree of intestinal inflammation and epithelial cell damage compared with control mice (Marini et al. 2003). Effects associated with inhibition of TNF included increased apoptosis of lamina propria mononuclear cells, while conversely suppressing the apoptosis of intestinal epithelial cells.

The collective data from this wide variety of intestinal inflammation models are substantial, and clearly supported further evaluation of the use of anti-TNF antibodies in patients with inflammatory bowel disease.

4.6 Psoriasis

The most definitive research on TNF neutralization in a psoriasis model was a xenotransplantation model in which human pre-psoriatic skin was engrafted onto immune-deficient mice (Boyman et al. 2004). Psoriatic skin lesions developed spontaneously on human skin grafts in AGR129 mice that lacked type I and type II IFN receptors and the recombination-activating gene 2. Approximately 6–8 weeks after engraftment, clinical (erythema, scaling) and histological (mononuclear cell infiltration, acanthosis) features of psoriasis appeared, and enhanced expression of Ki-67, major histocompability complex (MHC) class II antigen, TNF, IL-12, keratin 16, ICAM-1, and platelet/endothelial cell adhesion molecule (PECAM)-1 was detected. Neutralization of TNF significantly reduced papillomatosis and acanthosis indices, and was associated with a decrease in the number of T cells in the graft. These results suggest that development of psoriatic lesions and proliferation of resident T cells is dependent upon TNF.

5 Development of TNF-Specific Antibodies for Clinical Use

Convergence of a deeper understanding of the role of TNF as the primary mediator of pathogen-induced inflammation, along with advances in techniques to generate hybridoma-derived monoclonal antibodies and manipulate genes, spurred the rapid development of monoclonal antibodies for clinical testing and commercial use. In 1986, a murine monoclonal antibody (muromonab-CD3) that recognized the CD3 antigen found on human T cells was approved by the Food and Drug Administration for the treatment of kidney transplant rejection. However, patients were limited to a single 10- to 14-day dose regimen with this product since the majority of patients developed a significant immune response that prevented further treatment (Goldstein et al. 1986). The development of methods to chimerize or humanize antibody sequences significantly reduced murine antibody immunogenicity (Knight et al. 1995), and has allowed maintenance dosing with these types of antibody constructs in humans.

Three anti-TNF monoclonal antibodies have been developed to block the effects of TNF in patients with immune-mediated inflammatory diseases (Table 1). These include two approved mAbs (infliximab and adalimumab) and a pegylated Fab′ (certolizumab pegol) that is in late-stage clinical development.

5.1 Infliximab

A straightforward and simple improvement applied to monoclonal antibody technology was the generation of a chimeric molecule, in which the murine constant domains were replaced with corresponding human constant domains. This strategy was used to produce infliximab (previously called cA2), thus the binding characteristics of the fully murine antibody were identical to those of the chimeric antibody (Knight et al. 1993) and were combined with the functional properties of the human IgG1 Fc region (Scallon et al. 1995). Plasmids encoding the heavy and light chain genes for infliximab were used to transfect a myeloma cell line, and a high producing cell clone was selected. This mammalian cell line maintained proper posttranslational processing and glycosylation of the antibody.

Infliximab binds human TNF with high affinity and specificity and inhibits the bioactivity of both soluble and transmembrane TNF (Scallon et al. 2002). These stable, high avidity complexes (two or three infliximab molecules bound to each TNF trimer) prevent TNF binding to cellular receptors. No TNF-mediated bioactivity was observed when these complexes were incubated with target cells that typically respond to TNF. Furthermore, the expression of adhesion molecules by human endothelial cells was significantly reduced by the addition of infliximab, as much as 10 h after addition of TNF (Nakada et al. 1998).

5.2 Adalimumab

Human monoclonal antibodies such as adalimumab (also known as D2E7) have also been derived from a murine monoclonal antibody template using a guided phage display technique (Osbourn et al. 2005). The heavy chain of a mouse antibody directed against human TNF (MAK195) was cloned, paired with a repertoire of human light chains for display as Fab′ fragments, and screened for binding to human TNF. In parallel, a second library was prepared using the light chain from MAK195 combined with a repertoire of human heavy chains and screened in the same manner. The combined human light and heavy chains from the phage selected from these two libraries yielded an antibody that bound well to human TNF, and was affinity matured by site-specific mutagenesis in the complementarity determining regions (CDR) (Salfeld et al. 2000). Genes encoding the phage-derived human variable sequences were fused with human IgG1κ constant domain sequences and transfected into Chinese hamster ovary cells for selection of a production cell line. Despite its human origin, adalimumab is still reported to elicit an immune response in about 5% of RA patients (Humira® prescription label). Unique CDR sequences, as well as glycosylation, aggregation, route of administration, dose regimen, and formulation all influence the observed immune response (Clark 2000). Additionally, other clinical variables such as the timing of sample collection relative to dose administration can also significantly affect the reported antibody incidence.

Adalimumab has a reported affinity for human TNF of 100 pM (Santora et al. 2001). Mixtures of adalimumab and human TNF formed high molecular weight complexes that ranged in size from 600 to 5 000 kDa. The complex with the greatest thermal stability was 598 kDa and was postulated to comprise three molecules of adalimumab and three TNF trimers.

5.3 Certolizumab Pegol

Certolizumab pegol (formerly known as CDP-870) is a humanized anti-TNF monoclonal antibody derived from a murine monoclonal antibody by replacing the murine constant domains and framework sequences around each CDR with the corresponding human sequences (Kaushik and Moots 2005; Rose-John and Schooltink 2003). A Fab′ fragment of the humanized antibody is produced in an *Escherichia coli* expression system, and subsequently coupled with polyethylene glycol (PEG). Two 20 kDa PEG chains are attached via a maleimide linkage to the Fab′ fragment, extending the observed serum half-life in humans to approximately 14 days (Schreiber et al. 2005). The affinity and biologic potency of the pegylated Fab′ fragment for human TNF was similar to the intact antibody.

6 Pharmacokinetics of Anti-TNF Antibody Therapeutics

6.1 Infliximab

Infliximab is administered as an intravenous (IV) infusion for ≤2h, under various dosing regimens specific for each patient population. Analysis of single IV infusions ranging from 3 to 20 mg kg^{-1} demonstrated a linear relationship between the dose administered and the maximum serum concentration (Remicade$^{®}$ prescription label). The volume of distribution at steady state is independent of dose, indicating that infliximab is distributed primarily within the vascular compartment. High serum levels of infliximab are achieved within 1 h after infusion, with a median concentration of 68.6 µg mL^{-1} after a 3-mg kg^{-1} dose, and 219.1 µg mL^{-1} after a 10-mg kg^{-1} dose (St Clair et al. 2002). These high serum levels of infliximab effectively neutralize the local levels of TNF in the synovium, gut mucosa, and skin; an immediate response to therapy is observed in most responding patients.

Pharmacokinetic studies of patients with infliximab at doses ranging from 3 to 10 mg kg^{-1} in RA (Lipsky et al. 2000; Nestorov 2005; St Clair et al. 2004), 5 mg kg^{-1} in ankylosing spondylitis (AS) (Brandt et al. 2000; van der Heijde et al. 2005), psoriatic arthritis (Antoni et al. 2002), and CD (Baert et al. 1999; Farrell et al. 2000), 5 or 10 mg kg^{-1} in ulcerative colitis (Rutgeerts et al. 2005), and doses ranging from 3 to 5 mg kg^{-1} in plaque psoriasis showed that the median terminal half-life of infliximab ranged from 7.7 to 9.5 days (Scheinfeld 2004). The pharmacokinetics in pediatric patients with CD (6–17 years of age) were similar to those of adult CD patients, with a median terminal half-life of 10.9 days for a 5-mg kg^{-1} dose (Remicade$^{®}$ prescription label). Following an initial administration of infliximab, infusions at weeks 2 and 6 resulted in predictable concentration–time profiles following each treatment. Further, there was no systemic accumulation of infliximab upon repeated treatment with a dose of either 3 or 10 mg kg^{-1}, administered at 4- or 8-week intervals. The clearance of infliximab was nonlinear and was reduced in the presence of methotrexate (Markham and Lamb 2000; Schwab and Klotz 2001). The presence of antibodies to infliximab increased the clearance of infliximab. There were no major differences in clearance or volume of distribution in patient subgroups defined by age or weight. It remains unknown if there are differences in clearance or volume of distribution in patients with hepatic or renal impairment. There have been two population pharmacokinetic studies with infliximab to date, a single-dose study in patients with CD (Fasanmade et al. 2002) and a multiple-dose study in patients with AS (Xu et al. 2006). Overall, the pharmacokinetics of infliximab appear to be consistent across patient populations. In general, higher serum concentrations of infliximab are associated with greater clinical benefits (St Clair et al. 2004; Zhu et al. 2006).

6.2 Adalimumab

Adalimumab is administered every 2 weeks as a 40 mg subcutaneous (SC) injection for patients with psoriatic arthritis or AS, and patients with RA receive 40 mg every 1 or 2 weeks depending on disease severity (Humira$^{®}$ prescription label). Treatment with adalimumab was safe and well tolerated when administered as a single IV administration at doses up to 10 mg kg^{-1} in patients with active RA (den Broeder et al. 2002a). In addition to rheumatic diseases, adalimumab is currently being evaluated in clinical trials for the treatment of psoriasis, starting with an initial dose of 80 mg, followed by a maintenance dose of 40 mg administered either weekly or every 2 weeks (Chen et al. 2004).

The pharmacokinetics of adalimumab were observed to be linear over a dose range of 0.5 to 10 mg kg^{-1} following a single IV administration (Humira$^{®}$ prescription label). The volume of distribution at steady state (Vss) ranged from 4.7 to 6 L, and the systemic clearance was approximately 12 mL h^{-1}. The mean serum half-life ranged from 10 to 20 days. The steady-state concentration was approximately 5 µg mL^{-1} in the absence of methotrexate, and ranged from 8 to 9 µg mL^{-1} with concomitant methotrexate. A reduction in the clearance was observed in the presence of methotrexate (29% and 44% after single and multiple dosing, respectively) (Velagapudi et al. 2003). In long-term studies (longer than 2 years), there was no evidence of increased clearance over time. Serum adalimumab trough levels at steady state increased proportionally with dose following SC administration of 20, 40, and 80 mg either every week or every other week. The average absolute bioavailability was estimated to be 64% from three studies of single SC administrations of 40 mg (Humira$^{®}$ prescription label). Population pharmacokinetic analysis showed a trend toward a higher clearance of adalimumab in the presence of anti-adalimumab antibodies.

6.3 Certolizumab Pegol

Although not yet approved, certolizumab pegol has been studied for the treatment of both RA and CD. The optimal IV dose of certolizumab pegol in patients with RA was 5 mg kg^{-1} (Kaushik and Moots 2005). In a Phase II study of patients with RA, the peak plasma concentration occurred at the end of the infusion, and was proportional to the dose; the plasma concentration declined gradually thereafter (Choy et al. 2002). A similar pharmacokinetic profile was observed on redosing of certolizumab pegol as that of a single dose infusion. The plasma concentration profile was similar to that observed in healthy volunteers, with a half-life of 14 days. Antibodies to certolizumab pegol were low or undetectable after a single IV administration, but were detected in all treatment groups following a second cycle of treatment. A dose of 400 mg every 4 weeks has been proposed in patients with RA to achieve a clinical response (Kaushik and Moots 2005). In patients with moderate to severe CD, results from a dose ranging (100, 200, and 400 mg) study of SC administration of certolizumab pegol showed that this therapy was well tolerated when administered four times weekly (Schreiber et al. 2005).

7 Pharmacodynamics of Anti-TNF Antibody Therapeutics

Elevated levels of TNF have been found in the synovial fluid and tissues from patients with active RA, and in the intestinal biopsies and stool of patients with active CD. High levels of TNF have also been observed in tissues and/or serum from patients with other immune-mediated inflammatory diseases including AS, psoriasis, and ulcerative colitis. Therapeutic approaches aimed at blocking the activity of TNF are effective for controlling disease signs and symptoms and improving quality of life in these patients, as well as inhibiting radiographic damage in patients with RA. These profound clinical effects of TNF inhibition are believed to be due to the blockade of several mechanisms involved in inflammation that are activated by TNF.

7.1 Infliximab

Currently, the majority of data in the literature describing the pharmacodynamic effects of anti-TNF antibody therapies have focused on infliximab. Pharmacodynamic investigations have demonstrated that infliximab binds to, and inhibits, the intended target, TNF (Charles et al. 1999). As a result of infliximab binding to membrane-bound and soluble TNF with high affinity and avidity, it effectively blocks the biological activities of TNF as a pivotal inflammatory mediator. Infliximab forms stable immune complexes with TNF trimers; the resulting complexes are biologically inactive, and it is postulated that these complexes are cleared by the reticuloendothelial system of the liver. Despite its potent effects on systemic markers of inflammation, infliximab does not appear to induce a generalized suppression of the immune system, specifically in CD (Cornillie et al. 2001).

7.1.1 Markers Associated with Inflammation and Angiogenesis

The elevated levels of C-reactive protein (CRP) commonly observed in many patients with immune-mediated inflammatory diseases underscore the role of CRP as a prognostic marker for active inflammation, resulting in joint structural damage in patients with RA, and its potential value as an indicator of response to TNF blockade. Particularly noteworthy is the number of diverse immune-mediated inflammatory diseases for which infliximab has been shown to be both clinically effective and effective in reducing CRP levels. Infliximab has been shown to normalize CRP levels in patients with early RA (St Clair et al. 2004), refractory psoriatic arthritis (Feletar et al. 2004), AS (Brandt et al. 2000; Braun et al. 2005; van der Heijde et al. 2005), spondyloarthropathy (Antoni et al. 2002; Mandl and Jacobsson 2002), and CD (Baldassano et al. 2003; van Dullemen et al. 1995), as well as in patients with RA who had no clinical improvement but did have radiographic benefit (Smolen et al. 2005). Further, CRP levels have been shown to be associated with greater joint damage progression in early RA patients treated with MTX, but not associated with progression in patients treated with infliximab plus MTX (Smolen et al. 2006). However, in a recent study, CRP polymorphisms were associated with a differential response to infliximab in patients with CD (Willot et al. 2006).

In patients with CD, treatment with infliximab has been shown to reduce the levels of several disease-specific markers, including a significant reduction in inflammatory markers, such as IL-6 (van Dullemen et al. 1995). The levels of these markers often correlate with disease activity. When compared with patients who achieved remission after treatment with infliximab, patients with active CD had higher levels of IL-6, sIL-6R, sTNFR1, and sTNFR2 (Gustot et al. 2005). Detkova et al. observed a correlation between decreases in IL-10 levels and improvement in the CD activity index (CDAI) following infliximab treatment (Detkova et al. 2003). Also, reductions in serum levels of fibroblast growth factor (FGF) have been associated with decreases in perianal disease activity index and open fistula scores (Gao et al. 2004). Analyses of lamina propria mononuclear cells from the intestinal mucosa of patients with CD indicate that treatment with infliximab leads to a reduction in the number of cells that express TNF, IL-10, and IFN-γ (Plevy et al. 1997). Additional histological studies have provided evidence that infliximab treatment reduces the number of cells that stain positive for CD4, CD8, CD68, and MMP-9 (gelatinase B) in affected areas of the intestine, while also reducing the levels of detectable TNF, and other inflammatory markers, such as ICAM-1 (Baert et al. 1999; Geboes and Dalle 2002).

Infliximab has also been shown to induce caspase-3-dependent apoptosis of lamina propria T lymphocytes and peripheral monocytes in patients with steroid refractory CD (Lugering et al. 2001; ten Hove et al. 2002). Van den Brande et al. (2003) have shown that infliximab binds to transmembrane TNF on activated lamina propria T cells in patients with CD, resulting in apoptosis. Further, a significant increase in annexin V uptake has also been observed in active CD patients responding to infliximab therapy (Van den Brande et al. 2006). Additionally, the lamina propria T cells were identified in mucosal biopsies as target cells undergoing apoptosis in patients treated with infliximab. In T cell cultures from patients with CD, the production of IFN-γ was downregulated by infliximab (Agnholt and Kaltoft 2001). In contrast to the Van den Brande results, infliximab bound to the transmembrane form of TNF on activated T cells without inducing complement-mediated cytolysis or apoptosis, and without affecting proliferation. Infliximab has also been shown to reverse growth hormone resistance observed in patients with active inflammatory bowel disease through the suppression of systemic inflammation (Vespasiani Gentilucci et al. 2005).

In patients with RA, treatment with infliximab suppresses expression of markers related to inflammation (such as IL-6) and angiogenesis (such as vascular endothelial growth factor [VEGF]) (Charles et al. 1999; Strunk et al. 2006). Additionally, infliximab has been shown to reduce the synthesis of TNF, IL-1α, and IL-1β in the synovium within 2 weeks of treatment (Ulfgren et al. 2000). Also, patients with RA who were treated with infliximab had decreased serum levels of TNFR1, TNFR2, IL-1R antagonist, IL-6 and acute-phase proteins (serum amyloid A, haptoglobin, and fibrinogen) (Charles et al. 1999), IL-18 (Pittoni et al. 2002; van Oosterhout et al. 2005), as well as the chemokines GRO-α (Torikai et al. 2007), IL-8 (Visvanathan et al. 2007a), and CXCL16 (Kageyama et al. 2006). Low baseline serum levels of IL-2R have been associated with a clinical response to infliximab in patients with refractory RA (Kuuliala et al. 2006). Further, a recent study has shown that patients with RA who received infliximab therapy had decreased serum levels of sICAM-3 and sP-selectin (Gonzalez-Gay et al. 2006). Reduced levels of the cytokine

IL-18 have also been observed after infliximab treatment (Pittoni et al. 2002; van Oosterhout et al. 2005). The accumulation of CXCR3-positive T lymphocytes has been observed in the peripheral blood of RA patients treated with infliximab, suggesting altered lymphocyte trafficking (Aeberli et al. 2005). Treatment with infliximab has been shown to decrease activated p38 map kinase levels in CD4+ T cells in patients with RA (Garfield et al. 2005), and increase FOXP3 mRNA and protein expression by CD4+CD25hi regulatory T cells (Valencia et al. 2006). Infliximab therapy restored the suppressive function of the regulatory T cells (Ehrenstein et al. 2004), and appeared to induce a newly differentiated population of regulatory T cells (Nadkarni et al. 2007).

Elevated levels of anticyclic citrullinated peptide (CCP) antibodies have been associated with progression of structural damage in patients with RA (Meyer et al. 2003). Further, serum titers of anti-CCP antibodies and rheumatoid factor (RF) have been shown to decrease significantly after 6 months of treatment with infliximab (Ahmed et al. 2006; Alessandri et al. 2004). Decreases in anti-CCP antibody levels after initiation of treatment with infliximab were associated with decreases in IL-6 (Braun-Moscovici et al. 2006). After grouping the patients on the basis of their clinical response to infliximab, a significant decrease in serum anti-CCP antibodies and RF was observed only in those patients who had clinical improvement (Alessandri et al. 2004).

Infliximab therapy has also been shown to modulate inflammatory markers in patients with spondyloarthropathies. Treatment with infliximab resulted in a significant increase in IFN-γ and IL-2, and a transient decrease in IL-10 and natural killer (NK) T cells in patients who had high baseline values (Baeten et al. 2001). This switch in cytokine profile was observed in both the CD3+/CD8− and CD3+/CD8+ subsets. In psoriatic arthritis patients, a significant decrease in IL-6, VEGF, FGF, and E-selectin was observed after treatment with infliximab and reductions in VEGF, FGF, and MMP-2 were significantly correlated with improvement in psoriasis area and severity index (PASI) scores (Mastroianni et al. 2005). More recently, we have shown that treatment of AS patients with infliximab resulted in decreased serum levels of IL-6, VEGF, and CRP, and that these reductions were associated with an improvement in disease activity and spinal disease measures (Visvanathan et al. 2007b). Further, early decreases in IL-6 were associated with improvement in clinical measures in AS and psoriatic arthritis patients treated with infliximab (Visvanathan et al. 2006). Treatment with infliximab also resulted in decreases in the percentage of circulating CD4+ and CD8+ T cells expressing TNF or IFNγ in AS patients (Zou et al. 2003).

In a study of the mechanism of action of infliximab in the treatment of psoriasis vulgaris (Gottlieb et al. 2003), infliximab monotherapy was shown to disrupt the inflammatory processes associated with this dermatological disease. A reduction in the number of CD3-positive T cells and keratinocyte-derived ICAM-1 expression was demonstrated in lesional skin biopsies at weeks 2 and 10 after treatment initiation. Following treatment with infliximab, there was also a decrease in epidermal thickness and K16 and Ki67 expression levels, suggesting a role for TNF in the keratinocyte hyperproliferation observed in psoriasis.

7.1.2 Markers Associated with Bone and Cartilage Turnover

Several matrix metalloproteinases, including MMP-1 (interstitial collagenase) MMP-3 (stromelysin-1), and MMP-9 (gelatinase B), are up-regulated in inflammatory tissue, and TNF blockade with infliximab resulted in inhibition of these MMPs in patients with CD (Tchetverikov et al. 2005). More recently, Gao et al. observed decreased levels of MMP-9 and increased levels of MMP-2 in the sera of CD patients who responded to infliximab treatment (2007). Treatment with infliximab has been shown to provide a normalization of bone markers in patients with CD, with an increase in markers of bone formation (type-I procollagen N-terminal propeptide, bone-specific alkaline phosphatase, osteocalcin) and a decrease in markers of bone resorption (C-telopeptide of type-I collagen) in 30%–61% of patients (Franchimont et al. 2004).

In patients with RA, treatment with infliximab resulted in decreased levels of MMP-1, MMP-3 (Brennan et al. 1997), and MMP-9 (Klimiuk et al. 2004). Similar trends were observed in patients with spondyloarthropathies; infliximab treatment down-regulated MMPs and tissue inhibitors of metalloproteinases (TIMPs) in the synovium, and also resulted in a pronounced, rapid decrease in serum MMP-3 levels (Vandooren et al. 2004). More recently, we have shown that treatment of early RA patients with infliximab plus MTX not only resulted in a rapid decrease in inflammatory markers including MMP-3, but baseline levels of MMP-3 correlated with measures of clinical improvement at 1 year (Visvanathan et al. 2007a). Treatment with infliximab has also been shown to increase bone mineral density and modulate markers of bone metabolism in RA patients (Lange et al. 2005; Vis et al. 2006). Significant decreases in levels of the N-telopeptide of type I collagen (NTX) were observed 6 weeks after the initial treatment, and were maintained through 6 months. This decrease in NTX levels corresponded with an improvement in the number of swollen joints and modified Stanford Health Assessment Questionnaire (mHAQ) scores (Torikai et al. 2006). A recent small study of nine patients showed that infliximab therapy reduces the levels of serum cartilage oligomeric matrix protein (COMP) in patients with psoriatic arthritis, paralleling clinical improvement as measured by the American College of Rheumatology (ACR) response criteria (Cauza et al. 2006). Treatment of spondyloarthropathy patients with infliximab resulted in an increase in levels of procollagen type I N-terminal peptide (PINP) and insulin-like growth factor (IGF)-1, and a decrease in CTX-1 paralleled by an increase in bone mineral density, body weight, and lean mass (Briot et al. 2005).

7.1.3 Genes and Polymorphisms

Physiological responses to infliximab have been associated with multiple polymorphisms (Krejsa et al. 2006; Ranganathan 2005). In patients with CD, response to infliximab therapy has been associated with a single nucleotide polymorphism in the *FCGR3A* gene, which codes for the FcγRIIIa receptor (binds to the Fc portion of IgG) found on NK cells and macrophages (Louis et al. 2004). In patients with elevated CRP levels, the *FCGR3A* gene was an independent variable that influenced response to infliximab treatment. In two studies of patients with RA, the -308 polymorphism in the promoter for the *TNF* gene was associated with a good response to infliximab (Cuchacovich et al. 2004; Mugnier et al. 2003). Further, another study has shown that the 196 *TT* polymorphism in the *TNFRSF1B* gene was associated with a better response to infliximab therapy (Fabris et al. 2002). Due to the proximity of the *HLA DR* genes to the TNF locus, it is not surprising that HLA Class III microsatellites BAT2 and D6S273 have also been significantly associated with response to infliximab treatment in RA patients (Martinez et al. 2004). More recently, additional genes (cell adhesion, cell migration, cytochromes, proteasome-mediated proteolysis) have been associated with responses to infliximab therapy in RA patients (Lequerre et al. 2006); however, larger studies will be required to confirm these results.

7.2 Adalimumab

7.2.1 Markers Associated with Inflammation and Angiogenesis

Treatment with adalimumab resulted in a reduction in CRP, and this decrease correlated with improvement in radiological scores in RA patients after 2 years (den Broeder et al. 2002b). Decreases in serum levels of COMP, sICAM-1, MMPs, and HC gp-39, but not sE-selectin, were also observed in these patients. Further, baseline levels of COMP and sICAM-1 were predictive of radiological outcome in RA patients treated with adalimumab. In patients with RA, treatment with adalimumab therapy rapidly decreased the influx of leukocytes into inflamed joints but did not impair neutrophil chemotaxis or the production of reactive oxygen species (den Broeder et al. 2003). Circulating IL-7 levels were significantly reduced in RA patients that responded to adalimumab (van Roon et al. 2007).

A reduction in RF and anti-CCP antibody titers has been associated with clinical measures of response in patients treated with adalimumab (Atzeni et al. 2006). In a recent study, a reduction in serum concentrations of RF was observed after 12 weeks of treatment with adalimumab, whereas the anti-CCP antibody level remained constant (Semmler et al. 2007). Further, no significant changes in the activation levels of both NF-κB subunits were detected.

7.3 Certolizumab Pegol

7.3.1 Markers Associated with Inflammation and Angiogenesis

Minimal data have been reported on the pharmacodynamic effects of certolizumab pegol in patients with immune-mediated inflammatory diseases. Certolizumab pegol has been shown to have the unique property of not being capable of fixing complement and lysing cells, and therefore not activating other components of the immune system because of the lack of the IgG Fc domain (Kaushik and Moots 2005). Similar to the commercially available anti-TNF therapies, treatment with certolizumab pegol results in significant reductions in serum CRP levels in patients with CD, and to a lesser extent in patients with RA (Choy et al. 2002; Schreiber et al. 2005).

8 The Road Ahead for Anti-TNF Antibody Therapeutics

The postulated role of TNF in immune-mediated inflammatory diseases such as RA inflammatory bowel disease, and psoriasis has been confirmed in well-controlled clinical trials and to date, hundreds of thousands of patients have been successfully treated with infliximab and adalimumab. The impact of these breakthrough biologics on the patients' quality of life can be attributed to many scientists and clinicians, who continue to identify critical pathways and new targets that may further improve the benefits of these types of therapies, while minimizing unwanted side effects (Korzenik and Podolsky 2006; Myers et al. 2006; Strand et al. 2007), and to the patients who participate in these definitive clinical trials. With regard to the biology of TNF, there is persuasive data suggesting that activation of the TNFR1 receptor generates the proinflammatory properties of TNF, while the TNFR2 signaling pathway initiates the immunoregulatory actions attributed to TNF (Kollias 2005). This hypothesis suggests that blocking only TNF-mediated TNFR1 activation might be desirable, but this has not been tested in the clinic.

Researchers continue to develop new technologies to improve the efficiency of antibody selection and to further refine the specific properties of new, developing antibody therapeutics. These improvements range from transgenic mice engineered to produce human antibodies (Lonberg 2005) or new methods to enhance the affinity of existing antibodies (Rajpal et al. 2005), to the development of single domain antibodies (Holliger and Hudson 2005) whose unique small size and exceptional stability may allow topical, intranasal, or oral delivery options. In addition, a better characterization of patients who will respond to anti-TNF antibody therapies is of great importance. This can be achieved through more extensive studies examining relationships between pharmacodynamic markers and various clinical measures of response to anti-TNF treatment. Identification of associations between specific markers and a clinical response will aid in gaining a better understanding of the heterogeneity of individual patient populations, and their responses to anti-TNF therapies. Results from these types of studies will provide better insight into the profile of patients who will be the most likely to benefit from anti-TNF antibody therapy.

Despite new targets and technologies on the horizon, there is little doubt that anti-TNF antibodies will continue to be the biologic therapy of choice for immune-mediated inflammatory diseases for the foreseeable future. In addition, it is possible that other conditions with proinflammatory characteristics, such as Alzheimer's disease (Janelsins et al. 2005) or preterm labor (Sadowsky et al. 2006), may also be treatable with anti-TNF agents. The rigorous clinical testing and monitoring of commercially available anti-TNF therapies will enable a greater understanding of whether these agents can continue to expand their potential as effective therapies for other debilitating diseases and to improve patients' lives.

Acknowledgements We thank Rob Sarisky, Bernie Scallon, and Carrie Wagner for their critical review, and Rebecca E. Clemente and Mary Whitman for providing editorial support.

References

Aeberli D, Seitz M, Juni P, Villiger PM (2005) Increase of peripheral CXCR3 positive T lymphocytes upon treatment of RA patients with TNF-alpha inhibitors. Rheumatology (Oxford) 44:172–175

Aggarwal BB (2003) Signalling pathways of the TNF superfamily: a double-edged sword. Nat Rev Immunol 3:745–756

Aggarwal BB, Kohr WJ, Hass PE, Moffat B, Spencer SA, Henzel WJ, Bringman TS, Nedwin GE, Goeddel DV, Harkins RN (1985) Human tumor necrosis factor. Production, purification, and characterization. J Biol Chem 260:2345–2354

Agnholt J, Kaltoft K (2001) Infliximab downregulates interferon-gamma production in activated gut T-lymphocytes from patients with Crohn's disease. Cytokine 15:212–222

Ahmed MM, Mubashir E, Wolf RE, Hayat S, Hall V, Shi R, Berney SM (2006) Impact of treatment with infliximab on anticyclic citrullinated peptide antibody and rheumatoid factor in patients with rheumatoid arthritis. South Med J 99:1209–1215

Alessandri C, Bombardieri M, Papa N, Cinquini M, Magrini L, Tincani A, Valesini G (2004) Decrease of anti-cyclic citrullinated peptide antibodies and rheumatoid factor following anti-TNFalpha therapy (infliximab) in rheumatoid arthritis is associated with clinical improvement. Ann Rheum Dis 63:1218–1221

Antoni C, Dechant C, Hanns-Martin Lorenz PD, Wendler J, Ogilvie A, Lueftl M, Kalden-Nemeth D, Kalden JR, Manger B (2002) Open-label study of infliximab treatment for psoriatic arthritis: clinical and magnetic resonance imaging measurements of reduction of inflammation. Arthritis Rheum 47:506–512

Ashkenazi A, Dixit VM (1998) Death receptors: signaling and modulation. Science 281:1305–1308

Atzeni F, Sarzi-Puttini P, Dell' Acqua D, de Portu S, Cecchini G, Cruini C, Carrabba M, Meroni PL (2006) Adalimumab clinical efficacy is associated with rheumatoid factor and anti-cyclic citrullinated peptide antibody titer reduction: a one-year prospective study. Arthritis Res Ther 8:R3

Baert FJ, D'Haens GR, Peeters M, Hiele MI, Schaible TF, Shealy D, Geboes K, Rutgeerts PJ (1999) Tumor necrosis factor alpha antibody (infliximab) therapy profoundly down-regulates the inflammation in Crohn's ileocolitis. Gastroenterology 116:22–28

Baeten D, Van Damme N, Van den Bosch F, Kruithof E, De Vos M, Mielants H, Veys EM, De Keyser F (2001) Impaired Th1 cytokine production in spondyloarthropathy is restored by anti-TNFalpha. Ann Rheum Dis 60:750–755

Baldassano R, Braegger CP, Escher JC, DeWoody K, Hendricks DF, Keenan GF, Winter HS (2003) Infliximab (REMICADE) therapy in the treatment of pediatric Crohn's disease. Am J Gastroenterol 98:833–838

Baud V, Karin M (2001) Signal transduction by tumor necrosis factor and its relatives. Trends Cell Biol 11:372–377

Bazzoni F, Beutler B (1996) The tumor necrosis factor ligand and receptor families. N Engl J Med 334:1717–1725

Beutler B, Greenwald D, Hulmes JD, Chang M, Pan YC, Mathison J, Ulevitch R, Cerami A (1985a) Identity of tumour necrosis factor and the macrophage-secreted factor cachectin. Nature 316:552–554

Beutler B, Milsark IW, Cerami AC (1985b) Passive immunization against cachectin/tumor necrosis factor protects mice from lethal effect of endotoxin. Science 229:869–871

Bevilacqua MP, Gimbrone MA, Jr. (1987) Inducible endothelial functions in inflammation and coagulation. Semin Thromb Hemost 13:425–433

Black RA, Rauch CT, Kozlosky CJ, Peschon JJ, Slack JL, Wolfson MF, Castner BJ, Stocking KL, Reddy P, Srinivasan S, Nelson N, Boiani N, Schooley KA, Gerhart M, Davis R, Fitzner JN, Johnson RS, Paxton RJ, March CJ, Cerretti DP (1997) A metalloproteinase disintegrin that releases tumour-necrosis factor-alpha from cells. Nature 385:729–733

Bodmer M, Fournel MA, Hinshaw LB (1993) Preclinical review of anti-tumor necrosis factor monoclonal antibodies. Crit Care Med 21:S441–S446

Boyce BF, Schwarz EM, Xing L (2006) Osteoclast precursors: cytokine-stimulated immunomodulators of inflammatory bone disease. Curr Opin Rheumatol 18:427–432

Boyman O, Hefti HP, Conrad C, Nickoloff BJ, Suter M, Nestle FO (2004) Spontaneous development of psoriasis in a new animal model shows an essential role for resident T cells and tumor necrosis factor-alpha. J Exp Med 199: 731–736

Brandt J, Haibel H, Cornely D, Golder W, Gonzalez J, Reddig J, Thriene W, Sieper J, Braun J (2000) Successful treatment of active ankylosing spondylitis with the anti-tumor necrosis factor alpha monoclonal antibody infliximab. Arthritis Rheum 43:1346–1352

Braun J, Brandt J, Listing J, Zink A, Alten R, Burmester G, Gromnica-Ihle E, Kellner H, Schneider M, Sorensen H, Zeidler H, Sieper J (2005) Two year maintenance of efficacy and safety of infliximab in the treatment of ankylosing spondylitis. Ann Rheum Dis 64:229–234

Braun-Moscovici Y, Markovits D, Zinder O, Schapira D, Rozin A, Ehrenburg M, Dain L, Hoffer E, Nahir AM, Balbir-Gurman A (2006) Anti-cyclic citrullinated protein antibodies as a predictor of response to anti-tumor necrosis factor-alpha therapy in patients with rheumatoid arthritis. J Rheumatol 33:497–500

Brennan FM, Browne KA, Green PA, Jaspar JM, Maini RN, Feldmann M (1997) Reduction of serum matrix metalloproteinase 1 and matrix metalloproteinase 3 in rheumatoid arthritis patients following anti-tumour necrosis factor-alpha (cA2) therapy. Br J Rheumatol 36:643–650

Briot K, Garnero P, Le Henanff A, Dougados M, Roux C (2005) Body weight, body composition, and bone turnover changes in patients with spondyloarthropathy receiving anti-tumour necrosis factor {alpha} treatment. Ann Rheum Dis 64:1137–1140

Bunning RA, Russell RG (1989) The effect of tumor necrosis factor alpha and gamma-interferon on the resorption of human articular cartilage and on the production of prostaglandin E and of caseinase activity by human articular chondrocytes. Arthritis Rheum 32:780–784

Burke F (1999) Cytokines (IFNs, TNF-alpha, IL-2 and IL-12) and animal models of cancer. Cytokines Cell Mol Ther 5:51–61

Carswell EA, Old LJ, Kassel RL, Green S, Fiore N, Williamson B (1975) An endotoxin-induced serum factor that causes necrosis of tumors. Proc Natl Acad Sci USA 72:3666–3670

Cauza E, Hanusch-Enserer U, Frischmuth K, Fabian B, Dunky A, Kostner K (2006) Short-term infliximab therapy improves symptoms of psoriatic arthritis and decreases concentrations of cartilage oligomeric matrix protein. J Clin Pharm Ther 31:149–152

Charles P, Elliott MJ, Davis D, Potter A, Kalden JR, Antoni C, Breedveld FC, Smolen JS, Eberl G, deWoody K, Feldmann M, Maini RN (1999) Regulation of cytokines, cytokine inhibitors, and acute-phase proteins following anti-TNF-alpha therapy in rheumatoid arthritis. J Immunol 163:1521–1528

Chen DM, Gordon KB, Leonardi C, Menter MA (2004) Adalimumab efficacy and safety in patients with moderate to severe chronic plaque psoriasis: Preliminary findings from a 12-week dose ranging trial. J Am Acad Dermatol 50:Suppl:P2

Choy EH, Hazleman B, Smith M, Moss K, Lisi L, Scott DG, Patel J, Sopwith M, Isenberg DA (2002) Efficacy of a novel PEGylated humanized anti-TNF fragment (CDP870) in patients with rheumatoid arthritis: a phase II double-blinded, randomized, dose-escalating trial. Rheumatology (Oxford) 41:1133–1137

Clark M (2000) Antibody humanization: a case of the 'Emperor's new clothes'? Immunol Today 21:397–402

Cornillie F, Shealy D, D'Haens G, Geboes K, Van Assche G, Ceuppens J, Wagner C, Schaible T, Plevy SE, Targan SR, Rutgeerts P (2001) Infliximab induces potent anti-inflammatory and local immunomodulatory activity but no systemic immune suppression in patients with Crohn's disease. Aliment Pharmacol Ther 15: 463–473

Cuchacovich M, Ferreira L, Aliste M, Soto L, Cuenca J, Cruzat A, Gatica H, Schiattino I, Perez C, Aguirre A, Salazar-Onfray F, Aguillon JC (2004) Tumour necrosis factor-alpha (TNF-alpha) levels and influence of −308 TNF-alpha promoter polymorphism on the responsiveness to infliximab in patients with rheumatoid arthritis. Scand J Rheumatol 33:228–232

den Broeder A, van de Putte L, Rau R, Schattenkirchner M, Van Riel P, Sander O, Binder C, Fenner H, Bankmann Y, Velagapudi R, Kempeni J, Kupper H (2002a) A single dose, placebo controlled study of the fully human anti-tumor necrosis factor-alpha antibody adalimumab (D2E7) in patients with rheumatoid arthritis. J Rheumatol 29:2288–2298

den Broeder AA, Joosten LA, Saxne T, Heinegard D, Fenner H, Miltenburg AM, Frasa WL, van Tits LJ, Buurman WA, van Riel PL, van de Putte LB, Barrera P (2002b) Long term anti-tumour necrosis factor alpha monotherapy in rheumatoid arthritis: effect on radiological course and prognostic value of markers of cartilage turnover and endothelial activation. Ann Rheum Dis 61:311–318

den Broeder AA, Wanten GJ, Oyen WJ, Naber T, van Riel PL, Barrera P (2003) Neutrophil migration and production of reactive oxygen species during treatment with a fully human anti-tumor necrosis factor-alpha monoclonal antibody in patients with rheumatoid arthritis. J Rheumatol 30:232–237

Detkova Z, Kupcova V, Prikazska M, Turecky L, Weissova S, Jahnova E (2003) Different patterns of serum interleukin 10 response to treatment with anti-tumor necrosis factor alpha antibody (infliximab) in Crohn's disease. Physiol Res 52:95–100

Ehrenstein MR, Evans JG, Singh A, Moore S, Warnes G, Isenberg DA, Mauri C (2004) Compromised function of regulatory T cells in rheumatoid arthritis and reversal by anti-TNFalpha therapy. J Exp Med 200:277–285

Fabris M, Tolusso B, Di Poi E, Assaloni R, Sinigaglia L, Ferraccioli G (2002) Tumor necrosis factor-alpha receptor II polymorphism in patients from southern Europe with mild-moderate and severe rheumatoid arthritis. J Rheumatol 29:1847–1850

Farrell RJ, Shah SA, Lodhavia PJ, Alsahli M, Falchuk KR, Michetti P, Peppercorn MA (2000) Clinical experience with infliximab therapy in 100 patients with Crohn's disease. Am J Gastroenterol 95:3490–3497

Fasanmade AA, Zhu YW, Wagner C, Pendley C, Davis HM (2002) Population pharmacokinetics of single dose infliximab in patients with Crohn's disease. Clin Pharmacol Ther 71:P66

Feldmann M, Brennan FM, Paleolog E, Cope A, Taylor P, Williams R, Woody J, Maini RN (2004) Anti-TNFalpha therapy of rheumatoid arthritis: what can we learn about chronic disease? Novartis Found Symp 256: 53–69; discussion 69–73, 106–111, 266–109

Feldmann M, Maini RN (2001) Anti-TNF alpha therapy of rheumatoid arthritis: what have we learned? Annu Rev Immunol 19:163–196

Feletar M, Brockbank JE, Schentag CT, Lapp V, Gladman DD (2004) Treatment of refractory psoriatic arthritis with infliximab: a 12 month observational study of 16 patients. Ann Rheum Dis 63:156–161

Flynn JL, Goldstein MM, Chan J, Triebold KJ, Pfeffer K, Lowenstein CJ, Schreiber R, Mak TW, Bloom BR (1995) Tumor necrosis factor-alpha is required in the protective immune response against Mycobacterium tuberculosis in mice. Immunity 2:561–572

Franchimont N, Putzeys V, Collette J, Vermeire S, Rutgeerts P, De Vos M, Van Gossum A, Franchimont D, Fiasse R, Pelckmans P, Malaise M, Belaiche J, Louis E (2004) Rapid improvement of bone metabolism after infliximab treatment in Crohn's disease. Aliment Pharmacol Ther 20:607–614

Freeman BD, Natanson C (2000) Anti-inflammatory therapies in sepsis and septic shock. Expert Opin Investig Drugs 9:1651–1663

Gao Q, Hogezand RA, Lamers CB, Verspaget HW (2004) Basic fibroblast growth factor as a response parameter to infliximab in fistulizing Crohn's disease. Aliment Pharmacol Ther 20:585–592

Gao Q, Meijer MJ, Schluter UG, van Hogezand RA, van der Zon JM, van den Berg M, van Duijn W, Lamers CB, Verspaget HW (2007) Infliximab treatment influences the serological expression of matrix metalloproteinase (MMP)-2 and −9 in Crohn's disease. Inflamm Bowel Dis 13(6):693–702

Garfield BE, Krahl T, Appel S, Cooper SM, Rincon M (2005) Regulation of p38 MAP kinase in CD4+ lymphocytes by infliximab therapy in patients with rheumatoid arthritis. Clin Immunol 116:101–107

Geboes K, Dalle I (2002) Influence of treatment on morphological features of mucosal inflammation. Gut 50(Suppl 3):III37-III42

Georgopoulos S, Plows D, Kollias G (1996) Transmembrane TNF is sufficient to induce localized tissue toxicity and chronic inflammatory arthritis in transgenic mice. J Inflamm 46:86–97

Goldstein G, Fuccello AJ, Norman DJ, Shield CF, 3rd, Colvin RB, Cosimi AB (1986) OKT3 monoclonal antibody plasma levels during therapy and the subsequent development of host antibodies to OKT3. Transplantation 42:507–511

Gonzalez-Gay MA, Garcia-Unzueta MT, De Matias JM, Gonzalez-Juanatey C, Garcia-Porrua C, Sanchez-Andrade A, Martin J, Llorca J (2006) Influence of anti-TNF-alpha infliximab therapy on adhesion molecules associated with atherogenesis in patients with rheumatoid arthritis. Clin Exp Rheumatol 24:373–379

Gottlieb AB, Masud S, Ramamurthi R, Abdulghani A, Romano P, Chaudhari U, Dooley LT, Fasanmade AA, Wagner CL (2003) Pharmacodynamic and pharmacokinetic response to anti-tumor necrosis factor-alpha monoclonal antibody (infliximab) treatment of moderate to severe psoriasis vulgaris. J Am Acad Dermatol 48:68–75

Grell M, Becke FM, Wajant H, Mannel DN, Scheurich P (1998) TNF receptor type 2 mediates thymocyte proliferation independently of TNF receptor type 1. Eur J Immunol 28:257–263

Grell M, Douni E, Wajant H, Lohden M, Clauss M, Maxeiner B, Georgopoulos S, Lesslauer W, Kollias G, Pfizenmaier K, Scheurich P (1995) The transmembrane form of tumor necrosis factor is the prime activating ligand of the 80 kDa tumor necrosis factor receptor. Cell 83:793–802

Gustot T, Lemmers A, Louis E, Nicaise C, Quertinmont E, Belaiche J, Roland S, Van Gossum A, Deviere J, Franchimont D (2005) Profile of soluble cytokine receptors in Crohn's disease. Gut 54: 488–495

Haridas V, Darnay BG, Natarajan K, Heller R, Aggarwal BB (1998) Overexpression of the p80 TNF receptor leads to TNF-dependent apoptosis, nuclear factor-kappa B activation, and c-Jun kinase activation. J Immunol 160:3152–3162

Holliger P, Hudson PJ (2005) Engineered antibody fragments and the rise of single domains. Nat Biotechnol 23:1126–1136

Janelsins MC, Mastrangelo MA, Oddo S, LaFerla FM, Federoff HJ, Bowers WJ (2005) Early correlation of microglial activation with enhanced tumor necrosis factor-alpha and monocyte chemoattractant protein-1 expression specifically within the entorhinal cortex of triple transgenic Alzheimer's disease mice. J Neuroinflammation 2:23

Jelinek DF, Lipsky PE (1987) Enhancement of human B cell proliferation and differentiation by tumor necrosis factor-alpha and interleukin 1. J Immunol 139:2970–2976

Kageyama Y, Torikai E, Nagano A (2007) Anti-tumor necrosis factor-alpha antibody treatment reduces serum CXCL16 levels in patients with rheumatoid arthritis. Rheumatol Int 27:467–472

Karin M, Greten FR (2005) NF-kappaB: linking inflammation and immunity to cancer development and progression. Nat Rev Immunol 5:749–759

Kaushik VV, Moots RJ (2005) CDP-870 (certolizumab) in rheumatoid arthritis. Expert Opin Biol Ther 5:601–606

Keffer J, Probert L, Cazlaris H, Georgopoulos S, Kaslaris E, Kioussis D, Kollias G (1991) Transgenic mice expressing human tumour necrosis factor: a predictive genetic model of arthritis. Embo J 10:4025–4031

Klimiuk PA, Sierakowski S, Domyslawska I, Chwiecko J (2004) Effect of repeated infliximab therapy on serum matrix metalloproteinases and tissue inhibitors of metalloproteinases in patients with rheumatoid arthritis. J Rheumatol 31:238–242

Knight DM, Trinh H, Le J, Siegel S, Shealy D, McDonough M, Scallon B, Moore MA, Vilcek J, Daddona P, et al. (1993) Construction and initial characterization of a mouse-human chimeric anti-TNF antibody. Mol Immunol 30:1443–1453

Knight DM, Wagner C, Jordan R, McAleer MF, DeRita R, Fass DN, Coller BS, Weisman HF, Ghrayeb J (1995) The immunogenicity of the 7E3 murine monoclonal Fab antibody fragment variable region is dramatically reduced in humans by substitution of human for murine constant regions. Mol Immunol 32:1271–1281

Koch AE, Kunkel SL, Strieter RM (1995) Cytokines in rheumatoid arthritis. J Investig Med 43: 28–38

Kollias G (2005) TNF pathophysiology in murine models of chronic inflammation and autoimmunity. Semin Arthritis Rheum 34:3–6

Korner H, Cook M, Riminton DS, Lemckert FA, Hoek RM, Ledermann B, Kontgen F, Fazekas de St Groth B, Sedgwick JD (1997) Distinct roles for lymphotoxin-alpha and tumor necrosis factor in organogenesis and spatial organization of lymphoid tissue. Eur J Immunol 27:2600–2609

Korzenik JR, Podolsky DK (2006) Evolving knowledge and therapy of inflammatory bowel disease. Nat Rev Drug Discov 5:197–209

Krejsa C, Rogge M, Sadee W (2006) Protein therapeutics: new applications for pharmacogenetics. Nat Rev Drug Discov 5:507–521

Kumar A, Takada Y, Boriek AM, Aggarwal BB (2004) Nuclear factor-kappaB: its role in health and disease. J Mol Med 82:434–448

Kuuliala A, Nissinen R, Kautiainen H, Repo H, Leirisalo-Repo M (2006) Low circulating soluble interleukin 2 receptor level predicts rapid response in patients with refractory rheumatoid arthritis treated with infliximab. Ann Rheum Dis 65:26–29

Lange U, Teichmann J, Muller-Ladner U, Strunk J (2005) Increase in bone mineral density of patients with rheumatoid arthritis treated with anti-TNF-alpha antibody: a prospective open-label pilot study. Rheumatology (Oxford) 44:1546–1548

Legler DF, Micheau O, Doucey MA, Tschopp J, Bron C (2003) Recruitment of TNF receptor 1 to lipid rafts is essential for TNFalpha-mediated NF-kappaB activation. Immunity 18:655–664

Lejeune FJ, Lienard D, Matter M, Ruegg C (2006) Efficiency of recombinant human TNF in human cancer therapy. Cancer Immun 6:6

Lequerre T, Gauthier-Jauneau AC, Bansard C, Derambure C, Hiron M, Vittecoq O, Daveau M, Mejjad O, Daragon A, Tron F, Le Loet X, Salier JP (2006) Gene profiling in white blood cells predicts infliximab responsiveness in rheumatoid arthritis. Arthritis Res Ther 8:R105

Lipsky PE, van der Heijde DM, St Clair EW, Furst DE, Breedveld FC, Kalden JR, Smolen JS, Weisman M, Emery P, Feldmann M, Harriman GR, Maini RN (2000) Infliximab and methotrexate in the treatment of rheumatoid arthritis. Anti-Tumor Necrosis Factor Trial in Rheumatoid Arthritis with Concomitant Therapy Study Group. N Engl J Med 343:1594–1602

Lonberg N (2005) Human antibodies from transgenic animals. Nat Biotechnol 23:1117–1125

Louis E, El Ghoul Z, Vermeire S, Dall'Ozzo S, Rutgeerts P, Paintaud G, Belaiche J, De Vos M, Van Gossum A, Colombel JF, Watier H (2004) Association between polymorphism in IgG Fc receptor IIIa coding gene and biological response to infliximab in Crohn's disease. Aliment Pharmacol Ther 19:511–519

Lugering A, Schmidt M, Lugering N, Pauels HG, Domschke W, Kucharzik T (2001) Infliximab induces apoptosis in monocytes from patients with chronic active Crohn's disease by using a caspase-dependent pathway. Gastroenterology 121:1145–1157

Malik ST, Naylor MS, East N, Oliff A, Balkwill FR (1990) Cells secreting tumour necrosis factor show enhanced metastasis in nude mice. Eur J Cancer 26:1031–1034

Mandl T, Jacobsson L (2002) [Anti-TNF-α treatment–an effective complement in spondyloarthropathy.] Lakartidningen 99:5189–5193

Marini M, Bamias G, Rivera-Nieves J, Moskaluk CA, Hoang SB, Ross WG, Pizarro TT, Cominelli F (2003) TNF-alpha neutralization ameliorates the severity of murine Crohn's-like ileitis by abrogation of intestinal epithelial cell apoptosis. Proc Natl Acad Sci USA 100: 8366–8371

Marino MW, Dunn A, Grail D, Inglese M, Noguchi Y, Richards E, Jungbluth A, Wada H, Moore M, Williamson B, Basu S, Old LJ (1997) Characterization of tumor necrosis factor-deficient mice. Proc Natl Acad Sci USA 94:8093–8098

Markham A, Lamb HM (2000) Infliximab: a review of its use in the management of rheumatoid arthritis. Drugs 59:1341–1359

Martinez A, Salido M, Bonilla G, Pascual-Salcedo D, Fernandez-Arquero M, de Miguel S, Balsa A, de la Concha EG, Fernandez-Gutierrez B (2004) Association of the major histocompatibility complex with response to infliximab therapy in rheumatoid arthritis patients. Arthritis Rheum 50:1077–1082

Mastroianni A, Minutilli E, Mussi A, Bordignon V, Trento E, D'Agosto G, Cordiali-Fei P, Berardesca E (2005) Cytokine profiles during infliximab monotherapy in psoriatic arthritis. Br J Dermatol 153:531–536

Meyer O, Labarre C, Dougados M, Goupille P, Cantagrel A, Dubois A, Nicaise-Roland P, Sibilia J, Combe B (2003) Anticitrullinated protein/peptide antibody assays in early rheumatoid arthritis for predicting five year radiographic damage. Ann Rheum Dis 62:120–126

Micheau O, Tschopp J (2003) Induction of TNF receptor I-mediated apoptosis via two sequential signaling complexes. Cell 114:181–190

Moore RJ, Owens DM, Stamp G, Arnott C, Burke F, East N, Holdsworth H, Turner L, Rollins B, Pasparakis M, Kollias G, Balkwill F (1999) Mice deficient in tumor necrosis factor-alpha are resistant to skin carcinogenesis. Nat Med 5:828–831

Moss ML, Jin SL, Milla ME, Bickett DM, Burkhart W, Carter HL, Chen WJ, Clay WC, Didsbury JR, Hassler D, Hoffman CR, Kost TA, Lambert MH, Leesnitzer MA, McCauley P, McGeehan G, Mitchell J, Moyer M, Pahel G, Rocque W, Overton LK, Schoenen F, Seaton T, Su JL, Becherer JD, et al. (1997) Cloning of a disintegrin metalloproteinase that processes precursor tumour-necrosis factor-alpha. Nature 385:733–736

Mugnier B, Balandraud N, Darque A, Roudier C, Roudier J, Reviron D (2003) Polymorphism at position -308 of the tumor necrosis factor alpha gene influences outcome of infliximab therapy in rheumatoid arthritis. Arthritis Rheum 48:1849–1852

Mullin JM, Snock KV (1990) Effect of tumor necrosis factor on epithelial tight junctions and transepithelial permeability. Cancer Res 50:2172–2176

Myers WA, Gottlieb AB, Mease P (2006) Psoriasis and psoriatic arthritis: clinical features and disease mechanisms. Clin Dermatol 24:438–447

Nadkarni S, Mauri C, Ehrenstein MR (2007) Anti-TNF-alpha therapy induces a distinct regulatory T cell population in patients with rheumatoid arthritis via TGF-beta. J Exp Med 204:33–39

Nakada MT, Tam SH, Woulfe DS, Casper KA, Swerlick RA, Ghrayeb J (1998) Neutralization of TNF by the antibody cA2 reveals differential regulation of adhesion molecule expression on TNF-activated endothelial cells. Cell Adhes Commun 5:491–503

Nestorov I (2005) Clinical pharmacokinetics of TNF antagonists: how do they differ? Semin Arthritis Rheum 34:12–18

Neurath MF, Fuss I, Pasparakis M, Alexopoulou L, Haralambous S, Meyer zum Buschenfelde KH, Strober W, Kollias G (1997) Predominant pathogenic role of tumor necrosis factor in experimental colitis in mice. Eur J Immunol 27:1743–1750

Osbourn J, Groves M, Vaughan T (2005) From rodent reagents to human therapeutics using antibody guided selection. Methods 36:61–68

Pasparakis M, Alexopoulou L, Episkopou V, Kollias G (1996) Immune and inflammatory responses in TNF alpha-deficient mice: a critical requirement for TNF alpha in the formation of primary B cell follicles, follicular dendritic cell networks and germinal centers, and in the maturation of the humoral immune response. J Exp Med 184:1397–1411

Passeri G, Girasole G, Manolagas SC, Jilka RL (1994) Endogenous production of tumor necrosis factor by primary cultures of murine calvarial cells: influence on IL-6 production and osteoclast development. Bone Miner 24:109–126

Pennica D, Nedwin GE, Hayflick JS, Seeburg PH, Derynck R, Palladino MA, Kohr WJ, Aggarwal BB, Goeddel DV (1984) Human tumour necrosis factor: precursor structure, expression and homology to lymphotoxin. Nature 312:724–729

Perez C, Albert I, DeFay K, Zachariades N, Gooding L, Kriegler M (1990) A nonsecretable cell surface mutant of tumor necrosis factor (TNF) kills by cell-to-cell contact. Cell 63:251–258

Piguet PF, Grau GE, Vesin C, Loetscher H, Gentz R, Lesslauer W (1992) Evolution of collagen arthritis in mice is arrested by treatment with anti-tumour necrosis factor (TNF) antibody or a recombinant soluble TNF receptor. Immunology 77:510–514

Pikarsky E, Porat RM, Stein I, Abramovitch R, Amit S, Kasem S, Gutkovich-Pyest E, Urieli-Shoval S, Galun E, Ben-Neriah Y (2004) NF-kappaB functions as a tumour promoter in inflammation-associated cancer. Nature 431:461–466

Pittoni V, Bombardieri M, Spinelli FR, Scrivo R, Alessandri C, Conti F, Spadaro A, Valesini G (2002) Anti-tumour necrosis factor (TNF) alpha treatment of rheumatoid arthritis (infliximab) selectively down regulates the production of interleukin (IL) 18 but not of IL12 and IL13. Ann Rheum Dis 61:723–725

Pizarro TT, Arseneau KO, Bamias G, Cominelli F (2003) Mouse models for the study of Crohn's disease. Trends Mol Med 9:218–222

Plevy SE, Landers CJ, Prehn J, Carramanzana NM, Deem RL, Shealy D, Targan SR (1997) A role for TNF-alpha and mucosal T helper-1 cytokines in the pathogenesis of Crohn's disease. J Immunol 159:6276–6282

Powrie F, Leach MW, Mauze S, Menon S, Caddle LB, Coffman RL (1994) Inhibition of Th1 responses prevents inflammatory bowel disease in scid mice reconstituted with CD45RBhi CD4+ T cells. Immunity 1:553–562

Rajpal A, Beyaz N, Haber L, Cappuccilli G, Yee H, Bhatt RR, Takeuchi T, Lerner RA, Crea R (2005) A general method for greatly improving the affinity of antibodies by using combinatorial libraries. Proc Natl Acad Sci USA 102:8466–8471

Ranganathan P (2005) Pharmacogenomics of tumor necrosis factor antagonists in rheumatoid arthritis. Pharmacogenomics 6:481–490

Rose-John S, Schooltink H (2003) CDP-870. Celltech/Pfizer. Curr Opin Investig Drugs 4:588–592

Rothe M, Wong SC, Henzel WJ, Goeddel DV (1994) A novel family of putative signal transducers associated with the cytoplasmic domain of the 75 kDa tumor necrosis factor receptor. Cell 78:681–692

Rutgeerts P, Sandborn WJ, Feagan BG, Reinisch W, Olson A, Johanns J, Travers S, Rachmilewitz D, Hanauer SB, Lichtenstein GR, de Villiers WJ, Present D, Sands BE, Colombel JF (2005) Infliximab for induction and maintenance therapy for ulcerative colitis. N Engl J Med 353:2462–2476

Sadowsky DW, Adams KM, Gravett MG, Witkin SS, Novy MJ (2006) Preterm labor is induced by intraamniotic infusions of interleukin-1beta and tumor necrosis factor-alpha but not by interleukin-6 or interleukin-8 in a nonhuman primate model. Am J Obstet Gynecol 195:1578–1589

Saklatvala J (1986) Tumour necrosis factor alpha stimulates resorption and inhibits synthesis of proteoglycan in cartilage. Nature 322:547–549

Salfeld J, Allen D, Hoogenboom HR, Kaymakcalan Z, Labkovsky B, Mankovich J, McGuinness B, Roberts A, Sakorafas P, Schoenhaut D, Vaughan T, White M, Wilton A (2000) Human antibodies that bind human TNF alpha. US Patent 6,090,382

Santora LC, Kaymakcalan Z, Sakorafas P, Krull IS, Grant K (2001) Characterization of noncovalent complexes of recombinant human monoclonal antibody and antigen using cation exchange, size exclusion chromatography, and BIAcore. Anal Biochem 299:119–129

Scallon B, Cai A, Solowski N, Rosenberg A, Song XY, Shealy D, Wagner C (2002) Binding and functional comparisons of two types of tumor necrosis factor antagonists. J Pharmacol Exp Ther 301:418–426

Scallon BJ, Moore MA, Trinh H, Knight DM, Ghrayeb J (1995) Chimeric anti-TNF-alpha mono-clonal antibody cA2 binds recombinant transmembrane TNF-alpha and activates immune ef-fector functions. Cytokine 7:251–259

Scheinfeld N (2004) Off-label uses and side effects of infliximab. J Drugs Dermatol 3:273–284

Scheinin T, Butler DM, Salway F, Scallon B, Feldmann M (2003) Validation of the interleukin-10 knockout mouse model of colitis: antitumour necrosis factor-antibodies suppress the progres-sion of colitis. Clin Exp Immunol 133:38–43

Scheurich P, Thoma B, Ucer U, Pfizenmaier K (1987) Immunoregulatory activity of recombinant human tumor necrosis factor (TNF)-alpha: induction of TNF receptors on human T cells and TNF-alpha-mediated enhancement of T cell responses. J Immunol 138:1786–1790

Schreiber S, Rutgeerts P, Fedorak RN, Khaliq-Kareemi M, Kamm MA, Boivin M, Bernstein CN, Staun M, Thomsen OO, Innes A (2005) A randomized, placebo-controlled trial of certolizumab pegol (CDP870) for treatment of Crohn's disease. Gastroenterology 129:807–818

Schutze S, Machleidt T, Adam D, Schwandner R, Wiegmann K, Kruse ML, Heinrich M, Wickel M, Kronke M (1999) Inhibition of receptor internalization by monodansylcadaverine selectively blocks p55 tumor necrosis factor receptor death domain signaling. J Biol Chem 274:10203–10212

Schwab M, Klotz U (2001) Pharmacokinetic considerations in the treatment of inflammatory bowel disease. Clin Pharmacokinet 40:723–751

Scott KA, Moore RJ, Arnott CH, East N, Thompson RG, Scallon BJ, Shealy DJ, Balkwill FR (2003) An anti-tumor necrosis factor-alpha antibody inhibits the development of experimental skin tumors. Mol Cancer Ther 2:445–451

Seko Y, Cole S, Kasprzak W, Shapiro BA, Ragheb JA (2006) The role of cytokine mRNA stability in the pathogenesis of autoimmune disease. Autoimmun Rev 5:299–305

Semmler M, Seeck U, Neustadt B, Schulz M, Dotzlaw H, Neeck G, Eggert M (2007) No effects of adalimumab therapy on the activation of NF-kappaB in lymphocytes from patients with severe rheumatoid arthritis. Clin Rheumatol 26:1499–1504

Shealy DJ, Wooley PH, Emmell E, Volk A, Rosenberg A, Treacy G, Wagner CL, Mayton L, Griswold DE, Song XY (2002) Anti-TNF-alpha antibody allows healing of joint damage in polyarthritic transgenic mice. Arthritis Res 4:R7

Smith RA, Baglioni C (1987) The active form of tumor necrosis factor is a trimer. J Biol Chem 262:6951–6954

Smolen JS, Han C, Bala M, Maini RN, Kalden JR, van der Heijde D, Breedveld FC, Furst DE, Lip-sky PE (2005) Evidence of radiographic benefit of treatment with infliximab plus methotrexate in rheumatoid arthritis patients who had no clinical improvement: a detailed subanalysis of data from the anti-tumor necrosis factor trial in rheumatoid arthritis with concomitant therapy study. Arthritis Rheum 52:1020–1030

Smolen JS, Van Der Heijde DM, St Clair EW, Emery P, Bathon JM, Keystone E, Maini RN, Kalden JR, Schiff M, Baker D, Han C, Han J, Bala M (2006) Predictors of joint damage in patients with early rheumatoid arthritis treated with high-dose methotrexate with or without concomitant infliximab: results from the ASPIRE trial. Arthritis Rheum 54:702–710

St Clair EW, van der Heijde DM, Smolen JS, Maini RN, Bathon JM, Emery P, Keystone E, Schiff M, Kalden JR, Wang B, Dewoody K, Weiss R, Baker D (2004) Combination of infliximab and methotrexate therapy for early rheumatoid arthritis: a randomized, controlled trial. Arthritis Rheum 50:3432–3443

St Clair EW, Wagner CL, Fasanmade AA, Wang B, Schaible T, Kavanaugh A, Keystone EC (2002) The relationship of serum infliximab concentrations to clinical improvement in rheumatoid arthritis: results from ATTRACT, a multicenter, randomized, double-blind, placebo-controlled trial. Arthritis Rheum 46:1451–1459

Strand V, Kimberly R, Isaacs JD (2007) Biologic therapies in rheumatology: lessons learned, future directions. Nat Rev Drug Discov 6:75–92

Strunk J, Bundke E, Lange U (2006) Anti-TNF-alpha antibody Infliximab and glucocorticoids reduce serum vascular endothelial growth factor levels in patients with rheumatoid arthritis: a pilot study. Rheumatol Int 26:252–256

Sugarman BJ, Aggarwal BB, Hass PE, Figari IS, Palladino MA Jr, Shepard HM (1985) Recombinant human tumor necrosis factor-alpha: effects on proliferation of normal and transformed cells in vitro. Science 230:943–945

Szlosarek P, Charles KA, Balkwill FR (2006) Tumour necrosis factor-alpha as a tumour promoter. Eur J Cancer 42:745–750

Tchetverikov I, Lohmander LS, Verzijl N, Huizinga TW, TeKoppele JM, Hanemaaijer R, DeGroot J (2005) MMP protein and activity levels in synovial fluid from patients with joint injury, inflammatory arthritis, and osteoarthritis. Ann Rheum Dis 64:694–698

ten Hove T, van Montfrans C, Peppelenbosch MP, van Deventer SJ (2002) Infliximab treatment induces apoptosis of lamina propria T lymphocytes in Crohn's disease. Gut 50:206–211

Thorbecke GJ, Shah R, Leu CH, Kuruvilla AP, Hardison AM, Palladino MA (1992) Involvement of endogenous tumor necrosis factor alpha and transforming growth factor beta during induction of collagen type II arthritis in mice. Proc Natl Acad Sci USA 89:7375–7379

Torikai E, Kageyama Y, Suzuki M, Ichikawa T, Nagano A (2007) The effect of infliximab on chemokines in patients with rheumatoid arthritis. Clin Rheumatol 26(7):1088–1093

Torikai E, Kageyama Y, Takahashi M, Suzuki M, Ichikawa T, Nagafusa T, Nagano A (2006) The effect of infliximab on bone metabolism markers in patients with rheumatoid arthritis. Rheumatology (Oxford) 45:761–764

Tracey KJ, Beutler B, Lowry SF, Merryweather J, Wolpe S, Milsark IW, Hariri RJ, Fahey TJ, 3rd, Zentella A, Albert JD, et al. (1986) Shock and tissue injury induced by recombinant human cachectin. Science 234:470–474

Ulfgren AK, Andersson U, Engstrom M, Klareskog L, Maini RN, Taylor PC (2000) Systemic anti-tumor necrosis factor alpha therapy in rheumatoid arthritis down-regulates synovial tumor necrosis factor alpha synthesis. Arthritis Rheum 43:2391–2396

Valencia X, Stephens G, Goldbach-Mansky R, Wilson M, Shevach EM, Lipsky PE (2006) TNF downmodulates the function of human CD4+CD25hi T-regulatory cells. Blood 108:253–261

Van den Brande JM, Braat H, van den Brink GR, Versteeg HH, Bauer CA, Hoedemaeker I, van Montfrans C, Hommes DW, Peppelenbosch MP, van Deventer SJ (2003) Infliximab but not etanercept induces apoptosis in lamina propria T-lymphocytes from patients with Crohn's disease. Gastroenterology 124:1774–1785

Van den Brande JM, Koehler T, Zelinkova Z, Bennink RJ, Te Velde AA, Ten Kate F, van Deventer SJ, Peppelenbosch MP, Hommes DW (2006) Prediction of anti-TNF clinical efficacy by real-time visualisation of apoptosis in patients with Crohn's disease. Gut 56(4):461–463

van der Heijde D, Dijkmans B, Geusens P, Sieper J, DeWoody K, Williamson P, Braun J (2005) Efficacy and safety of infliximab in patients with ankylosing spondylitis: results of a randomized, placebo-controlled trial (ASSERT). Arthritis Rheum 52:582–591

van Dullemen HM, van Deventer SJ, Hommes DW, Bijl HA, Jansen J, Tytgat GN, Woody J (1995) Treatment of Crohn's disease with anti-tumor necrosis factor chimeric monoclonal antibody (cA2). Gastroenterology 109:129–135

van Oosterhout M, Levarht EW, Sont JK, Huizinga TW, Toes RE, van Laar JM (2005) Clinical efficacy of infliximab plus methotrexate in DMARD naive and DMARD refractory rheumatoid arthritis is associated with decreased synovial expression of TNF alpha and IL18 but not CXCL12. Ann Rheum Dis 64:537–543

van Roon JA, Hartgring SA, Wenting-van Wijk M, Jacobs KM, Tak PP, Bijlsma JW, Lafeber FP (2007) Persistence of IL-7 activity and IL-7 levels upon TNFα blockade in patients with rheumatoid arthritis. Ann Rheum Dis 66:664–669

Vandooren B, Kruithof E, Yu DT, Rihl M, Gu J, De Rycke L, Van Den Bosch F, Veys EM, De Keyser F, Baeten D (2004) Involvement of matrix metalloproteinases and their inhibitors in peripheral synovitis and down-regulation by tumor necrosis factor alpha blockade in spondylarthropathy. Arthritis Rheum 50:2942–2953

Velagapudi RB, Noertersheuser PA, Awni WM, Fischkoff SA, Kupper H, Granneman GR, van de Putte LBA, Keystone EC (2003) Effect of methotrexate coadministration on the pharmacokinetics of Adaliumab (Humira, Abbott) following a single intravenous injection. Arthritis Rheum 51(Suppl):S141

Vespasiani Gentilucci U, Caviglia R, Picardi A, Carotti S, Ribolsi M, Galati G, Petitti T, Afeltra A, Cicala M (2005) Infliximab reverses growth hormone resistance associated with inflammatory bowel disease. Aliment Pharmacol Ther 21:1063–1071

Vis M, Havaardsholm EA, Haugeberg G, Uhlig T, Voskuyl AE, van de Stadt RJ, Dijkmans BA, Woolf AD, Kvien TK, Lems WF (2006) Evaluation of bone mineral density, bone metabolism, osteoprotegerin and receptor activator of the NFkappaB ligand serum levels during treatment with infliximab in patients with rheumatoid arthritis. Ann Rheum Dis 65:1495–1499

Visvanathan S, Marano C, Braun J, Kavanaugh A, Yan S, Gathany T, Han J, Zhou B, Baker D, Wagner C (2006) Comparison of the effect of infliximab on inflammation and bone forma-tion biomarkes and associations with clinical response in ankylosing spondylitis and psoriatic arthritis. Arthritis Rheum 54(Suppl):S792

Visvanathan S, Marini JC, Smolen JS, St Clair EW, Pritchard C, Shergy W, Pendley C, Baker D, Bala M, Gathany T, Wagner C (2007a) Changes in biomarkers of inflammation and bone turnover and associations with clinical efficacy following infliximab plus methotrexate therapy in patients with early rheumatoid arthritis. J Rheumatol 34:1465–1474

Visvanathan S, Wagner C, Marini JC, van der Heijde D, Baker D, Gathany T, Han J, Braun J (2007b) Inflammatory biomarkers, disease activity, and spinal disease measures in patients with ankylosing spondylitis after treatment with infliximab. Ann Rheum Dis doi:10.1136/ard.2007.071605

Watkins PE, Warren BF, Stephens S, Ward P, Foulkes R (1997) Treatment of ulcerative colitis in the cottontop tamarin using antibody to tumour necrosis factor alpha. Gut 40:628–633

Williams RO, Feldmann M, Maini RN (1992) Anti-tumor necrosis factor ameliorates joint disease in murine collagen-induced arthritis. Proc Natl Acad Sci USA 89:9784–9788

Willot S, Vermeire S, Ohresser M, Rutgeerts P, Paintaud G, Belaiche J, De Vos M, Van Gossum A, Franchimont D, Colombel JF, Watier H, Louis E (2006) No association between C-reactive protein gene polymorphisms and decrease of C-reactive protein serum concentration after in-fliximab treatment in Crohn's disease. Pharmacogenet Genomics 16:37–42

Xu Z, Fasanmade A, Pendley C, Williamson P, Xu W, Jang H, Davis HM, Zhou H (2006) Popula-tion pharmacokinetics of infliximab, an anti-tumor necrosis factor-alpha monoclonal antibody in patients with ankylosing spondylitis: a randomized double blind Phase III trial. Arthritis Rheum 54(Suppl):S475

Zhang YH, Lin JX, Vilcek J (1990) Interleukin-6 induction by tumor necrosis factor and interleukin-1 in human fibroblasts involves activation of a nuclear factor binding to a kappa B-like sequence. Mol Cell Biol 10:3818–3823

Zhu Y, Menter A, Jang H, Zhou H (2006) Pharmacokinetics and Pharmacodynamics of Infliximab in a Phase III Trial in Patients with Plaque-type Psoriasis American Academy of Dermatology, San Francisco, CA

Zou J, Rudwaleit M, Brandt J, Thiel A, Braun J, Sieper J (2003) Down-regulation of the nonspecific and antigen-specific T cell cytokine response in ankylosing spondylitis during treatment with infliximab. Arthritis Rheum 48:780–790

Therapeutic Anti-VEGF Antibodies

S. Lien and H.B. Lowman(✉)

1 Introduction 132
2 VEGF in Angiogenesis 132
3 Production and Characterization of an Anti-VEGF
   Antibody: A4.6.1 133
4 Humanization and the Development of Bevacizumab 134
   4.1 Preclinical Studies with Bevacizumab 139
   4.2 Clinical Studies with Bevacizumab 140
5 Humanization and the Development of Ranibizumab 140
   5.1 Preclinical Studies with Ranibizumab 143
   5.2 Clinical Studies with Ranibizumab 144
6 Next Generation Anti-VEGF Antibodies 144
7 Conclusion 145
References 146

Abstract Vascular endothelial growth factor (VEGF-A) is a key cytokine in the development of normal blood vessels as well as the development of vessels in tumors and other tissues undergoing abnormal angiogenesis. Here, we review the molecular engineering of two humanized antibodies derived from a common mouse anti-VEGF antibody – bevacizumab, a full-length IgG1 approved for the treatment of specified cancer indications, and ranibizumab, an affinity-matured antibody Fab domain approved for use in age-related macular degeneration (AMD). In clinical trials and as FDA-approved therapeutics, these two anti-VEGF antibodies, bevacizumab (Avastin® anti-VEGF antibody) and ranibizumab (Lucentis® anti-VEGF antibody), have demonstrated therapeutic utility in blocking VEGF-induced angiogenesis.

H.B. Lowman

Antibody Engineering, Protein Engineering, and Immunology Departments, Genentech, Inc., 1 DNA Way, South San Francisco, CA 94080, USA

e-mail: hbl@gene.com

Y. Chernajovsky, A. Nissim (eds.) *Therapeutic Antibodies. Handbook of Experimental Pharmacology 181.*
© Springer-Verlag Berlin Heidelberg 2008

1 Introduction

The idea of a tumor-derived blood vessel growth stimulating factor was first postulated in 1939 due to observations of a strong neovascular response induced by transplanted tumors (Ide et al. 1939). The authors proposed that the induction of such a factor, and hence newly developed vasculature, would allow rapidly growing tumors to receive nutrients. It was not until 1989, however, that this factor was cloned from medium conditioned by bovine pituitary cells (Ferrara and Henzel 1989). The factor was named vascular endothelial growth factor (VEGF), in recognition of its potent mitogenic effects on endothelial cells.

2 VEGF in Angiogenesis

VEGF, also known as VEGF-A, is a homodimeric glycoprotein of 36–46 kDa with significant homology to the A and B chains of placental-derived growth factor, PDGF (Leung et al. 1989). The VEGF family consists of VEGF-A, VEGF-B, VEGF-C, VEGF-D, VEGF-E, and placental growth factor, PlGF. Each of these proteins represents a distinct gene product with distinct receptor interactions, as opposed to the various isoforms of VEGF-A described below. While VEGF-A availability is the rate-limiting step in normal and pathological blood vessel growth (Ferrara et al. 2003), VEGF-C and VEGF-D regulate lymphatic angiogenesis (Stacker et al. 2002). The current review will focus on inhibition of VEGF-A activity, henceforth referred to as VEGF.

The human VEGF gene is organized into eight exons (Houck et al. 1991; Tischer et al. 1991). Alternative splicing results in four main VEGF isoforms: VEGF121 (i.e., VEGF-A isoform with residues 1–121), VEGF165, VEGF189, and VEGF206 (Leung et al. 1989), which differ in their bioavailability. VEGF121, which lacks the heparin-binding domain, is a freely diffusible protein. VEGF189 and VEGF206 are nearly completely retained in the extracellular matrix (Houck et al. 1992; Park et al. 1993). VEGF165 is secreted but remains bound to the cell surface and the extracellular matrix due to its heparin binding ability. The bound isoforms may be released by heparin or heparinase, or by plasmin cleavage at the C-terminus. Plasmin cleavage generates a bioactive fragment consisting of the first 110 amino acids (VEGF110; Houck et al. 1992). There is now much evidence to suggest that VEGF165 is the most physiologically relevant isoform (reviewed in Ferrara (2004)).

Expression of VEGF is induced by a variety of factors. As its biology would suggest, VEGF mRNA is upregulated in conditions of hypoxia (Dor et al. 2001). Increased VEGF signaling can occur in the hypoxic environment of aberrant tumor vasculature, or due to mutation of other elements in the hypoxia induced pathway such as hypoxia-inducible factor 1, the von Hippel-Lindau tumor suppressor gene, the PTEN tumor suppressor gene, and/or the Forkhead transcription factor FOXO4. VEGF mRNA transcription and stability is also influenced by other growth factors, hormones, and oncogenes, including estrogen, nitric oxide, FGF, PDGF, TNF-alpha, EGF, IL-1 alpha, IL-6, Ras, and wnt (reviewed in Ferrara (2004)).

Signaling occurs through two VEGF receptor tyrosine kinases: Flt-1/VEGFR1 (de Vries et al. 1992; Shibuya et al. 1990) and Flk-1/KDR/VEGFR2 (Millauer et al. 1993; Quinn et al. 1993; Terman et al. 1992). Growing evidence supports the idea that VEGFR1 plays an important role in hematopoiesis while VEGFR2 on endothelial cells is the major mediator of the mitogenic, migratory, survival, angiogenic, and vascular permeability enhancing effects of VEGF (reviewed in Ferrara (2004)). Neuropilin 1 and neuropilin 2, molecules previously shown to bind the collapsin/semaphorin family, are also receptors for the heparin-binding isoforms of VEGF. Neuropilin 1 is thought to present VEGF165 to VEGFR2 in a manner that potentiates VEGFR2 signaling (Soker et al. 1998).

3 Production and Characterization of an Anti-VEGF Antibody: A4.6.1

In 1971, Judah Folkman proposed that anti-angiogenesis might be an effective anticancer strategy (Folkman 1971). Subsequently, human VEGF-A was identified (Ferrara and Henzel 1989), and it was demonstrated that VEGF was upregulated in many human cancers, including glioblastoma, colorectal cancer, nonsmall-cell lung cancer, renal cell cancer, pancreatic cancer, ovarian cancer, acute myeloid leukemia, multiple myeloma, Hodgkin's disease, and Non-Hodgkin's Lymphoma (reviewed in Ranieri et al. (2006)). The numbers of malignancies in which VEGF levels have been correlated with survival, as well as the demonstration that the growth of tumors beyond 0.2–2 mm depends on angiogenesis (Gimbrone et al. 1972), underlines the widespread utility of an agent capable of preventing VEGF signaling.

To address this need, Ferrara and coworkers generated murine monoclonal antibodies using recombinant human VEGF165 as the immunogen (Kim et al. 1992). They isolated four antibodies of IgG1 isotype with high affinity for human VEGF (K_D's of 0.4–2.2 nM). Competition binding experiments revealed that the antibodies could be divided into two classes: antibodies A3.13.1 and B2.6.2 recognized one epitope, while antibodies A4.6.1 and B4.3.1 recognized another. Since A4.6.1 and B2.6.2 had the highest affinities to VEGF, they were characterized further.

Subsequent experiments showed that B2.6.2 recognized a discontinuous epitope, whereas A4.6.1 appeared to recognize a continuous epitope. Furthermore, A4.6.1 bound VEGF121, VEGF165, and VEGF189, while B2.6.2 bound only VEGF165 and VEGF189. The antibodies also differed in their ability to inhibit VEGF activity. A4.6.1 was a far more effective inhibitor of VEGF activity in an in vitro bovine adrenal cortex endothelial cell proliferation assay, an in vivo vascular permeability assay, and an in vivo embryonic chicken angiogenesis assay (Kim et al. 1992). The results suggested that A4.6.1 had potent VEGF neutralizing activities.

The utility of this antibody in pathological models was demonstrated by treatment of immunodeficient mice bearing human tumor cell line xenografts (Borgstrom et al. 1996; Kim et al. 1993; Melnyk et al. 1996; Warren et al. 1995), and by treatment of cynomolgous monkeys with laser-induced retinal ischemia (Adamis et al.

1996). Treatment with as little as 0.05 mg ($\sim$2 mg kg^{-1}) of A4.6.1, given twice weekly intraperitoneally, was enough to inhibit growth of human rhabdomyosarcoma, glioblastoma multiforme, leiomyosarcoma (Kim et al. 1993), and colon carcinoma cell lines (Warren et al. 1995). Treatment with 0.1 mg twice weekly resulted in decreased tumor burden in a liver metastatic model of colon carcinoma (Warren et al. 1995) and reduction of metastasis in an epidermoid carcinoma model (Melnyk et al. 1996). Results were similar regardless of whether the antibody treatment was initiated at the time of tumor implantation or 1 week later (Kim et al. 1993). Treatment of the cell lines with A4.6.1 in vitro had no effect on growth, demonstrating that the effect was not due to autocrine VEGF activity or direct cytotoxicity of the antibody (Kim et al. 1993; Melnyk et al. 1996; Warren et al. 1995).

Ocular neovascularization, a characteristic of diabetic retinopathy and age-related macular degeneration (AMD), is associated with leakage and bleeding of vessels within the subretinal space. Intraocular levels of VEGF have been shown to correlate temporally, spatially, and quantitatively with new blood vessel formation (Alon et al. 1995; Stone et al. 1995). Furthermore, intraocular VEGF levels are elevated in diabetic retinopathy, iris revascularization, and retinopathy of prematurity (Adamis et al. 1994; Aiello et al. 1994; Malecaze et al. 1994). When iris neovascularization was induced in cynomolgous monkeys by laser retinal vein occlusion, 5 of 8 control eyes developed symptoms within 4–7 days. In contrast, iris neovascularization was not seen in any of the eight eyes treated with A4.6.1 (Adamis et al. 1996). Collectively, these results suggested that VEGF did indeed play a large role in ocular neovascularization and that anti-VEGF treatment might be a useful approach to therapy.

4 Humanization and the Development of Bevacizumab

Murine-derived antibodies are generally not used for human therapeutic purposes due to their potential immunogenicity. Antibody A4.6.1 was therefore humanized by a process of CDR grafting and framework mutations (Presta et al. 1997). This procedure had been successfully performed previously for trastuzumab, an anti-HER2 antibody (Carter et al. 1992). CDR residues were identified based on sequence (Kabat et al. 1991) and structural (Chothia et al. 1989) hypervariability and grafted into the consensus sequence of the human heavy chain subgroup III and light chain subgroup kI immunoglobulin variable-domain frameworks (Fig. 1; Kabat et al. 1991) ELISA assays of the CDR-grafted antibody showed that it was 1,000-fold reduced in binding to VEGF compared to the original antibody. Comparisons of the human and murine framework residues and the use of judicious mutations resulted in a humanized antibody with seven framework residue mutations in the heavy chain variable region and one framework residue mutation in the light chain variable region as compared to the human consensus sequence (Table 1, Fig. 2). The humanized antibody (bevacizumab) had an affinity within twofold of the parent antibody, A4.6.1 (Fig. 3), but showed no reduction in VEGF bioactivity (Presta et al. 1997).

```
                        10          20          30          40
MB1.6       DIQLTQSPSSLSASVGDRVTITC [SASQDISNYLN] WYQQKP
                 *
Hu2.0       DIQMTQSPSSLSASVGDRVTITC [SASQDISNYLN] WYQQKP
               **       *       * *
A4.6.1      DIQMTQTTSSLSASLGDRVIISC [SASQDISNYLN] WYQQKP
               **       *       * *
Fab 1       DIQMTQSPSSLSASVGDRVTITC [SASQDISNYLN] WYQQKP

Fab 12      DIQMTQSPSSLSASVGDRVTITC [SASQDISNYLN] WYQQKP
                 *
Y0317       DIQLTQSPSSLSASVGDRVTITC [SASQDISNYLN] WYQQKP
                 *                     *    *      *
hum ki      DIQMTQSPSSLSASVGDRVTITC [RASQSISNYLA] WYQQKP

                        50          60          70          80
MB1.6       GKAPKLLIY [FTSSLHS] GVPSRFSGSGSGTDYTLTISSLQP
                                              *
Hu2.0       GKAPKLLIY [FTSSLHS] GVPSRFSGSGSGTDFTLTISSLQP
            ****  *                          **      *  *
A4.6.1      DGTVKVLIY [FTSSLHS] GVPSRFSGSGSGTDYSLTISNLEP
            ****  *                          **      *  *
Fab 1       GKAPKLLIY [FTSSLHS] GVPSRFSGSGSGTDFTLTISSLQP
                 *
Fab 12      GKAPKVLIY [FTSSLHS] GVPSRFSGSGSGTDFTLTISSLQP

Y0317       GKAPKVLIY [FTSSLHS] GVPSRFSGSGSGTDFTLTISSLQP
              *     **     *
hum ki      GKAPKLLIY [AASSLES] GVPSRFSGSGSGTDFTLTISSLQP

                                 90    100
MB1.6       EDFATYYC [QQYSTVPWT] FGQGTKVEIKR

Hu2.0       EDFATYYC [QQYSTVPWT] FGQGTKVEIKR
               *                    *    *
A4.6.1      EDIATYYC [QQYSTVPWT] FGGGTKLEIKR
              *                     *    *
Fab 1       EDFATYYC [QQYSTVPWT] FGQGTKVEIKR

Fab 12      EDFATYYC [QQYSTVPWT] FGQGTKVEIKR

Y0317       EDFATYYC [QQYSTVPWT] FGQGTKVEIKR
                         ***
hum ki      EDFATYYC [QQYNSLPWT] FGQGTKVEIKR
```

Fig. 1 (a) Light chain amino acid sequences of MB1.6, Hu2.0, A4.6.1, Fab-1, Fab-12, Y0317, and human consensus sequences of light chain subgroup kappa I (hum kI) and heavy chain subgroup III (hum III). CDR loops are enclosed in brackets. Asterisks denote differences between sequences. Residue numbering is according to Kabat et al. (1991)

```
                    10          20           30          40
MB1.6      EVQLVESGGGLVQPGGSLRLSCAAS [GYTFTNYGMN] WIRQA
                                                      *
Hu2.0      EVQLVESGGGLVQPGGSLRLSCAAS [GYTFTNYGMN] WVRQA
            *    *   ** *   *** *   *                  *
A4.6.1     EIQLVQSGPELKQPGETVRISCKAS [GYTFTNYGMN] WVKQA
            *    *   ** *   *** *   *                  *
Fab 1      EVQLVESGGGLVQPGGSLRLSCAAS [GYTFTNYGMN] WVRQA
                                          *   *
Fab 12     EVQLVESGGGLVQPGGSLRLSCAAS [GYTFTNYGMN] WVRQA
                                          *   *
Y0317      EVQLVESGGGLVQPGGSLRLSCAAS [GYDFTHYGMN] WVRQA
                                       ** ** * *
hum III    EVQLVESGGGLVQPGGSLRLSCAAS [GFTFSSYAMS] WVRQA

                     50    a      60          70          80
MB1.6      PGKGLEWVG [WINTYTGEPTYAADFKR] RFTISADTSSNTVYL
                                                 * * *   *
Hu2.0      PGKGLEWVG [WINTYTGEPTYAADFKR] RFTISRDNSKNTLYL
              * *                             * *** ** *
A4.6.1     PGKGLKWMG [WINTYTGEPTYAADFKR] RFTFSLETSASTAYL
              * *                             * *** ** *
Fab 1      PGKGLEWVG [WINTYTGEPTYAADFKR] RFTISRDNSKNTLYL
                                              * * *   * *
Fab 12     PGKGLEWVG [WINTYTGEPTYAADFKR] RFTFSLDTSKSTAYL
Y0317      PGKGLEWVG [WINTYTGEPTYAADFKR] RFTFSLDTSKSTAYL
              *    * **** ***    *** *       * * *   * *
hum III    PGKGLEWVS [VISGDGGSTYYADSVKG] RFTISRDNSKNTLYL

             abc     90       100abcde          110
MB1.6      QMNSLRAEDTAVYYCAK [YPHYYGSSHWYFDV] WGQGTLVTVSS
                            *
Hu2.0      QMNSLRAEDTAVYYCAR [YPHYYGSSHWYFDV] WGQGTLVTVSS
             *** ***    * *   *                    *   *
A4.6.1     QISNLKNDDTATYFCAK [YPHYYGSSHWYFDV] WGAGTTVTVSS
             *** ***    * *   *                    *   *
Fab 1      QMNSLRAEDTAVYYCAR [YPHYYGSSHWYFDV] WGQGTLVTVSS
                            *
Fab 12     QMNSLRAEDTAVYYCAK [YPHYYGSSHWYFDV] WGQGTLVTVSS
                                 *    *
Y0317      QMNSLRAEDTAVYYCAK [YPYYYGTSHWYFDV] WGQGTLVTVSS
                            *    **** ***
hum III    QMNSLRAEDTAVYYCAR [-----------FDY] WGQGTLVTVSS
```

Fig. 1 (b) Heavy chain amino acid sequences of the variable domains

The crystal structure of the Fab portion of bevacizumab was solved in complex with VEGF (Fig. 4; Muller et al. 1998), elucidating the importance of the framework mutations as well as the specificity of the antibody. In the heavy chain variable domain, residues 49, 69, 71, and 78 (residue numbers are indicated in the numbering system of Kabat) were buried or partially buried and affected binding by influencing

Table 1 Humanized anti-VEGF Fab constructs generated during bevacizumab development[1]

Variant	Template	Changes	Purpose
Chim-Fab	Chimeric Fab	Murine variable, human constant domains	Standard transfer of variable domains
Fab-1	Human FR	CDR swap:murine CDRs in human FR with VH:S49G[2]	Humanization starting point
Fab-2	–	Chim-Fab light chain, Fab-1 heavy chain	See effect of heavy chain CDR swap
Fab-3	–	Fab-1 light chain, Chim-Fab heavy chain	See effect of light chain CDR swap
Fab-4	Fab-1	VH: R71L VH: N73T	CDR H2 conformation framework change
Fab-5	Fab-4	VL: L46V	VL-VH interface
Fab-6	Fab-5	VH: L78A	CDR H1 conformation
Fab-7	Fab-5	VH: I69F	CDR H2 conformation
Fab-8	Fab-5	VH: I69F VH: L78A	CDR H2 conformation CDR H1 conformation
Fab-9	Fab-8	VH: G49A	CDR H2 conformation
Fab-10	Fab-8	VH: N76S	Framework change
Fab-11	Fab-10	VH: K75A	Framework change
Fab-12	Fab-10	VH: R94K	CDR H3 conformation

[1] Data taken from Presta et al. (1997)

[2] The human subgroup III heavy chain consensus sequence was defined as having Ser at position 49; however, Ala and Gly are also commonly found in human antibody sequences at this position; the murine A4.6.1 sequence contained G49

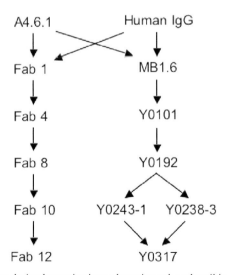

Fig. 2 Significant clones during humanization to bevacizumab and ranibizumab

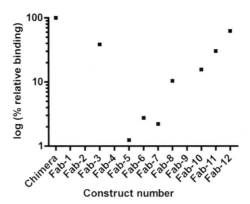

Fig. 3 Binding affinities during antibody A4.6.1 humanization leading to bevacizumab. Approximate changes in affinity of the humanized anti-VEGF Fab constructs relative to the binding of the chimeric Fab as measured by ELISA (Presta et al. 2007) are plotted against construct number. VEGF binding was undetectable for Fabs −1, −2, −4, and −9

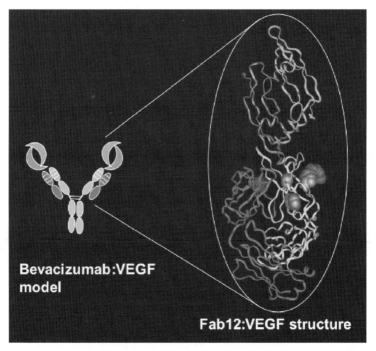

Fig. 4 Bevacizumab structure. The relationship of this Fab:VEGF complex to that of the full-length bevacizumab IgG in complex with VEGF is shown at *left*. At *right* is shown a ribbon diagram of the Fab fragment Fab-12 (heavy chain in *cyan*, light chain in *magenta*), in complex with the dimer form of VEGF-A (fragment 8–109, with one monomer in *orange* and the other in *green*) from the crystal structure of Muller et al. (1998) (PDB accession number 1BJ1). Framework residues that were changed during humanization are shown in space-filling form (spherical atoms): L46V in the light chain, and I69F, R71L, N73T, N76S, L78A, and R94K in the heavy chain

CDR loop conformations. Residues 73 and 76 were located in a non-CDR loop adjacent to CDRs H1 and H2 and interacted directly with VEGF. A lysine was required at H94, instead of the usual human arginine. The presence of a lysine allowed favorable packing interactions with two tyrosines, Y27 and Y32 of CDR H1. Both Y27 and Y32 are important for VEGF binding, as demonstrated by alanine-scanning mutagenesis. In the light chain variable domain, only L46 had to be changed to the murine residue (Val). In the Fab structure, residue 46 is buried and interacts directly with CDR H3, suggesting that it is required to maintain the conformation of this loop.

Alanine-scanning mutagenesis of VEGF revealed that the epitope for antibody binding overlapped the epitope for binding to VEGFR1 (Muller et al. 1998; Wiesmann et al. 1997). Bevacizumab, therefore, prevents VEGF bioactivity by steric hindrance of receptor binding. Alanine-scanning also revealed the basis for the species specificity of bevacizumab binding. G88 of human VEGF is bound in a deep pocket formed by the sidechains of residues from CDR L3, CDR H2, and CDR H3 (Muller et al. 1998). Murine VEGF contains a serine at position 88 and is therefore unable to bind bevacizumab due to steric hindrance.

4.1 Preclinical Studies with Bevacizumab

Following humanization, the anti-VEGF activity of bevacizumab was compared directly to that of A4.6.1. The two antibodies were shown to be equipotent in in vitro bovine capillary endothelial cell proliferation assays. Furthermore, both antibodies efficiently suppressed the growth of human rhabdomyosarcoma and breast carcinoma xenografts in nude mice at 0.5 and 5 mg kg^{-1} doses (Presta et al. 1997). Other preclinical studies of bevacizumab, as a single agent or in combination with cytotoxic therapies, are reviewed in Gerber and Ferrara (2005).

The pharmacokinetics of bevacizumab after intravenous administration have been studied in several species and are consistent with those of other humanized antibodies. Bevacizumab is cleared from circulation in a similar manner to endogenous antibodies. The terminal elimination half-life was 1–2 weeks in all species tested (Lin et al. 1999). Safety studies were performed in cynomolgus monkeys (Ryan et al. 1999). This species was chosen since cynomolgus monkey VEGF is identical to human VEGF at the protein level (Shima et al. 1996). After administration of bevacizumab for 4–13 weeks, young adult cynomolgus monkeys showed apparent mechanism-of-action-related effects such as physeal dysplasia and suppression of angiogenesis in the female reproductive tract. Both effects were reversible with cessation of treatment. No other treatment-related effects were seen, even at doses up to 50 mg kg^{-1} (Ryan et al. 1999).

The pharmacokinetics, ocular tissue distribution, and safety of the Fab fragment of bevacizumab (known as Fab-12) have also been studied following intravitreal administration. ^{125}Iodine labeling studies in rhesus monkeys showed that the intravitreal half-life of a Fab fragment of bevacizumab was 3.2 days, compared with 5.6 days for a full-length antibody (trastuzumab). The Fab reached the retinal pigment epithelial layer within 1 h and was detectable within this layer for up to 7 days. In contrast, the full-length antibody was unable to penetrate the inner limiting membrane of the retina. Systemic exposure to the full-length antibody was variable but low, whereas the Fab fragment was not detected in the plasma at any time point. No adverse treatment-related effects were noted in this study (Mordenti et al. 1999).

4.2 Clinical Studies with Bevacizumab

Phase I clinical trials of bevacizumab began in 1997. FDA approval was first granted on the 26th of February 2004, following a successful phase III trial for treatment of metastatic colorectal cancer. In a randomized controlled trial of 813 patients with first-line metastatic colorectal cancer, the median duration of survival was 20.3 months in patients who received bevacizumab plus chemotherapy, compared to 15.6 months in those patients receiving chemotherapy alone (Hurwitz et al. 2004). FDA approval was then granted on the 11th of October 2006, for use of bevacizumab in combination with carboplatin and paclitaxel chemotherapy in metastatic, nonsquamous, nonsmall-cell lung cancer. Combination therapy resulted in a 25% improvement in survival compared to chemotherapy alone (Sandler and Herbst 2006). Many other clinical trials are currently under way, for indications including renal cell cancer, metastatic breast cancer, and cervical cancer (reviewed in Ranieri et al. 2006). Bevacizumab has the potential to significantly improve the standard of patient treatment in a wide variety of indications.

The most common side effects of bevacizumab treatment are hypertension, proteinuria, bleeding, and thrombosis (Zondor and Medina 2004). In most cases, hypertension during treatment can be managed with antihypertensive medications. Patients with proteinuria have been generally asymptomatic. Bleeding, thrombosis, and complications with wound healing are the most significant side effects of bevacizumab therapy. Importantly, there were no reported incidents of patients developing antibodies to bevacizumab (Ferrara 2004), suggesting that the humanization of A4.6.1 was successful.

5 Humanization and the Development of Ranibizumab

Preclinical and clinical studies show that VEGF is involved in the ocular neovascularisation associated with age-related macular degeneration (AMD) and diabetic retinopathy (Ferrara and Alitalo 1999). Anti-VEGF therapy is a promising new treatment for these conditions, particularly with the development of ranibizumab. Ranibizumab is a Fab fragment of an anti-VEGF antibody distinct from bevacizumab. Its smaller size allows penetration into the retina (Gaudreault et al. 2005) and more rapid clearance from the circulation than a full length antibody (cf. Gaudreault et al. 2005, Lin et al. 1999). Ranibizumab also has a higher affinity for VEGF than does bevacizumab (Chen et al. 1999; Ferrara et al. 2004), allowing it to more efficiently inhibit VEGFR binding before it is cleared.

Clearance of a VEGF inhibitor is likely to reduce the incidence of treatment-related side effects. There is evidence that VEGF has multiple important roles in vivo. Safety studies in cynomolgus monkeys demonstrated that VEGF plays a part in bone growth, cyclic endometrial development, and placental vascularization (Ryan et al. 1999). VEGF has also been shown to be important in wound healing and psoriasis (Detmar et al. 1995), monocyte chemotaxis (Clauss et al. 1990), B cell production (Hattori et al. 2001), and neuronal function (Storkebaum et al. 2004). Given these findings and the known side effects of anti-VEGF therapy (hypertension, thrombotic events, and proteinuria), the use of an agent with rapid systemic clearance is particularly important for elderly or wound-healing compromised patients.

The origin of ranibizumab was A4.6.1, the same murine anti-human VEGF antibody that gave rise to bevacizumab. However, the humanization processes for bevacizumab and ranibizumab were quite different (Fig. 2). While bevacizumab was the product of site-directed mutagenesis of a CDR graft from A4.6.1, humanization to ranibizumab involved both phage display and site-directed mutagenesis. Initially, the CDRs of A4.6.1 were grafted into a phage-displayed Fab construct, hu2.0 (Fig. 1), with the C-terminal region of the Fab fused to a portion of the gene-3 protein of bacterophage M13 (Baca et al. 1997). Framework-region libraries were constructed and panned to yield a humanized Fab, MB1.6 (Fig. 1; Table 2), that bound VEGF with greater than 125-fold improved affinity than the CDR graft. Introduction of a single additional mutation, L46V, selected by rational design further improved

Table 2 Humanized anti-VEGF Fab constructs generated during ranibizumab development

Variant	Template	Changes
Chim-Fab	Chimeric Fab	Murine variable, human constant domains
Fab 12[1]	Human FR	VL: L46V VH: I69F, R71L, N73T, N76S, L78A, R94K
Hu2.0[2]	Human FR Fab phage vector	CDR swap with VH:S49G (see Table 1) and T221L in the C_H1 domain for fusion to M13 phage gene-3 protein
MB1.6[2]	Hu2.0	VL: M4L, F71Y VH: V37I, R71A, N73T, K75S, L78V, R94K
Y0101[3]	MB1.6	VL: L46V, Y71F VH: I37V, I69F, A71L, S75K, N76S, V79A
Y0192[3]	Y0101	VL: S24R, S26N, Q27E, D28Q, I29L VH: M34I
Y0243-1[4]	Y0192	VH: T28D, N31H, I34M
Y0238-3[4]	Y0192	VH: H97Y, S100aT
Y0317[4]	Y0192	VL: R24S, N26S, E27Q, Q28D, L29I VH: T28D, N31H, I34M, H97Y, S100aT

[1] Data taken from Presta et al. (1997)

[2] Data taken from Baca et al. (1997)

[3] Data taken from Muller et al. (1998)

[4] Data taken from Chen et al. (1999)

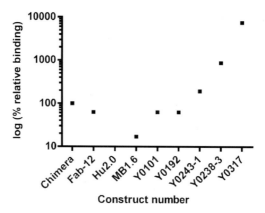

Construct number

Fig. 5 Binding affinities during antibody MB1.6 affinity maturation leading to ranibizumab. Approximate changes in affinity of the humanized anti-VEGF Fab constructs relative to the binding of the chimeric Fab as measured by BIAcore studies (Baca et al. 1997; Muller et al. 1998; Chen et al. 1999) are plotted against construct number

the affinity to within sixfold of a human/murine chimera of A4.6.1 (Baca et al. 1997). Additional framework changes yielded MB1.6, which had similar affinity to Fab-12 and was used as the basis of clone Y0101 (Table 2; Muller et al. 1998). Y0101 was a phage displayed Fab with framework mutations identified during the humanization of bevacizumab (Presta et al. 1997), and two mutations from MB1.6 (Baca et al. 1997). Unfortunately, this variant expressed poorly. Further phage display efforts produced clone Y0192, which was significantly improved in expression (Muller et al. 1998).

Alanine scanning mutagenesis of Y0192 and a crystal structure highlighted the importance of the heavy-chain CDRs H1, H2, and H3 for VEGF binding (Muller et al. 1998). Directed phage display libraries were therefore created and panned, with resulting marked improvements in affinity (Table 2; Fig. 5). Mutations isolated from CDR H1 and H3 libraries were combined to create ranibizumab, also known as Y0317 or rhuFAb V2, a Fab with greater than 100-fold affinity improvement over Fab 12 as measured by surface plasmon resonance. Cell proliferation assays were used to confirm the increased biological potency of the affinity matured antibody (Chen et al. 1999).

The binding epitopes of Fab 12 and Y0317 were shown to be similar by affinity measurements of VEGF alanine scanning mutants and crystal structures of the Fab:VEGF complexes (Fig. 4, Fig. 6) (Chen et al. 1999; Muller et al. 1998). One notable difference was the presence of two additional hydrogen bonds in the complex between VEGF and Y0317 due to the CDR H3 mutation H97Y in the latter. The tyrosine substitution resulted in exclusion of a water molecule present in the Fab 12 structure, an increase in buried surface area, and additional hydrogen bonds, all of which may contribute to increased binding energy and slower complex-dissociation kinetics. The H97Y substitution was indeed shown to be the amino acid substitution contributing the largest portion of the increase in binding affinity to VEGF. Thus, the

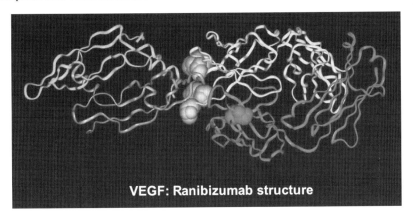

Fig. 6 Ranibizumab structure. The structure of ranibizumab (Y0317 Fab; heavy chain in *cyan*; light chain in *magenta*) in complex with VEGF (fragment 8-109; with one monomer in *orange* and the other in *green*) is shown based on the crystal structure reported in Chen et al. (1999) (PDB accession number 1CZ8). Heavy-chain CDR residues changed during affinity maturation of the Y0101 parental antibody are shown in space-filling form: T28D and N31H in CDR-H1 and H97Y and S100aT in CDR-H3. Also shown in space-filling form is the site M4L in the light chain variable framework region, which differs from bevacizumab. The site of one constant-domain change, made for cloning convenience, as compared to bevacizumab is near the C-terminus (bottom of the figure) of the heavy chain. This residue, T221L, is not shown in this figure

structural data correlated well with the 14-fold affinity improvement measured with this single mutation (Chen et al. 1999).

5.1 Preclinical Studies with Ranibizumab

The utility of an anti-VEGF for treatment of choroidal neovascularization has been demonstrated in a number of models (Adamis et al. 1996; Bashshur et al. 2006; Krzystolik et al. 2002; Michels et al. 2005; Rosenfeld et al. 2005a). However, because of concerns about the systemic inhibition of VEGF, the safety and pharmacokinetics of intravitreal injections of ranibizumab were of interest. Ranibizumab delivered intravitreally was demonstrated to penetrate all layers of the rabbit retina (Gaudreault et al. 1999), in contrast to a full length antibody (trastuzumab), which could not penetrate the inner limiting membrane of the retina in rhesus monkeys (Mordenti et al. 1999). Further, pharmacokinetic studies in cynomolgus monkeys showed that after a single intravitreal injection of ranibizumab, the Fab was present at biologically effective retinal levels for about a month, while serum levels were less than 1000th of the ocular levels. Any tissue distribution of ranibizumab was therefore below the limit of detection (Gaudreault et al. 2005). Combination treatment with ranibizumab and verteporfin therapy also demonstrated benefits in nonhuman primates (Husain et al. 2005; Kim et al. 2006). Verteporfin is a small-molecule dye that has been previously used in photodynamic therapy for AMD, in which the dye is infused systemically and red light is used to activate its cytotoxic action locally on vascular structures in the eye (Schmidt-Erfurth and Michels 2003).

5.2 Clinical Studies with Ranibizumab

A phase 1 study in patients with AMD found that the maximum tolerated dose was 0.5 mg when injected intravitreally. The major dose limiting toxicity was due to intraocular inflammation (Rosenfeld et al. 2005b). However, in a dose-escalating study, clinically significant inflammation was not seen at doses of up to 2 mg per eye. There were no notable differences in clinical outcomes between study groups receiving different maximal doses, but this trial was insufficiently powered to detect small treatment benefits (Rosenfeld et al. 2006a). Significantly, no patients developed antibodies to ranibizumab in either study, suggesting that the substitution of new CDR and framework residues did not create significant new immunogenic determinants (Rosenfeld et al. 2006b, 2005a).

In December 2005, Genentech submitted a Biologics License Application to the FDA for the use of ranibizumab in the treatment of neovascular AMD based on the results of two phase three trials (Rosenfeld et al. 2006b; Rosenfeld et al. 2006c; Brown et al. 2006). In both trials, patients treated with ranibizumab demonstrated significantly better visual acuity than control patients at 1 and 2 year time-points. Adverse events were similar to those seen in earlier trials, with low rates of serious ocular adverse events, although slightly increased rates of myocardial infarction and stroke were noted at higher ranibizumab dose (Rosenfeld et al. 2006b). It is important to note that ranibizumab therapy is the first treatment for neovascular AMD that improves vision for most patients. When compared with verteporfin at 12 months (Brown et al. 2006), ranibizumab treatment led to 94.3–96.4% of patients losing fewer than 15 letters in visual acuity (0.3 and 0.5 mg doses, respectively) vs. 64.3% of patients losing fewer than 15 letters in the verteporfin group. Mean visual acuity increased by 8.5–11.3 letters (low and high doses) in the ranibizumab groups, while it decreased by 9.5 letters in the verteporfin group. Improvement in acuity was stable for at least 2 years. FDA approval for ranibizumab therapy was given on June 30, 2006.

6 Next Generation Anti-VEGF Antibodies

Next generation anti-VEGF antibodies might have improved VEGF affinity or might more efficiently block VEGF activity through binding to a novel epitope. Structural studies (Wiesmann et al. 1997) and alanine scanning mutagenesis (Li et al. 2000; Muller et al. 1997; Pan et al. 2002) show that VEGF receptors 1 and 2 bind similar epitopes on VEGF. Bevacizumab and ranibizumab bind to an epitope that only partially overlaps the receptor binding site. It, therefore, appears that bevacizumab inhibits receptor binding by steric hindrance (Wiesmann et al. 1997). Thus, it is possible that mutations, which may arise in vivo, could abrogate bevacizumab binding without impacting receptor interaction.

The site of bevacizumab binding can be explained by considering the origin of the antibody. Mice were immunized with human VEGF to produce A4.6.1, the progenitor of bevacizumab. Since self-reactive antibodies are disfavored by immune tolerance in vivo, antibodies raised by the hybridoma technique will tend to bind to regions of the immunizing antigen distinct from that of any corresponding host protein. The sequence of the receptor binding regions of human and mouse VEGF are not completely conserved (Claffey et al. 1992; Leung et al. 1989). Thus, bevacizumab binding is centered around G88 (where the mouse sequence contains a Ser), located at the periphery of the receptor binding epitope (Wiesmann et al. 1997).

To identify a larger set of antibody specificities for a variety of therapeutic targets, phage-displayed synthetic antibody libraries that mimic the diversity of natural human antibodies have been developed at Genentech (Lee et al. 2004). Panning these libraries against VEGF resulted in novel, high affinity, antibodies capable of blocking both murine and human VEGF activity (Liang et al. 2006). Structural and functional analysis of these antibodies in complex with VEGF showed that their binding epitopes closely matched the epitope for VEGFR1 (Fuh et al. (2006)). Therefore, hypothetical mutations in VEGF that prevent the binding of these antibodies may also prevent VEGF:receptor interaction.

An additional desirable quality for new anti-VEGF antibodies is an ability to bind both mouse and human VEGF. This allows testing of the antibodies in a greater variety of model systems before progression to primate studies and address the contribution of host VEGF to xenograft growth. The antibodies isolated from synthetic phage display libraries possess this quality (Liang et al. 2006). Some of these novel antibodies had equivalent anti-VEGF activity to bevacizumab (B20 family of variants), while others had equivalent anti-VEGF activity to ranibizumab (G6 family). These novel reagents therefore not only allow an examination of the effects of host vs. tumor VEGF contribution to tumor growth in mouse models, but also a comparison of epitope and affinity effects upon efficacy and safety in mouse models (Liang et al. 2006; Gerber et al. 2007).

7 Conclusion

Bevacizumab (Avastin® anti-VEGF antibody) is a full-length, high-affinity IgG1 produced through humanization of antibody A4.6.1 from mice immunized with human VEGF. In vivo, bevacizumab may benefit from avidity effects to bind tightly to VEGF, effectively blocking VEGF receptor binding and signaling. This blockade results from steric hindrance of the ligand–receptor interaction since the antibody epitope overlaps – and is not identical to – the epitope of the VEGF receptors VEGFR-1 and VEGFR-2. As an intravenously injected molecule, the full-length antibody is maintained at high concentrations in the blood and binds circulating VEGF in the vasculature. As a cancer therapeutic, bevacizumab is being investigated in a growing number of oncology indications and in combination with other therapies to more fully define its safety and efficacy. For example, some patients with metastatic colorectal have demonstrated prolonged survival over several years with treatment using bevacizumab in combination with chemotherapy, and the drug has generally remained well tolerated (Hurwitz et al. 2006).

Ranibizumab (Lucentis® anti-VEGF antibody) is the Fab form of Y0317, another humanized antibody variant based on A4.6.1. Ranibizumab was affinity-matured using phage display, and differs at five residues in the variable domains and one residue in the constant domain from bevacizumab. These changes led to ~100-fold higher binding affinity to VEGF and enabled the monomeric (Fab) form of this antibody to very effectively block VEGF binding to its receptors. The lower molecular weight (~48 kDa) of ranibizumab as compared to bevacizumab (~150 kDa) may enhance the activity of this molecule in blocking VEGF within retinal tissue following intraocular injection. At the same time, because of the unique route of delivery, the rapid systemic clearance of the Fab from the circulation allows for the maintenance of therapeutic drug concentrations at the site of disease with low systemic concentrations. Such clearance may be important for limiting possible side effects such as hemorrhagic events that are potentially associated with systemic exposure to VEGF inhibitors (Liew and Mitchell 2007). Ranibizumab is currently being investigated in additional eye diseases and in combination with other therapies, and long-term studies are underway to evaluate further its safety and efficacy.

References

Adamis AP, Miller JW, Bernal MT, D'Amico DJ, Folkman J, Yeo TK, Yeo KT (1994) Increased vascular endothelial growth factor levels in the vitreous of eyes with proliferative diabetic retinopathy. Am J Ophthalmol 118:445–450

Adamis AP, Shima DT, Tolentino MJ, Gragoudas ES, Ferrara N, Folkman J, D'Amore PA, Miller JW (1996) Inhibition of vascular endothelial growth factor prevents retinal ischemia-associated iris neovascularization in a nonhuman primate. Arch Ophthalmol 114:66–71

Aiello LP, Avery RL, Arrigg PG, Keyt BA, Jampel HD, Shah ST, Pasquale LR, Thieme H, Iwamoto MA, Park JE et al. (1994) Vascular endothelial growth factor in ocular fluid of patients with diabetic retinopathy and other retinal disorders. N Engl J Med 331:1480–1487

Alon T, Hemo I, Itin A, Pe'er J, Stone J, Keshet E (1995) Vascular endothelial growth factor acts as a survival factor for newly formed retinal vessels and has implications for retinopathy of prematurity. Nat Med 1:1024–1028

Baca M, Presta LG, O'Connor SJ, Wells JA (1997) Antibody humanization using monovalent phage display. J Biol Chem 272:10678–10684

Bashshur ZF, Bazarbachi A, Schakal A, Haddad ZA, El Haibi CP, Noureddin BN (2006) Intravitreal bevacizumab for the management of choroidal neovascularization in age-related macular degeneration. Am J Ophthalmol 142:1–9

Borgstrom P, Hillan KJ, Sriramarao P, Ferrara N (1996) Complete inhibition of angiogenesis and growth of microtumors by anti-vascular endothelial growth factor neutralizing antibody: Novel concepts of angiostatic therapy from intravital videomicroscopy. Cancer Res 56:4032–4039

Brown DM, Kaiser PK, Michels M, Soubrane G, Heier JS, Kim RY, Sy JP, Schneider S (2006) Ranibizumab versus verteporfin for neovascular age-related macular degeneration. New Eng J Med 355:1432–1444

Carter P, Presta L, Gorman CM, Ridgway JB, Henner D, Wong WL, Rowland AM, Kotts C, Carver ME, Shepard HM (1992) Humanization of an anti-p185HER2 antibody for human cancer therapy. Proc Natl Acad Sci USA 89:4285–4289

Chen Y, Wiesmann C, Fuh G, Li B, Christinger HW, McKay P, de Vos AM, Lowman HB (1999) Selection and analysis of an optimized anti-VEGF antibody: Crystal structure of an affinity-matured Fab in complex with antigen. J Mol Biol 293:865–881

Chothia C, Lesk AM, Tramontano A, Levitt M, Smith-Gill SJ, Air G, Sheriff S, Padlan EA, Davies D, Tulip WR et al. (1989) Conformations of immunoglobulin hypervariable regions. Nature 342:877–883

Claffey KP, Wilkison WO, Spiegelman BM (1992) Vascular endothelial growth factor. Regulation by cell differentiation and activated second messenger pathways. J Biol Chem 267:16317–16322

Clauss M, Gerlach M, Gerlach H, Brett J, Wang F, Familletti PC, Pan YC, Olander JV, Connolly DT, Stern D (1990) Vascular permeability factor: A tumor-derived polypeptide that induces endothelial cell and monocyte procoagulant activity, and promotes monocyte migration. J Exp Med 172:1535–1545

de Vries C, Escobedo JA, Ueno H, Houck K, Ferrara N, Williams LT (1992) The fms-like tyrosine kinase, a receptor for vascular endothelial growth factor. Science 255:989–991

Detmar M, Yeo KT, Nagy JA, Van de Water L, Brown LF, Berse B, Elicker BM, Ledbetter S, Dvorak HF (1995) Keratinocyte-derived vascular permeability factor (vascular endothelial growth factor) is a potent mitogen for dermal microvascular endothelial cells. J Invest Dermatol 105:44–50

Dor Y, Porat R, Keshet E (2001) Vascular endothelial growth factor and vascular adjustments to perturbations in oxygen homeostasis. Am J Physiol Cell Physiol 280:C1367–C1374

Ferrara N (2004) Vascular endothelial growth factor: Basic science and clinical progress. Endocr Rev 25:581–611

Ferrara N, Alitalo K (1999) Clinical applications of angiogenic growth factors and their inhibitors. Nat Med 5:1359–1364

Ferrara N, Gerber HP, LeCouter J (2003) The biology of VEGF and its receptors. Nat Med 9:669–676

Ferrara N, Henzel WJ (1989) Pituitary follicular cells secrete a novel heparin-binding growth factor specific for vascular endothelial cells. Biochem Biophys Res Commun 161:851–858

Ferrara N, Hillan KJ, Gerber HP, Novotny W (2004) Discovery and development of bevacizumab, an anti-VEGF antibody for treating cancer. Nat Rev Drug Discov 3:391–400

Folkman J (1971) Tumor angiogenesis: Therapeutic implications. N Eng J Med 285:1182–1186

Fuh G, Wu P, Liang WC, Ultsch M, Lee CV, Moffat B, Wiesmann C (2006) Structure-function studies of two synthetic anti-vascular endothelial growth factor Fabs and comparison with the Avastin Fab. J Biol Chem 281:6625–6631

Gaudreault J, Fei D, Rusit J, Suboc P, Shiu V (2005) Preclinical pharmacokinetics of Ranibizumab (rhuFabV2) after a single intravitreal administration. Invest Ophthalmol Vis Sci 46:726–733

Gaudreault J, Webb W, Van Hoy M (1999) Pharmacokinetics and retinal distribution of AMD rhuFab V2 after intravitreal administration in rabbits. AAPS Pharm Sci Suppl 1:2142

Gerber HP, Ferrara N (2005) Pharmacology and pharmacodynamics of bevacizumab as monotherapy or in combination with cytotoxic therapy in preclinical studies. Cancer Res 65:671–680

Gerber HP, Wu X, Yu L, Wiesmann C, Liang XH, Lee CV, Fuh G, Olsson C, Damico L, Xie D, Meng YG, Gutierrez J, Corpuz R, Li B, Hall L, Rangell L, Ferrando R, Lowman H, Peale F, Ferrara N (2007) Mice expressing a humanized form of VEGF-A may provide insights into the safety and efficacy of anti-VEGF antibodies. Proc Natl Acad Sci USA 104:3478–3483

Gimbrone MA, Leapmaan SB, Cotran RS, Folkman J (1972) Tumor dormancy in vivo by prevention of neovascularization. J Exp Med 136:261–276

Hattori K, Dias S, Heissig B, Hackett NR, Lyden D, Tateno M, Hicklin DJ, Zhu Z, Witte L, Crystal RG, Moore MA, Rafii S (2001) Vascular endothelial growth factor and angiopoietin-1 stimulate postnatal hematopoiesis by recruitment of vasculogenic and hematopoietic stem cells. J Exp Med 193:1005–1014

Houck KA, Ferrara N, Winer J, Cachianes G, Li B, Leung DW (1991) The vascular endothelial growth factor family: Identification of a fourth molecular species and characterization of alternative splicing of RNA. Mol Endocrinol 5:1806–1814

Houck KA, Leung DW, Rowland AM, Winer J, Ferrara N (1992) Dual regulation of vascular endothelial growth factor bioavailability by genetic and proteolytic mechanisms. J Biol Chem 267:26031–26037

Hurwitz H, Fehrenbacher L, Novotny W, Cartwright T, Hainsworth J, Heim W, Berlin J, Baron A, Griffing S, Holmgren E, Ferrara N, Fyfe G, Rogers B, Ross R, Kabbinavar F (2004) Bevacizumab plus irinotecan, fluorouracil, and leucovorin for metastatic colorectal cancer. N Eng J Med 350:2335–2342

Hurwitz HI, Honeycutt W, Haley S, Favaro J (2006) Long-term treatment with bevacizumab for patients with metastatic colorectal cancer: Case report. Clin Colorectal Cancer 6:66–69

Husain D, Kim I, Gauthier D, Lane AM, Tsilimbaris MK, Ezra E, Connolly EJ, Michaud N, Gragoudas ES, O'Neill CA, Beyer JC, Miller JW (2005) Safety and efficacy of intravitreal injection of ranibizumab in combination with verteporfin PDT on experimental choroidal neovascularization in the monkey. Arch Ophthalmol 123:509–516

Ide AG, Baker NH, Warren SL (1939) Vascularization of the Brown Pearce rabbit epithelioma transplant as seen in the transparent ear chamber. Am J Roentgenol 42:891–899

Kabat EA, Wu TT, Perry H, Gottesmann KS, Foeller C (1991) Sequences of proteins of immunological interest. Public Health Service, National Institutes of Health, Bethesda, MD

Kim IK, Husain D, Michaud N, Connolly EJ, Lane AM, Durrant K, Hafezi-Moghadam A, Gragoudas ES, O'Neill CA, Beyer JC, Miller JW (2006) Effect of the intravitreal injection of ranibizumab in combination with verteporfin PDT on normal primate retina and choroids. Invest Ophthalmol Vis Sci 47:357–363

Kim KJ, Li B, Houck K, Winer J, Ferrara N (1992) The vascular endothelial growth factor proteins: Identification of biologically relevant regions by neutralizing monoclonal antibodies. Growth Factors 7:53–64

Kim KJ, Li B, Winer J, Armanini M, Gillett N, Phillips HS, Ferrara N (1993) Inhibition of vascular endothelial growth factor-induced angiogenesis suppresses tumor growth in vivo. Nature 362:841–844

Krzystolik MG, Afshari MA, Adamis AP, Gaudreault J, Gragoudas ES, Michaud NA, Li W, Connolly E, O'Neill CA, Miller JW (2002) Prevention of experimental choroidal neovascularization with intravitreal anti-vascular endothelial growth factor antibody fragment. Arch Ophthalmol 120:338–346

Lee CV, Liang WC, Dennis MS, Eigenbrot C, Sidhu SS, Fuh G (2004) High-affinity human antibodies from phage-displayed synthetic Fab libraries with a single framework scaffold. J Mol Biol 340:1073–1093

Leung DW, Cachianes G, Kuang WJ, Goeddel DV, Ferrara N (1989) Vascular endothelial growth factor is a secreted angiogenic mitogen. Science 246:1306–1309

Li B, Fuh G, Meng G, Xin X, Gerritsen ME, Cunningham B, de Vos AM (2000) Receptor-selective variants of human vascular endothelial growth factor. Generation and characterization. J Biol Chem 275:29823–29828

Liang WC, Wu X, Peale FV, Lee CV, Meng YG, Gutierrez J, Fu L, Malik AK, Gerber HP, Ferrara N, Fuh G (2006) Cross-species vascular endothelial growth factor (VEGF)-blocking antibodies completely inhibit the growth of human tumor xenografts and measure the contribution of stromal VEGF. J Biol Chem 281:951–961

Liew G, Mitchell P (2007) Ranibizumab for neovascular age-related macular degeneration. N Eng J Med 356:747–750

Lin YS, Nguyen C, Mendoza JL, Escandon E, Fei D, Meng YG, Modi NB (1999) Preclinical pharmacokinetics, interspecies scaling, and tissue distribution of a humanized monoclonal antibody against vascular endothelial growth factor. J Pharmacol Exp Ther 288:371–378

Malecaze F, Clamens S, Simorre-Pinatel V, Mathis A, Chollet P, Favard C, Bayard F, Plouet J (1994) Detection of vascular endothelial growth factor messenger RNA and vascular endothelial growth factor-like activity in proliferative diabetic retinopathy. Arch Ophthalmol 112:1476–1482

Melnyk O, Shuman MA, Kim KJ (1996) Vascular endothelial growth factor promotes tumor dissemination by a mechanism distinct from its effect on primary tumor growth. Cancer Res 56:921–924

Michels S, Rosenfeld PJ, Puliafito CA, Marcus EN, Venkatraman AS (2005) Systemic bevacizumab (Avastin) therapy for neovascular age-related macular degeneration twelve-week results of an uncontrolled open-label clinical study. Ophthalmology 112:1035–1047

Millauer B, Wizigmann-Voos S, Schnurch H, Martinez R, Moller NP, Risau W, Ullrich A (1993) High affinity VEGF binding and developmental expression suggest Flk-1 as a major regulator of vasculogenesis and angiogenesis. Cell 72:835–846

Mordenti J, Cuthbertson RA, Ferrara N, Thomsen K, Berleau L, Licko V, Allen PC, Valverde CR, Meng YG, Fei DT, Fourre KM, Ryan AM (1999) Comparisons of the intraocular tissue distribution, pharmacokinetics, and safety of 125I-labeled full-length and Fab antibodies in rhesus monkeys following intravitreal administration. Toxicol Pathol 27:536–544

Muller YA, Chen Y, Christinger HW, Li B, Cunningham BC, Lowman HB, de Vos AM (1998) VEGF and the Fab fragment of a humanized neutralizing antibody: Crystal structure of the complex at 2.4 Å resolution and mutational analysis of the interface. Structure 6:1153–1167

Muller YA, Christinger HW, Keyt BA, de Vos AM (1997) The crystal structure of vascular endothelial growth factor (VEGF) refined to 1.93 Å resolution: Multiple copy flexibility and receptor binding. Structure 5:1325–1338

Pan B, Li B, Russell SJ, Tom JY, Cochran AG, Fairbrother WJ (2002) Solution structure of a phage-derived peptide antagonist in complex with vascular endothelial growth factor. J Mol Biol 316:769–787

Park JE, Keller GA, Ferrara N (1993) The vascular endothelial growth factor (VEGF) isoforms: Differential deposition into the subepithelial extracellular matrix and bioactivity of extracellular matrix-bound VEGF. Mol Biol Cell 4:1317–1326

Presta LG, Chen H, O'Connor SJ, Chisholm V, Meng YG, Krummen L, Winkler M, Ferrara N (1997) Humanization of an anti-vascular endothelial growth factor monoclonal antibody for the therapy of solid tumors and other disorders. Cancer Res 57:4593–4599

Quinn TP, Peters KG, De Vries C, Ferrara N, Williams LT (1993) Fetal liver kinase 1 is a receptor for vascular endothelial growth factor and is selectively expressed in vascular endothelium. Proc Natl Acad Sci USA 90:7533–7537

Ranieri G, Patruno R, Ruggieri E, Montemurro S, Valerio P, Ribatti D (2006) Vascular endothelial growth factor (VEGF) as a target of bevacizumab in cancer: From the biology to the clinic. Curr Med Chem 13:1845–1857

Rosenfeld PJ, Heier JS, Hantsbarger G, Shams N (2006a) Tolerability and efficacy of multiple escalating doses of ranibizumab (Lucentis) for neovascular age-related macular degeneration. Ophthalmology 113:623–632

Rosenfeld PJ, Moshfeghi AA, Puliafito CA (2005a) Optical coherence tomography findings after an intravitreal injection of bevacizumab (avastin) for neovascular age-related macular degeneration. Ophthalmic Surg Lasers Imaging 36:331–335

Rosenfeld PJ, Schwartz SD, Blumenkranz MS, Miller JW, Haller JA, Reimann JD, Greene WL, Shams N (2005b) Maximum tolerated dose of a humanized anti-vascular endothelial growth factor antibody fragment for treating neovascular age-related macular degeneration. Ophthalmology 112:1048–1053

Rosenfeld PJ, Rich RM, Lalwani GA (2006b) Ranibizumab: Phase III clinical trial results. Ophthalmol Clin North Am 19:361–372

Rosenfeld PJ, Brown DM, Heier JS, Boyer DS, Kaiser PK, Chung CY, Kim RY (2006c) Ranibizumab for neovascular age-related macular degeneration. New Eng J Med 355:1419–1431

Ryan AM, Eppler DB, Hagler KE, Bruner RH, Thomford PJ, Hall RL, Shopp GM, O'Neill CA (1999) Preclinical safety evaluation of rhuMAbVEGF, an antiangiogenic humanized monoclonal antibody. Toxicol Pathol 27:78–86

Sandler A, Herbst R (2006) Combining targeted agents: blocking the epidermal growth factor and vascular endothelial growth factor pathways. Clin Cancer Res 12:4421s–4425s

Schmidt-Erfurth UM, Michels S (2003) Changes in confocal indocyanine green angiography through two years after photodynamic therapy with verteporfin. Ophthalmology 110:1306–1314

Shibuya M, Yamaguchi S, Yamane A, Ikeda T, Tojo A, Matsushime H, Sato M (1990) Nucleotide sequence and expression of a novel human receptor-type tyrosine kinase gene (flt) closely related to the fms family. Oncogene 5:519–524

Shima DT, Gougos A, Miller JW, Tolentino M, Robinson G, Adamis AP, D'Amore PA (1996) Cloning and mRNA expression of vascular endothelial growth factor in ischemic retinas of Macaca fascicularis. Invest Ophthalmol Vis Sci 37:1334–1340

Soker S, Takashima S, Miao HQ, Neufeld G, Klagsbrun M (1998) Neuropilin-1 is expressed by endothelial and tumor cells as an isoform-specific receptor for vascular endothelial growth factor. Cell 92:735–745

Stacker SA, Achen MG, Jussila L, Baldwin ME, Alitalo K (2002) Lymphangiogenesis and cancer metastasis. Nat Rev Cancer 2:573–583

Stone J, Itin A, Alon T, Pe'er J, Gnessin H, Chan-Ling T, Keshet E (1995) Development of retinal vasculature is mediated by hypoxia-induced vascular endothelial growth factor (VEGF) expression by neuroglia. J Neurosci 15:4738–4747

Storkebaum E, Lambrechts D, Carmeliet P (2004) VEGF: Once regarded as a specific angiogenic factor, now implicated in neuroprotection. Bioessays 26:943–954

Terman BI, Dougher-Vermazen M, Carrion ME, Dimitrov D, Armellino DC, Gospodarowicz D, Bohlen P (1992) Identification of the KDR tyrosine kinase as a receptor for vascular endothelial cell growth factor. Biochem Biophys Res Commun 187:1579–1586

Tischer E, Mitchell R, Hartman T, Silva M, Gospodarowicz D, Fiddes JC, Abraham JA (1991) The human gene for vascular endothelial growth factor. Multiple protein forms are encoded through alternative exon splicing. J Biol Chem 266:11947–11954

Warren RS, Yuan H, Matli MR, Gillett NA, Ferrara N (1995) Regulation by vascular endothelial growth factor of human colon cancer tumorigenesis in a mouse model of experimental liver metastasis. J Clin Invest 95:1789–1797

Wiesmann C, Fuh G, Christinger HW, Eigenbrot C, Wells JA, de Vos AM (1997) Crystal structure at 1.7 Å resolution of VEGF in complex with domain 2 of the Flt-1 receptor. Cell 91:695–704

Zondor SD, Medina PJ (2004) Bevacizumab: an angiogenesis inhibitor with efficacy in colorectal and other malignancies. Ann Pharmacother 38:1258–1264

Humanized Antihuman IL-6 Receptor Antibody, Tocilizumab

N. Nishimoto(✉) and T. Kishimoto

1 Introduction 152
2 Structure of Tocilizumab. 152
3 Immunopharmacological Characteristics of Tocilizumab 153
    3.1   Mechanism of Action 153
    3.2   Pharmacokinetics 154
    3.3   Pharmacological Characteristics 154
4 Clinical Utility of Tocilizumab. 155
5 Conclusion 158
References 159

Abstract Interleukin-6 (IL-6) is a pleiotropic cytokine that regulates immune responses and inflammatory reactions. Overproduction of IL-6 has been shown to play a role in inflammatory autoimmune diseases such as rheumatoid arthritis (RA), and juvenile idiopathic arthritis (JIA) and, therefore, an agent blocking IL-6 actions can be a therapy of these diseases. IL-6 belongs to a cytokine family, which shares the cytokine receptor subunit glycoprotein (gp) 130. This family also includes IL-11, oncostatin-M, and leukemia inhibitory factor (LIF). In the IL-6 receptor (IL-6R) system, both a membrane-bound IL-6R and a soluble form of IL-6R are able to mediate IL-6 signals into the cells through the interaction of gp130. Tocilizumab is a humanized antihuman IL-6 receptor antibody designed using genetic engineering technology. Tocilizumab recognizes both the membrane-bound and the soluble form IL-6R and specifically blocks IL-6 actions. Tocilizumab is expected to ameliorate the autoimmune inflammatory diseases with IL-6 overproduction and has been clinically developed as a therapeutic agent for RA, systemic-onset and articular types of JIA, Crohn's disease, etc. Tocilizumab has been shown to be effective not only

N. Nishimoto

Laboratory of Immune Regulation, Graduate School of Frontier Biosciences, Osaka University, 1–3 Yamadaoka, Suita City, Osaka 565-0871, Japan

e-mail: norihiro@fbs.osaka-u.ac.jp

Y. Chernajovsky, A. Nissim (eds.) *Therapeutic Antibodies. Handbook of Experimental Pharmacology 181.*

for improving signs and symptoms but also for preventing joint destruction of RA. Immunopharmacology and clinical benefit of tocilizumab in RA is addressed.

1 Introduction

Interleukin-6 (IL-6) is a multifunctional cytokine that regulates immune responses and inflammatory reactions, and is likely to mediate the autoimmune, inflammatory, and joint destruction aspects of rheumatoid arthritis (RA) (Nishimoto 2006). Thus, agents that block the actions of IL-6 are potential therapeutic options for RA treatment. Tocilizumab is a humanized antihuman IL-6 receptor antibody designed using genetic engineering technology (Sato et al. 1993). Since it specifically blocks the actions of IL-6, it is effective in treating conditions resulting from excessive IL-6 production. Moreover, it was approved in April 2005 as the world's first drug for Castleman's disease (Nishimoto et al. 2005), an atypical lymphoproliferative disorder (trade name: ACTEMRA® 200 for intravenous infusion). Tocilizumab has also been developed as a treatment for RA, juvenile idiopathic arthritis (Yokota et al. 2005), and Crohn's disease (Ito et al. 2004). This review describes the immunopharmacology and clinical utility of tocilizumab mainly in RA.

2 Structure of Tocilizumab

Tocilizumab is a genetically-engineered monoclonal antibody, humanized from a mouse antihuman IL-6 receptor antibody using the CDR grafting method (Sato

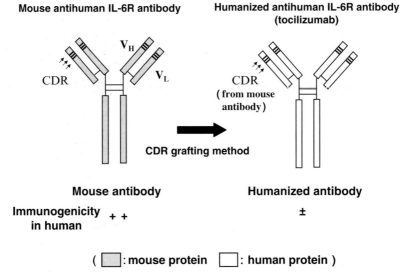

Fig. 1 Humanized antihuman IL-6 receptor (tocilizumab). Antigenicity in humans is reduced by humanizing a mouse antihuman IL-6 receptor with the CDR grafting method (Sato et al. 1993)

et al. 1993) (Fig. 1). It was initially called MRA for myeloma receptor antibody, because of potential applications in multiple myeloma treatments (Sato et al. 1993; Nishimoto et al. 1994), but was then renamed tocilizumab. Humanization of tocilizumab has resulted in decreased antigenicity in the human body. Therefore, the drug's half-life is prolonged and repetitive treatment with tocilizumab rarely causes production of neutralizing antibodies compared with mouse antibodies or mouse and human chimeric antibodies.

3 Immunopharmacological Characteristics of Tocilizumab

3.1 Mechanism of Action

Tocilizumab recognizes the IL-6 binding site of the human IL-6 receptor (IL-6R) and inhibits IL-6 signaling through competitive blockade of IL-6 binding (Fig. 2). Despite being an IgG1 antibody, a regular dose of tocilizumab in humans causes no antibody-dependent cellular cytotoxicity or complement-dependent cytotoxicity in cells that express IL-6R.

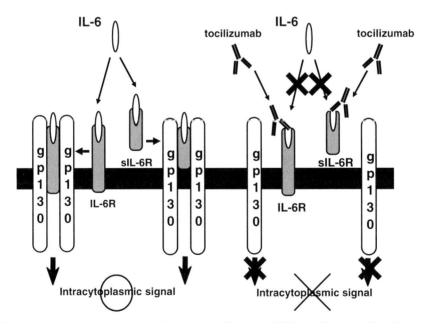

Fig. 2 IL-6 receptor system and mechanism for tocilizumab inhibition of IL-6 signaling. IL-6 triggers dimerization of signal-transducing gp130 molecules on the cell membrane when binding with membrane IL-6 receptors (IL-6R) or soluble receptors (sIL-6R) in body fluids, thus transmitting signals into the cells. Tocilizumab recognizes both IL-6R on the cell membrane and sIL-6R, and blocks IL-6 signaling

Soluble IL-6 receptors (sIL-6R), on the other hand, are found in body fluids such as blood and synovial fluid. Unlike tumor necrosis factor (TNF), whose signals are blocked by soluble TNF receptors, IL-6 signals are transmitted into the cell by sIL-6R. This mechanism is called trans-signaling (Scheller et al. 2006) and occurs when IL-6 binds sIL-6R, assembles with gp130 molecules on the cell membrane, and triggers formation of the high affinity IL-6R complex. Tocilizumab recognizes both IL-6R on the cell membrane and sIL-6R, and inhibits IL-6 signaling by preventing ligand-receptor binding (Mihara et al. 2005).

3.2 Pharmacokinetics

The pharmacokinetics of tocilizumab were examined in detail by conducting a phase I study of healthy adults and a phase I/II study of RA patients (Nishimoto et al. 2003). The phase I/II study was conducted with 15 RA patients who had previously had an insufficient response to one or more doses of disease modifying antirheumatic drugs or immunosuppressants, or had side effects that led to discontinued treatment. Patients underwent repetitive treatment with 2, 4, or $8\,mg\,kg^{-1}$ body weight of tocilizumab at 2-week intervals for a total of three times, and the pharmacokinetics were examined. Figure 3A shows changes in blood-level tocilizumab during repetitive treatment, indicating nonlinear pharmacokinetics in the $2-8\,mg\,kg^{-1}$ dose range. The half-life of tocilizumab (t1/2) was dose-dependent and prolonged as dosage increased from 2 to $8\,mg\,kg^{-1}$, as well as when the number of doses increased through repetitive treatment (Fig. 3B). In addition, the half-life at the third $8\,mg\,kg^{-1}$ dose was about 240 h, close to the half-life of human immunoglobin (Ig) G1. Blood-level area under the curve (AUC) of tocilizumab also increased an average of $19.9\,mg\,hr\,ml^{-1}$ (Nishimoto et al. 2003).

3.3 Pharmacological Characteristics

Blood-level tocilizumab in the second posttreatment week was absent in most patients who received $2\,mg\,kg^{-1}$ tocilizumab at 2-week intervals, while it tended to accumulate in most patients who received 4 or $8\,mg\,kg^{-1}$. These patients were completely negative for CRP and serum amyloid A (Fig. 4A). On the other hand, those who showed no blood-level tocilizumab were positive for CRP and serum amyloid A (Nishimoto et al. 2003).

CRP and serum amyloid A are acute-phase proteins produced by the liver as a result of IL-6, IL-1, and TNF stimulation. Infliximab and etanercept, TNF inhibitors, also reduce CRP, but only a limited number of patients became completely negative for CRP (Charles et al. 1999). Production of CRP and serum amyloid A clearly requires IL-6, as IL-6 inhibition resulted in negative values for these markers. Therefore, it is important to maintain blood-level tocilizumab to inhibit the actions of IL-6.

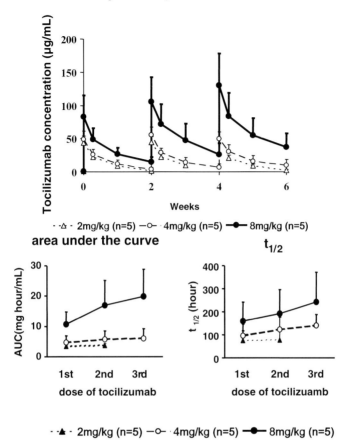

Fig. 3 Pharmacokinetics of tocilizumab. (**A**) Changes in blood-level tocilizumab. (**B**) Blood-level area under the curve (AUC) and blood half-life (t1/2) (adapted from Nishimoto et al. 2003) Repetitive treatment increases both AUC and t1/2

CRP may serve as an alternate indicator for sufficient blood levels of tocilizumab (Nishimoto et al. 2003).

4 Clinical Utility of Tocilizumab

Choy et al. have conducted a British phase I study with 45 patients treated with a single dose of 0.1, 1, 5, or $10\,\mathrm{mg\,kg^{-1}}$ tocilizumab, or placebo (Choy et al. 2002). This study evaluated tocilizumab safety and RA disease activity in the second posttreatment week using the American College of Rheumatology (ACR) improvement criteria. The ACR20 rate was 56% for the $5\,\mathrm{mg\,kg^{-1}}$ tocilizumab group and 0% for placebo group, indicating a significant difference. However, no significant

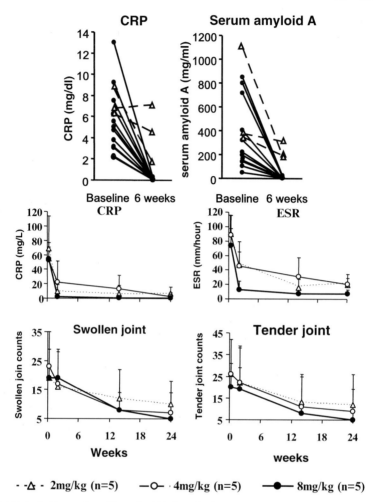

Fig. 4 Clinical effects of tocilizumab. (**A**) Quantitative changes in acute-phase proteins in the blood: acute-phase proteins, CRP, and serum amyloid A were normalized in patients with measurable blood-level tocilizumab (*filled circle*). Normalization of CRP and serum amyloid A was not observed in patients who did not maintain blood-level tocilizumab (*open triangle*). (**B**) Improved clinical findings: treatment with tocilizumab quantitatively improved swollen and painful joints, as well as CRP values and erythrocyte sedimentation rates (ESR) (adapted from Nishimoto et al. 2003)

difference in ACR20 rate was observed between other tocilizumab groups and the placebo group. The results of this study also confirmed an adequate level of safety with no serious side effects.

In the Japanese 24-week phase I/II study, patients that did not show serious side effects, had improved CRP or erythrocyte sedimentation rate (ESR) in the second week following the third dose, were further treated with tocilizumab if the patients were willing to continue the tocilizumab therapy, and also if the principal investigator physician decided that the patients required to receive the treatment. Of all the patients, the ACR20 response rate at the sixth week was 60% and 86% at the sixth month (Nishimoto et al. 2003). In addition, the ACR50 rate was 13% at the sixth week and 33% at the sixth month. The findings of this open study suggested that tocilizumab has large treatment effects on RA disease activity (Fig. 4B), which lead to a phase II study.

A randomized, multicenter, double-blind, placebo-controlled trial of tocilizumab was conducted in a Japanese late phase II study, with 164 patients who previously had an insufficient response to one or more doses of antirheumatic or immunosup-pressant drugs. Patients underwent intravenous therapy with either 4 or $8\,\mathrm{mg\,kg^{-1}}$ tocilizumab, or placebo given at 4-week intervals for a total of three times. RA disease activity was evaluated in the fourth posttreatment week (Nishimoto et al. 2004). The ACR20 response rate of $8\,\mathrm{mg\,kg^{-1}}$ tocilizumab was 78%, while that of placebo was only 11%, thus confirming clinical utility of tocilizumab in a double-blind study (Fig. 5).

Evaluation of drug safety showed no significant difference in adverse event rates between 4 and $8\,\mathrm{mg\,kg^{-1}}$ tocilizumab, and placebo groups. Laboratory findings, however, indicated a dose-dependent increase of total cholesterol values in 44% of patients treated with tocilizumab. This increase stabilized at around $240\,\mathrm{mg\,dl^{-1}}$, and HDL cholesterol also increased in a similar way. Long-term safety evaluation is necessary to know whether or not the increased total cholesterol value indicates a higher risk of cardiovascular diseases. It has been reported that TNF inhibition also

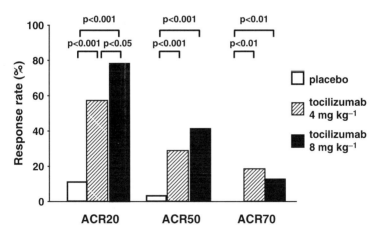

Fig. 5 Disease activity evaluation by ACR improvement criteria. Treatment with tocilizumab significantly improved RA disease activity when compared with the placebo treatment (adapted from Nishimoto et al. 2004). ACR improvement criteria: ACR20 is defined as improvement by 20% or more in tender and swollen joint counts and 20% improvement in 3 of the 5 remaining ACR core set measures: patient and physician global assessments, pain, disability, and an acute-phase reactant (CRP or ESR). Likewise, ACR50 is achieved with improvement by 50% or more and ACR70 with improvement by 70% or more

resulted in an increase in total cholesterol, suggesting that this effect may be due to a decrease in RA disease activity (Seriolo et al. 2006).

Tocilizumab monotherapy, with no combinatory use of methotrexate, resulted in an insignificant number of patients developing antinuclear antibodies or anti-DNA antibodies, which are frequently observed with anti-TNF antibody treatment. Moreover, the anti-tocilizumab antibody was observed only in 2% of the patients treated with tocilizumab, reconfirming the advantages of humanized antibodies. As IL-6 is a cytokine that induces antibody production, IL-6 inhibition may reduce the production of neutralizing antibodies. In terms of treatment strategy, it is highly advantageous that methotrexate is not required.

Serious adverse events have been observed in patients with infectious diseases treated with $8\,mg\,kg^{-1}$ tocilizumab. A patient with Epstein-Barr virus (EBV) reactivation died about 2 months later from subsequent hemophagocytic syndrome. This patient manifested conditions similar to those of chronic active EBV infection, with fluctuation in abnormal liver function tests and CRP increase, which inversely correlated with the number of peripheral leukocytes. Plasma EBV DNA was detected prior to study participation, but later findings indicated that this patient also had Hodgkin's disease prior to the study (Ogawa et al. 2006). Subsequent studies examined more than 200 patients treated with tocilizumab, of which none had plasma EBV DNA. While the EBV reactivation mechanism is currently unclear, a careful pretreatment examination is necessary in tocilizumab therapy to determine whether or not the patient has an infectious disease.

The above studies indicate that tocilizumab is effective in reducing RA disease activity, even as a monotherapy, and has a tolerability within the permissible range. An $8\,mg\,kg^{-1}$ dose at 4-week intervals appears to be the optimum regimen.

Maini et al. have conducted a European phase II study on the combinatory treatment of tocilizumab with methotrexate (Maini et al. 2006). This study yielded results that confirm the effectiveness of tocilizumab as a monotherapy. No difference was observed in the ACR20 rate between monotherapy with $8\,mg\,kg^{-1}$ tocilizumab and combinatory treatment with $8\,mg\,kg^{-1}$ tocilizumab and methotrexate. However, a synergistic effect was observed in combinatory treatment with $4\,mg\,kg^{-1}$ or a lower dose of tocilizumab and methotrexate.

A Japanese phase III trial was conducted to examine the preventive effects of tocilizumab on progressive joint destruction. This study evaluated the 1-year change in the van der Heijde's modified Sharp score (i.e., a quantitative radiographic evaluation of bone erosion and joint space narrowing in hand and foot joints of RA patients). The results indicate that tocilizumab is also effective in preventing progressive joint destruction (Nishimoto et al. 2005).

5 Conclusion

Ongoing clinical trials have shown the effectiveness of tocilizumab in treating RA, and the drug is currently undergoing the application process for approval in Japan. Although no direct comparison data with TNF inhibitors are available, it is notable that tocilizumab is highly effective even in a monotherapy. Future studies include long-term safety evaluation and the examination of differential applications of IL-6 inhibition treatment and TNF or IL-1 inhibition treatments. These studies based on the biological functions of target molecules will elucidate how each treatment takes part in the strategy of RA treatment.

References

Charles P, Elliott MJ, Davis D, Potter A, Kalden JR, Antoni C, Breedveld FC, Smolen JS, Eberl G, deWoody K, Feldmann M, Maini RN (1999) Regulation of cytokines, cytokine inhibitors, and acute-phase proteins following anti-TNF-alpha therapy in rheumatoid arthritis. J Immunol 163:1521–1528

Choy EH, Isenberg DA, Garrood T, Farrow S, Ioannou Y, Bird H, Cheung N, Williams B, Price R, Yoshizaki K, Nishimoto N, Kishimoto T, Panay GS (2002) Therapeutic benefit after blocking interleukin-6 activity in rheumatoid arthritis with an anti-interleukin-6 receptor monoclonal antibody. Arthritis Rheum 46:3143–3150

Ito H, Takazoe M, Fukuda Y, Hibi T, Kusugami K, Andoh A, Matsumoto T, Yamamura T, Azuma J, Nishimoto N, Yoshizaki K, Shimoyama T, Kishimoto T (2004) A pilot randomized trial of a human anti-interleukin-6 receptor monoclonal antibody in active Crohn's disease. Gastroenterol 126:989–996

Maini RN, Taylor PC, Szechinski J, Pavelka K, Broll J, Balint G, Emery P, Raemen F, Petersen J, Smolen J, Thomson D, Kishimoto T CHARISMA Study Group (2006) Double-blind randomized controlled clinical trial of the interleukin-6 receptor antagonist, tocilizumab, in European patients with rheumatoid arthritis who had an incomplete response to methotrexate. Arthritis Rheum 54:2817–2829

Mihara M, Kasutani K, Okazaki M, Nakamura A, Kawai S, Sugimoto M, Matsumoto Y, Ohsugi Y (2005) Tocilizumab inhibits signal transduction mediated by both mIL-6R and sIL-6R, but not by the receptors of other members of IL-6 cytokine family. Int Immunopharmacol 5:1731–1740

Nishimoto N, Ogata A, Shima Y, Tani Y, Ogawa H, Nakagawa M, Sugiyama H, Yoshizaki K, Kishimoto T (1994) Oncostatin M, leukemia inhibitory factor, and interleukin-6 induce the proliferation of human plasmacytoma cells via the common signal transducer, gp130. J Exp Med 179:1343–1347

Nishimoto N, Yoshizaki K, Maeda K, Kuritani T, Deguchi H, Sato B, Imai N, Suemura M, Kakei T, Takagi N, Kishimoto T (2003) Toxicity, Pharmacokinetics, and Dose-Finding Study of Repetitive Treatment with the Humanized Anti-Interleukin 6 Receptor Antibody MRA in Rheumatoid Arthritis. Phase I/II Clinical Study. J Rheumatol 30:1426–1435

Nishimoto N, Yoshizaki K, Miyasaka N, Yamamoto K, Kawai S, Takeuchi T, Hashimoto J, Azuma J, Kishimoto T (2004) Treatment of rheumatoid arthritis with humanized anti-interleukin 6 receptor antibody. Arthritis Rheum 50:1761–1769

Nishimoto N, Kanakura Y, Aozasa K, Johkoh T, Nakamura M, Nakano S, Nakano N, Ikeda Y, Sasaki T, Nishioka K, Hara M, Taguchi H, Kimura Y, Kato Y, Asaoku H, Kumagai S, Kodama F, Nakahara H, Hagihara K, Yoshizaki K, Kishimoto T (2005) Humanized anti-interleukin-6 receptor antibody treatment of multicentric Castleman's disease. Blood 106:2627–2632

Nishimoto N, Hashimoto J, Miyasaka N, Yamamoto K, Kawai S, Takeuchi T, Murata N, van der Heijde D, Kishimoto T (2007) Study of active controlled monotherapy used for rheumatoid arthritis, an IL-6 inhibitor (SAMURAI): evidence of clinical and radiographic benefit from an X-ray reader-blinded randomised controlled trial of tocilizumab. Ann Rheum Dis 66:1162–1167

Nishimoto N (2006) Interleukin-6 in rheumatoid arthritis. Curr Opin Rheumatol 18:277–281

Ogawa J, Harigai M, Akashi T, Nagasaka K, Suzuki F, Tominaga S, Miyasaka N (2006)
    Exacerbation of chronic active Epstein-Barr virus infection in a patient with rheumatoid
    arthritis receiving humanised anti-interleukin-6 receptor monoclonal antibody. Ann Rheum Dis
    65:1667–1669
Sato K, Tsuchiya M, Saldanha J, Koishihara Y, Ohsugi Y, Kishimoto T, Bendig MM (1993)
    Reshaping a human antibody to inhibit the interleukin 6-dependent tumor cell growth.
    Cancer Res 53:851–856
Scheller J, Ohnesorge N, Rose-John S (2006) Interleukin-6 trans-signalling in chronic inflamma-
    tion and cancer. Scand J Immunol 63:321–329
Seriolo B, Paolino S, Sulli A, Fasciolo D, Cutolo M (2006) Effects of anti-TNF-alpha treatment on
    lipid profile in patients with active rheumatoid arthritis. Ann N Y Acad Sci 1069:414–419
Yokota S, Miyamae T, Imagawa T, Iwata N, Katakura S, Mori M, Woo P, Nishimoto N,
    Yoshizaki K, Kishimoto T (2005) Therapeutic efficacy of humanized recombinant anti-IL
    6-receptor antibody for children with systemic-onset juvenile idiopathic arthritis. Arthritis
    Rheum 52:818–825

Part IV
Antibodies to Cell Markers

Anti-CD20 Monoclonal Antibody in Rheumatoid Arthritis and Systemic Lupus Erythematosus

F. Goldblatt and D.A. Isenberg(✉)

1   Introduction 164
2   Anti-CD 20 Monoclonal Antibody Treatment
     of Rheumatoid Arthritis 166
     2.1   Role of B Cells in the Pathogenesis
            of Rheumatoid Arthritis 166
     2.2   Trials of Rituximab in Rheumatoid Arthritis 167
3   Anti-CD20 Monoclonal Antibody (Rituximab) for the Treatment of Systemic Lupus
     Erythematosus 174
     3.1   Role of B Cells in Pathogenesis of Systemic Lupus Erythematosus 174
     3.2   Trials of Rituximab in Systemic Lupus Erythematosus 175
4   Future B Cell Targeted Therapies 177
     4.1   Epratuzumab 177
     4.2   Anti-B Lymphocyte Stimulator Monoclonal Antibody 177
5   Conclusion 178
References 178

Abstract Rheumatoid arthritis (RA) and systemic lupus erythematosus (SLE) are both chronic autoimmune rheumatic diseases. In the last few years, evolution in the understanding of RA and SLE pathogenesis and underlying molecular mechanisms has resulted in development and availability of novel therapies. In particular, the recent acknowledgement of a more significant role for B cells in the pathogenesis of RA, in contrast to the view that it was predominantly a T cell disorder, provided rationale for trials of B cell depletion therapy with the chimeric anti-CD20 monoclonal antibody rituximab. The efficacy and favourable safety profile of rituximab have resulted in the recent approval by the European Medicines Agency for

F. Goldblatt, D.A. Isenberg

Centre for Rheumatology, Department of Medicine, University College London Hospital, 3rd Floor Central, 250 Euston Road, London NW1 2PQ, UK

e-mail: fgoldblatt@ntlworld.com and d.isenberg@ucl.ac.uk

Y. Chernajovsky, A. Nissim (eds.) *Therapeutic Antibodies. Handbook of
Experimental Pharmacology 181.*
© Springer-Verlag Berlin Heidelberg 2008

its usage in patients with RA unresponsive to conventional therapies. The salient features from the pivotal open and randomised controlled trials are reviewed in this chapter. Given the recognition of B cell dysfunction as central to SLE pathogenesis, the use of anti-CD20 antibody therapy for this patient group has also been established. Results of the open trials have been encouraging, particularly in patients not responding to usual therapies, and a randomised controlled trial is underway.

1 Introduction

In recent years a number of exciting new therapies have been developed for rheumatoid arthritis (RA) and systemic lupus erythematosus (SLE), reflecting advances in the understanding of disease pathogenesis and molecular mechanisms. Various biological modifiers, including anti-tumour necrosis factor-α (TNF-α) agents and interleukin-1 receptor antagonists have been developed in recognition of the important role of these pro-inflammatory cytokines in RA. Based on an increased appreciation of the likely pathogenic role for B cells autoimmune diseases such as RA and SLE, targeted therapy against B cells has also been explored. Therapeutic B cell depletion with the anti-CD20 monoclonal antibody rituximab was initially licensed in 1997 for treatment of relapsed low grade B cell follicular NHL and over 700,000 patients have now been treated for this condition. Following this success, experimental use in autoimmune disorders was undertaken, with initial promise demonstrated in chronic idiopathic thrombocytopenic purpura (ITP) (Stasi et al. 2001). B cell depletion therapy for RA has now undergone open and randomised controlled trials and has been recently approved by the European Medicines Agency for usage in patients with RA unresponsive to conventional therapies (Leandro et al. 2002a; Edwards et al. 2004; Emery et al. 2006). Similarly, there have been a number of open studies of B cell depletion therapy for treatment of refractory SLE, and there are two ongoing phase II/III trials currently evaluating safety and efficacy in patients with severely active disease and nephritis. Importantly, however, there has not yet been a large double blind randomised control trial and it is imperative this be performed in the near future. This chapter summarises the role of B cells in pathogenesis of RA and SLE, the current knowledge of the mechanism of B cell depletion by rituximab and the main clinical trials of anti-CD20 monoclonal antibody treatment for RA and SLE. Salient features of new B cell targeted therapies, epratuzumab and anti-B Lymphocyte Stimulator (BLys) monoclonal antibody therapy will be briefly discussed.

   Whilst other anti-human CD20 monoclonal antibodies exist, including a fully humanised antibody (Phase I/II controlled trial recently completed recruitment) and radioisotope conjugated antibody, rituximab is currently the most extensively studied and hence will form the basis of this chapter. Rituximab is a chimeric monoclonal antibody directed against human CD20, fusing variable regions of a murine anti-human CD20 B cell hybridoma with the constant region of human immunoglobulin IgG_1K. B cell ontogeny is characterised by a series of changing surface phenotypes and the CD20 surface marker (a 33–37 kDa membrane-associated phosphoprotein) expressed during intermediate stages of development is lost on terminal differentiation to the immunoglobulin producing plasma cell. This exclusivity and high specificity makes CD20 an attractive pharmacological target. Other beneficial features are that free CD20 antigen is not present in circulation, it does not self modulate its expression, is not shed or internalised after antibody binding and there are no endogenous molecules known to interfere with its function (Press et al. 1987). Rituximab rapidly depletes peripheral blood CD20 positive B cells via complement-mediated and antibody dependent cell-mediated cytotoxicity (ADCC), induction of apoptosis and inhibition of cell growth (Maloney et al. 2002). It is not yet certain which of the possible mechanisms of action is most important in vivo. Rituximab also down regulates CD40ligand, CD40 and CD80, resulting in changes to T cell function (Sfikakis et al. 2005; Tokunaga et al. 2005). B cell depletion usually reaches a nadir by 1 month and re-population generally starts by 6 months, generally coinciding with the clinical responses. Interestingly, marked variability between individual responses has been observed, with a proportion of patients never adequately depleting and hence failing to achieve clinical response, whilst others remain depleted and in clinical remission for over 2 years. Various reasons for inadequate depletion have been proposed, including genetic polymor-phisms of the FcRγIIIa (Anolik et al. 2003; Weng and Levy 2003) or defective com-plement; however, neither fully explains all the patients in this subgroup and future research to predict rituximab responders will be of interest. Following rituximab therapy, peripheral B cell re-population is reported to be dependent on the forma-tion of naïve B cells (Leandro et al. 2006), although it still remains to be verified whether tolerance is re-established to autoantigens and if so, does it persist or does it become lost because of the underlying genetic mechanisms that resulted in the initial development of the autoimmune disease? A recent publication demonstrated that patients who experience an earlier disease relapse tended to have a higher num-ber of circulating memory B cells at re-population compared to those with a later disease relapse (Leandro et al. 2006). Whilst it remains uncertain whether autoim-mune memory is attributable to long-lived plasma cells and/or continued stimulation of autoreactive memory B cells by self antigen, it is known that elimination of both populations is probably necessary to obtain re-establishment of B cell tolerance and further studies should clarify the situation.

When treating patients with rituximab, some practical issues require consi-deration. First, awareness of rare fatal infusion reactions, which typically occur 30–120 min after onset of the first infusion, is necessary. Symptoms include fever and chills, flushing, tachycardia, chest pressure, nausea and vomiting, with more serious reactions including hypoxia, cardiovascular collapse, myocardial infarc-tion and cardiogenic shock. Fortunately, these infusion reactions tend to occur less frequently during treatment of patients with autoimmune diseases than in patients with underlying malignancies, and also appear to be reduced by corticosteroid pre-medication (Cohen et al. 2006). Whilst published infection rates with rituximab have been surprisingly low and of unremarkable type, treating doctors should remain vigilant for potential typical and atypical infectious complications. As anticipated, following rituximab treatment, a failure to respond to vaccination has been observed although further studies are required to determine duration of this effect. In addition, patients with non-malignant autoimmune disease, in particular those with SLE, have shown higher human anti-chimeric antibodies (HACA) levels than patients with non-Hodgkin's lymphoma (Looney et al. 2004), and studies are being performed to determine whether the addition of methotrexate might suppress the formation of these HACA. Whether these antibodies are a contra-indication to re-treatment remains in doubt, and it is not yet certain if they reduce the therapeutic effectiveness of the drug or result in more adverse events. Many of these queries should be resolved with results from longer-term studies currently underway.

2 Anti-CD 20 Monoclonal Antibody Treatment of Rheumatoid Arthritis

2.1 Role of B Cells in the Pathogenesis of Rheumatoid Arthritis

The role of T cells in the immunopathogenesis of RA is well established. Evidence suggests that interaction between an unknown exogenous or endogenous antigen via antigen presenting cells and CD4+ T helper cells is involved in the induction of the immune response in RA. T cells with the appropriate T cell receptor, complex with processed antigenic peptides to become activated, resulting in a series of events including production of IL-2, leading to the clonal expansion of T cells and the enlargement and expression of a number of surface molecules such as TNF-α and receptor activator of NF-κB ligand (RANKL). Subsequent recruitment and activation of monocytes and macrophages occurs with secretion of pro-inflammatory cytokines, in particular TNF-α and IL-1 into the synovial cavity. Release of these cytokines mediates tissue destruction by activation of chondrocytes and fibroblasts, which release collagenases and metalloproteinases with resultant cartilage loss and bone erosion (Panayi 2005). However, contrary to this long held view that RA is a predominantly T cell mediated disease, there is an emerging acceptance of the role of B cells in disease aetiology. This is supported by the development, trials and success of B cell depletion therapies in patients with RA.

B lymphocyte dysregulation with the production of rheumatoid factor and other autoantibodies, formation of immune complexes and release of destructive mediators are known to contribute to RA pathogenesis (Mannik and Nardella 1985). Approximately 80% of patients develop RF antibodies and seropositive RA is associated with more aggressive articular disease and a higher frequency of extra-articular manifestations. It is thought that B cells with RF specificity migrate into the synovium activating T cells by presentation of a complex of antigen and IgG via the HLA-DR4 molecule and stimulating secretion of pro-inflammatory cytokines and co-stimulatory signals for T cell clonal expansion (Edwards and Cambridge 2001; Takemura et al. 2001; Keystone 2005). It was hypothesised that by eliminating this B cell antigen presentation to synovial T cells with rituximab, T cell activation and T cell dependent synovial inflammation would decrease. In addition, the ability of IgG RF B cells to self perpetuate, due to secretion of own antigen, provided rationale for the proposal that eradication of these cell clones may result in prolonged disease remission (Edwards et al. 1999). These theories were later elegantly supported by an experiment using transplantation of human synovial tissue from RA patients into SCID mice, which showed that the increase in synovial tissue graft cytokine production required the presence of B cells in lymphoid follicles (Takemura et al. 2001). Following rituximab therapy and subsequent B cell depletion, production of IFN-gamma and IL-1 were suppressed and arthritis failed to develop.

2.2 Trials of Rituximab in Rheumatoid Arthritis

2.2.1 The Initial Study and Open Trials of Rituximab in Rheumatoid Arthritis

Efficacy and response to new rheumatic medications is generally defined by either an outcome measure of the American College of Rheumatology (ACR) (Felson et al. 1995) or EULAR disease activity score 28 criteria (DAS28) (Prevoo et al. 1995). ACR criteria assesses the percentage improvement from baseline with regards: number of tender and swollen joints, patient pain (Visual Analogue Scale), global assessments by patient and physician (Visual Analogue Scales), self assessed physical disability and levels of acute phase reactants (Table 1). ACR20 is most often used, although ACR50 and ACR70 (reflecting larger percentage improvements from baseline) are being increasingly utilized and generally considered more clinically relevant. DAS28 is calculated using the formula $0.56\sqrt{TEN28} + 0.28\sqrt{SW28} + 0.70[\ln(ESR)] + 0.014(VAS)$ with TEN = number of tender joints, SW = number of swollen joints, ESR = erythrocyte sedimentation rate (mm/hour) and VAS = patient assessment of disease activity (mm) (Table 2).

B cell depletion in RA was initially trialled by Edwards and Cambridge in 5 patients resistant to at least five disease modifying anti-rheumatic drugs (DMARDS), based on the rationale that B cells contributed significantly to the pathogenesis of the disease (Edwards and Cambridge 2001). The small open labelled study combined rituximab infusions (600 mg days 2, 8, 15 and 22), cyclophosphamide (2×750 mg IVI days 4 and 17) and 60 mg oral prednisolone daily for 11–22 days then tapered to baseline dose. B cells were undetectable shortly after infusion and remained depressed for 6 months. All patients achieved ACR50 responses at 6 months

Table 1 American College of Rheumatology preliminary definition of 20% improvement in rheumatoid arthritis (ACR20)

Measure of Disease Activity	Requirement
Tender joint count	≥20% improvement
Swollen joint count	≥20% improvement
Patient's assessment of pain	
Patient's global assessment of disease activity	
Physician global assessment of disease activity	≥20% improvement in
Patient's assessment of physical function	three of the five measures
Markers of inflammation	

Table 2 Evaluation of the European League Against Rheumatism Modified Disease Activity Score (DAS28)

Current DAS28	DAS28: Difference to Initial Value		
	>1.2	>0.6≤1.2	≤0.6
≤3.2 Inactive	Good improvement	Moderate improvement	No improvement
>3.2≤5.1 Moderate	Moderate improvement	Moderate improvement	No improvement
>5.1 Very active	Moderate improvement	No improvement	No improvement

and three had ACR70. Clinical benefit persisted to approximately 12 months. Two patients who relapsed at 7 and 9 months, respectively, were retreated with a modified schedule of B cell depletion with good results. This study was extended to include 22 seropositive RA patients with disease resistant to multiple DMARDs (Leandro et al. 2002a). Patients were treated with varying protocols of rituximab, cyclophosphamide and/or high dose prednisolone to further assess dose response and requirement for additive therapies. Optimal treatment was determined as rituximab $\geq 600 \, \text{mg m}^{-2}$ plus cyclophosphamide. Apart from infrequent mild infusion reactions; no major adverse events attributable to therapy were reported. Rheumatoid factor titres and anti-cyclic citrullinated peptide (CCP) antibodies were depressed in all responders for 3–6 months, in contrast to total immunoglobulin which hardly declined. More detailed analysis of serological changes post B lymphocyte depletion therapy in 22 of the treated patients are shown in Table 3, and interestingly, mean anti-pneumococcal antibodies and anti-tetanus IgG did not decrease significantly (Cambridge et al. 2003). Sixteen of this University College London (UCL) cohort have now been followed for over 5 years (Edwards et al. 2005). Patients have been treated with up to four courses of rituximab, with mean duration of response being 15 months. Complications have included eight serious respiratory events, not clearly defined as infectious or due to infusion reactions, and reduction in IgM, IgA and IgG to below the lower limit of normal in a proportion of the patients. Two deaths, one from infection after changing to an anti-TNF-α agent and one from pre-existing cerebrovascular disease, have occurred. Analysis of the quantitative and phenotypic reconstitution of peripheral B cells in 24 of the UCL cohort revealed that re-population with mainly naïve B cells occurred at a mean of 8 months post treatment. Relapse of RA was only observed following peripheral repopulation with CD19+ cells, in half of the patients this occurred at the time of B cell repopulation and in the other half at a variable time post repopulation. Patients who relapsed at time of B cell re-emergence tended to repopulate with a higher frequency of CD27+ memory B cells than those who relapsed later, suggesting that less extensive B cell depletion in solid tissues may be associated with an earlier relapse of RA (Leandro et al. 2006).

A number of other open studies using slightly variable protocols have been published. These also demonstrated good clinical responses to rituximab (DAS28 < 2.6 or ACR20 and ACR50), reduction in rheumatoid factor levels parallel to disease

Table 3 Serologic parameters in patients before treatment and at nadir

Parameter, response to therapy	Pretreatment value (number of patients per group)	Lowest level attained after treatment	$P^{\dagger}$
IgM-RF			
Responders (15)	126 ± 78.2	50 ± 38.2	0.00006
Non-responders (5)	122 ± 16.8	90 ± 15.4	NS
IgG-RF			
Responders (10)	77 ± 25.9	15.5 ± 12.6	0.002
Non-responders (3)	50 ± 24.1	24.5 ± 13.5	NS
IgA-RF			
Responders (13)	147 ± 194.32	78 ± 86.1	0.0002
Non-responders (5)	158 ± 28.2	118 ± 18.5	NS
Anti-CCP			
Responders (8)	950 ± 340.9	236 ± 122.1	0.008
Non-responders (4)	$2,282 \pm 1,145$	$1,350 \pm 894$	NS
CRP			
Responders (15)	37.9 ± 8.4	$2 \pm 1.3^{\ddagger}$	0.00006
Non-responders (7)	39.7 ± 18	13.7 ± 5.4	NS

Responders were defined as having American College of Rheumatology $\geq 20\%$ improvement at 6 months. Values are the median $\pm$ SEM IU ml^{-1}, except values for C-reactive protein (CRP), which are the median $\pm$ SEM mg l^{-1}. IgM-RF = Immunoglobulin M Rheumatoid Factor; IgG $-$ RF = Immunoglobulin G Rheumatoid Factor; IgA $-$ RF = Immunoglobulin A Rheumatoid Factor; CCP = cyclic citrullinated peptide; NS = not significant.
[†] Pretreatment values vs. values at nadir for each group of patients tested, using Wilcoxon signed rank test with significance level of 0.1%
[‡] $P = 0.009$ vs. non-responders by Wilcoxon rank sum test
Reproduced with permission (Cambridge et al. 2003)

activity and absence of serious adverse events (De Vita et al. 2002; Kneitz et al. 2004).

2.2.2 Phase IIa Trial

A multicentre randomised double blind controlled study was performed to confirm these earlier open trial observations (Edwards et al. 2004). One hundred sixty one patients with seropositive RA, active despite at least 10 mg/week methotrexate were treated with either of the following:

1. Placebos for rituximab and cyclophosphamide + oral methotrexate ≥ 10 mg/week
2. One gram IVI rituximab days 1 and 15 + placebos for methotrexate and cyclophosphamide
3. One gram IVI rituximab days 1 and 15 + 750 mg IVI cyclophosphamide days 3 and 17 + placebo for methotrexate
4. One gram IVI rituximab days 1 and 15 + methotrexate ≥ 10 mg/week + placebo for cyclophosphamde

All received 17 days of corticosteroids as 100 mg IV methylprednisolone prior to rituximab and cyclophosphamide (or placebo) infusions together with 60 mg oral prednislone on days 2, days 4–7 and 30 mg daily on days 8–14. Anti-emetics and folinic acid were given to all patients and responses were defined according to criteria of the ACR and EULAR.

At week 24, 43% and 41% of patients given full dose rituximab + methotrexate and rituximab + cyclophosphamde, respectively, achieved ACR50 responses, which was significantly higher than that in the methotrexate alone group ($P = 0.005$ each) (Fig. 1). On exploratory analysis at 48 weeks, the ACR50 effect of rituximab and either methotrexate or cyclophosphamide remained significantly greater than compared to methotrexate alone ($P = 0.002$ and $P = 0.01$ respectively). The ACR50 response of the rituximab monotherapy group was higher than the control group; however this did not reach statistical significance. Patients in all rituximab groups showed significant improvement over methotrexate alone as measured by disease activity scores (DAS) and EULAR criteria ($P \leq 0.002$ and $P \leq 0.004$).

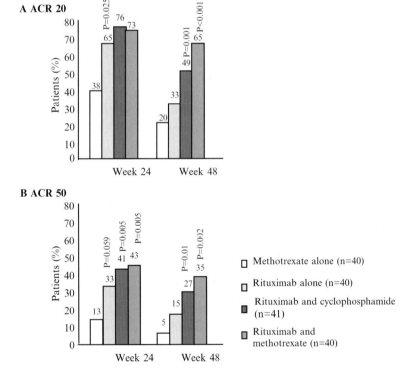

Fig. 1 American College of Rheumatology Clinical Responses at weeks 24 and 48 ACR 20 denotes at least a 20% improvement in disease symptoms according to the American College of Rheumatology (ACR) core set of outcome measures, ACR 50 a 50% improvement. *P* values are for comparisons with the methotrexate-monotherapy (control) group. Reproduced and adapted with permission (Edwards et al. 2004)

Table 4 Summary of adverse events

Adverse event	Methotrexate group (N = 40)	Rituximab groups (N = 40) No. of patients (%)	Rituximab–Cyclophosphamide group (N = 41)	Rituximab–Methotrexate group (N = 40)
Any Event				
Up to week 24	32 (80)	32 (80)	30 (73)	34 (85)
Up to week 48	34 (85)	36 (90)	35 (85)	35 (88)
Serious adverse event				
Up to week 24	3 (8)	2 (5)	6 (15)	3 (8)
Up to week 48	4 (10)	4 (10)	7 (17)	4 (10)
Any event associated with the first infusion	12 (30)	18 (45)	13 (32)	13 (33)
Specific event[a]				
Hypotension[b]	7 (18)	12 (30)	12 (29)	7 (18)
Exacerbation of RA	16 (40)	6 (15)	6 (15)	2 (5)
Hypertension[b]	6 (15)	6 (15)	3 (7)	10 (25)
Nasopharyngitis	6 (15)	4 (10)	2 (5)	4 (10)
Arthralgia	3 (8)	3 (8)	1 (2)	4 (10)
Rash	1 (3)	4 (10)	4 (10)	1 (3)
Back pain	2 (5)	4 (10)	3 (7)	0
Cough	0	5 (13)	1 (2)	2 (5)
Prutitus	0	4 (10)	4 (10)	0
Nausea	1 (3)	2 (5)	4 (10)	0
Dyspnea	0	4 (10)	0	0

[a] Adverse events that occurred in at least 10% of patients in any treatment group up to and including week 24 are shown

[b] A change of more than 30 mmHg in systolic or diastolic blood pressure from the pressure at screening was classified as hypotension or hypertension

Reproduced with permission (Edwards et al. 2004)

Near complete B cell depletion persisted throughout the 24 week study period. Rheumatoid factor titres decreased in all treatment groups although by 24 weeks had returned to baseline in the control group. Despite B cell depletion, total and immunoglobulin isotype levels did not drop below the normal range and anti-tetanus antibody titres were also unchanged. Changes in inflammatory markers reflected clinical disease and five of 117 patients who received rituximab developed HACA without significant clinical manifestations. About 30–45% of patients in all groups reported events associated with the first infusion, including transient hypo- or hypertension, pruritus and rash. Adverse events were similarly reported in all treatment groups, although serious adverse events were more common in the rituximab + cyclophosphamide group (Table 4). Serious infections occurred in one of the methotrexate group, 2 patients in the rituximab monotherapy group and 2 given rituximab + cyclophosphamide. Two further serious infections were reported in the extension to 48 weeks. This was a pivotal study that provided strong evidence that rituximab may offer another effective treatment option to patients with active RA despite methotrexate treatment.

2.2.3 Phase IIb Trial: Dose-Ranging Assessment International Clinical Evaluation of Rituximab in Rheumatoid Arthritis (DANCER)

A second larger multicentre randomised double blind placebo controlled trial aimed to determine the optimal rituximab dose and the role for concomitant corticosteroids in patients resistant to treatment with DMARDs, including biologic agents (Emery et al. 2006). Four hundred sixty five patients with active, poorly responsive disease were recruited, including those with seronegative disease. The study was of complex design with nine treatment groups consisting of various combinations of the following:

1. Rituximab infusion administered on days 1 and 15 as either (a) placebo; (b) 500 mg; or (c) 1,000 mg
2. Corticosteroids administered as either (a) placebo; (b) 100 mg methylprednisolone IVI days 1 and 15 or (c) 100 mg methylprednisolone IVI days 1 and 15 plus 60 mg oral prednisolone days 2–7 and 30 mg oral prednisolone days 8–14

All patients received methotrexate (10–25 mg/week). The primary endpoint was ACR20 at 24 weeks, although ACR50 and 70 responses were also assessed. The response rate was significantly superior for rituximab ($2\times$ infusions of either 500 mg or 1,000 mg) vs. placebo; ACR20 (55 and 54%, respectively, compared with placebo 28%; $P < 0.0001$), ACR50 (33, 34 and 13% of patients, respectively, $P < 0.001$) and ACR70 (13, 20 and 5% of patients ($P < 0.05$). Corticosteroids did not influence efficacy, however, IV methylprednisolone at infusion reduced the frequency and intensity of first infusion associated reactions by one third. Serious adverse events occurred in all groups (2.7, 7.3 and 6.8% in placebo, 500 mg rituximab and 1,000 mg rituximab, respectively). Six serious infections were reported, two in placebo and four in the rituximab treated groups. This study confirmed the safety and efficacy for both dosages of rituximab in patients with RA and suggested that whilst corticosteroids do not enhance treatment efficacy they may reduce infusion related reactions.

2.2.4 Phase III Trial: Randomised Evaluation of Long-term Efficacy of Rituximab in RA (REFLEX)

This phase III multicentre, randomised double-blind placebo controlled study aimed to determine the efficacy and safety of treatment with rituximab plus methotrexate (MTX) in patients with active rheumatoid arthritis (RA), who had an inadequate response to anti-TNF-α therapies (Cohen et al. 2006). Five hundred twenty patients on a stable dose of methotrexate, who failed to respond to one or more anti-TNF-α agent, were randomised at a 3:2 ratio to receive either two infusions of 1,000 mg rituximab or placebo (days 1 and 15). All received 100 mg methylprednislone pre-infusion and additional corticosteroids between infusions. The primary efficacy endpoint was ACR20 at 24 weeks, with secondary endpoints of ACR50, ACR70, DAS 28 and EULAR response criteria, after which patients were followed for an overall duration of 24 months. X-ray data were collected using the Genant-modified Sharp radiographic scores and additional information obtained via the Health Assessment Questionnaire (HAQ), Short Form 36 (SF-36) Functional Assessment of Chronic Illness Therapy-Fatigue (FACIT-F) and Disability Index (DI) instruments.

Significantly more patients receiving rituximab achieved ACR20 (51% vs. 18%), ACR50 (27% vs. 5%) and ACR70 (12% vs. 1%) compared to patients receiving methotrexate alone ($P < 0.0001$ for each) (Fig. 2a). Similarly, significantly more patients treated with rituximab demonstrated moderate to good EULAR responses (65% vs. 22%) ($P < 0.0001$) (Fig. 2b), reduction in RF titres and decreased CRP and ESR levels. Whilst fewer RF negative patients reached ACR20 than RF positive patients, there remained a significant difference between each group and placebo (RF negative $P < 0.0009$ and RF positive $P < 0.0001$). This treatment effect in the RF negative patients further suggests that in addition to acting through mechanisms involving RF and other autoantibody production, rituximab may also function via several different pathogenic pathways affecting T cell activation and cytokine production. Clinically valid improvements in SF-36, HAQ and FACIT-F were evident and a trend to less radiological progression was seen. Whether

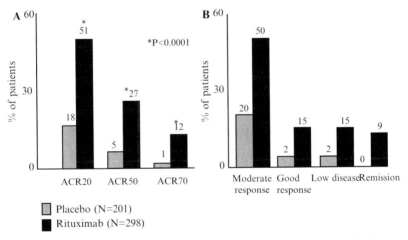

Fig. 2 Responses to treatment at week 24 in the intent-to-treat population. (**a**) Percentages of patients achieving a response according to the American College of Rheumatology 20% improvement criteria (ACR20), 50% improvement criteria (ACR50) and 70% improvement criteria (ACR70). The ACR20, ACR50 and ACR70 responses in rituximab treated patients were statistically significant ($P<0.0001$) compared with those in the placebo treated patients. (**b**) Percentages of patients achieving a response according to the European League Against Rheumatism (EULAR) criteria at week 24. EULAR responses defined as follows: moderate represents a Disease Activity Score 28 – joint assessment for swelling and tenderness (DAS28) of <5.1 and an improvement from 0.6 to 1.2; good represents a DAS28 score of <3.2 and an improvement of >1.2; low disease activity represents a DAS28 score of ≤3.2; remission represents a DAS28 score of <2.6. The EULAR moderate and good responses in the rituximab group (65%) were statistically significant ($P<0.0001$) compared with the placebo group (22%). Numbers above the bars are the numerical percentages represented by the bars. Reproduced with permission (Cohen et al. 2006)

rituximab can actually reduce progression of joint erosion and damage requires further evaluation and will be reported after longer term follow-up studies are completed. Adverse events were comparable to previous studies, including mild-moderate infusion reactions occurring with the first infusion of rituximab, which resulted in the withdrawal of five patients. The incidence of infections was slightly higher in the rituximab treated group (41%) compared to the placebo group (38%) and typically consisted of upper respiratory tract infections, bronchitis, sinusitis and urinary tract infections. Seven serious infections occurred in the rituximab group and three in the placebo group; however, there were no reports of tuberculosis or opportunistic infections in the study period.

This study has expanded the previous efficacy and safety profile of rituximab and demonstrated that rituximab is a therapeutic option for RA patients who have responded inadequately to one or more anti-TNF-α agents.

3 Anti-CD20 Monoclonal Antibody (Rituximab) for the Treatment of Systemic Lupus Erythematosus

3.1 Role of B Cells in Pathogenesis of Systemic Lupus Erythematosus

Patients with systemic lupus erythematosus may develop heterogeneous clinical manifestations ranging from non-specific symptoms such as fatigue and arthralgia to life threatening renal or cerebral disease. SLE is characterised immunologically by a variety of autoantibodies to deoxyribonucleic acid (DNA), ribonucleic acid (RNA), other nuclear antigens (e.g. Ro, La) and cytoplasmic antigens, with pathogenicity most closely linked to anti-dsDNA and anti-Ro autoantibodies (Hagelberg et al. 2002; Rahman et al. 2002; Buyon and Clancy 2003). Although the exact aetiopathogenesis of SLE remains uncertain, there is consensus that its aetiology is dependent upon a combination of environmental, hormonal, genetic and immunological factors. Whilst many facets of the immune system including pathogenic T cells, cytokines and autoantibodies may play a role, experimental evidence indicates that loss of B cell tolerance and B cell dysfunction is a central feature, thus providing a rationale for trials to further evaluate the anti-CD20 monoclonal antibody rituximab for treatment of SLE (Chan et al. 1999b).

In patients with SLE, autoreactive T cells are necessary to activate B cells, which are then further stimulated to proliferate and produce autoantibodies by the elevated levels of pro-inflammatory cytokines, including TNF-α, interleukin (IL)-6, IL-10 and interferon (IFN)-γ (Davas et al. 1999; Tokano et al. 1999). Furthermore, the autoantibody production may be enhanced by T and B cell interaction via co-stimulatory molecules that generate anti-apoptotic signals or stimulated by the failure to efficiently remove the apoptotic cells (Herrmann et al. 1998; Taylor et al. 2000). Cytokine imbalance between IL-10 and IL-12 (Houssiau et al. 1995; Liu and Jones 1998) results in further B cell activation and inhibition of T cell function (Emilie and Mariette 2001). IL-12 levels are down-regulated by IL-10, with lower levels correlating with increased disease activity and nephritis (Liu and Jones 1998; Min et al. 2001). Interestingly, B cells also appear to have an autoantibody independent role in SLE, including presentation of self antigen to T cells and regulation of T cell activation (Chan et al. 1999a). An antibody-independent role is also supported by clinical recent studies, which demonstrate significant improvement in SLE disease activity following rituximab induced B cell depletion even in the absence of substantial antibody reduction (Anolik et al. 2004; Looney et al. 2004).

3.2 Trials of Rituximab in Systemic Lupus Erythematosus

3.2.1 Open Phase I/II Trials

Increasingly, rituximab is being studied in patients with SLE unresponsive or poorly responsive to conventional therapies. Several small uncontrolled series have suggested merit for B cell depletion in this cohort, although formal placebo controlled studies remain outstanding. An early phase I/II trial of rituximab for patients with mild to moderately active SLE without severe organ involvement reported tolerance and efficacy using a dose escalation protocol of between a single $100\,mg\,m^{-2}$ dose and four weekly $375\,mg\,m^{-2}$ doses with 40 mg oral prednisolone pre-treatment (Anolik 2002). Twelve patients were initially treated, later extended to 18 (Looney et al. 2004), demonstrating that higher dosage resulted in more prolonged and consistent B cell depletion. Effective B cell depletion was associated with significant improvements in the Systemic Lupus Activity Measure (SLAM) score by 1 month, which persisted for 12 months. Interestingly, despite these significant improvements as assessed by the SLAM, corrections in anti-dsDNA antibody titres and complement occurred variably, although they were altered in the in two patients who had complete and prolonged B cell depletion. In patients in whom B cells did not deplete well, SLAM scores did not improve, and in some HACAs developed. Development of HACAs was associated with lower doses of rituximab, less depletion of B cells, higher baseline SLAM scores, homozygosity for the low affinity allele FcγRIIIa and African American ancestry. As part of these studies, evaluation of discrete peripheral B cell subsets in the patients after B cell depletion demonstrated improvements in B cell homeostasis and tolerance, despite persistence of autoantibodies, supporting an antibody-independent role for B cells in SLE pathogenesis (Anolik et al. 2004). Of interest, another phase I/II open study using full dose rituximab also reported excellent B cell depletion in six of seven patients without evidence of serological changes (Albert et al. 2003).

Six patients with more severe active disease were investigated in an open study using a combination of two doses of 500 mg rituximab, two 750 mg infusions of cyclophosphamide and high dose oral corticosteroids. One patient was unresponsive at 3 months and then lost to follow up. All the remaining patients improved clinically in their systemic, cutaneous and joint symptoms as assessed by the British Isles Lupus Assessment Group (BILAG), and a proportion showed improvement in haematological parameters, C3 levels and anti-dsDNA titres (Leandro et al. 2002b). The BILAG index distinguishes disease activity in eight organs or systems and is based on the principle of the physician's intention to treat (Hay et al. 1993). In the patients with nephritis, improvement in urine protein to creatinine ratio was observed. Extended review demonstrated that two of the five patients continued disease free and without immunosuppressive agents for 2 and 3 years post B cell depletion, respectively. Relapse occurred in the remaining patients simultaneously or post B cell repopulation. Similarly encouraging results were published by the same group who used two doses of 1,000 mg rituximab, two doses of 750 mg cyclophosphamide and high dose corticosteroids over 2 weeks for 14 patients with treatment 'resistant' active renal lupus (WHO class IV or V), including failure with intravenous cyclophosphamide (Leandro et al. 2003). Reponses of six of the most 'homogenous' patients with lupus nephritis were analysed, and reductions in disease activity, improvement in renal function and immunological and haematological indices were reported. Apart from mild infusion reactions, adverse events were minimal. Vigna-Perez and colleagues Vigna-Perez et al. (2006) also studied the clinical and immunological effects of rituximab in 22 patients with active disease and lupus nephritis (mainly WHO class III or IV) refractory to conventional therapies. Twenty patients depleted sufficiently and significant reductions in disease activity (MEX-SLEDAI) and proteinuria $(p < 0.05)$ were achieved. No significant changes in dsDNA antibody levels or complement levels were detected. There was one patient death due to an opportunistic infection and no other serious adverse events were observed. This study also examined the effect of rituximab on regulatory T lymphocytes, demonstrating a transient rise in various subsets, including $T_{REG}(CD4 + CD25^{bright})$ and Tr1 $(CD4 + IL - 10+)$ cells accompanied by an increase in the suppressor function of T_{REG} lymphocytes. Apoptosis of T cells were also increased, and further work is required to elucidate the mechanism responsible.

In 2005, Leandro and colleagues Leandro et al. (2005) reported the long-term follow-up data of 24 patients with severe SLE who had received rituximab in an open study (usually 1 g IV 2 weeks apart) accompanied by two 750 mg cyclophosphamide infusions and two methylprednisolone infusions of 250 mg each. Disease activity was assessed every 1–2 months using the BILAG system and estimates of anti-dsDNA antibodies and serum C3 levels. In accordance with this groups' usual practice, concomittant immunosuppressive agents were stopped when B cell depletion was given. One patient did not deplete and one repopulated at 3 months requiring re-treatment. Manifestations such as arthralgia/arthritis, fatigue, serositis, nephritis, thrombocytopenia and haemolytic anaemia responded particularly well. From the time of B cell depletion to 6 months post therapy, the mean global BILAG score, serum C3 and dsDNA binding all significantly improved $(P < 0.00001,$ $P < 0.0005$ and $P < 0.002$, respectively). The period of B cell depletion ranged from 3–8 months, except for one patient who remains depleted over 5 years. Treatment was well tolerated in the majority of patients. A review of repeated B cell depletion therapy for patients with refractory SLE reported a median clinical benefit of 12 months and a favourable safety profile, which augurs well for longer term treatment (Ng et al. 2006). There has been a single report of use of humanised anti-CD20 monoclonal antibody for the treatment of a patient with severe treatment resistant SLE, which described remarkable clinical and serological improvement despite the presence of a HACA following rituximab use (Tahir et al. 2005).

Together, these open studies support the notion that rituximab therapy seems to offer an alternative option for lupus patients with active systemic disease, who have failed or are only partially responsive to conventional treatments. Future studies should help clarify the observed variability in the degree of B cell depletion that is achieved with rituximab in patients with SLE and also in the association between B cell depletion, levels of circulating antibodies and patient response. Trials to establish optimal dosing regimens, requirements for adjuvant therapies and long-term tolerability are in progress but most importantly, we eagerly await publication of a large double blind randomised control trial.

4 Future B Cell Targeted Therapies

4.1 Epratuzumab

Epratuzumab is a humanised monoclonal antibody recognising the pan B cell surface marker CD22. In addition to being a target on B cells, the CD22 molecule is involved in intracellular signalling and also modifies signalling via other surface molecules, including the B cell receptor. Genetic studies have demonstrated that CD22 polymorphisms are linked to SLE, making it an attractive therapeutic target for autoimmune diseases. The benefit of epratuzumab may be twofold; either via B cell depletion and/or modification of B cell function. In a recently published open study of 14 patients with moderately active SLE, patients received intravenous two weekly $360\,mg\,m^{-2}$ epratuzumab with four doses with anti-histamine/analgesic premedication (Dorner et al. 2006). No steroids were administered with the treatment. Regular evaluation over 18 weeks demonstrated a $\geq 50\%$ reduction in BILAG scores, although due to small numbers statistical significance could not be shown. The medication was well tolerated and an approximately 35–40% decrease in B cell was achieved with epratuzumab without significant changes in T cells, immunoglobulins or autoantibodies. As in other reports of its use, therapeutic practice with epratuzumab is complicated by inconsistent and unpredictable effects of the drug in individual patients. Further evaluation requires larger controlled studies before more widespread utilisation.

4.2 Anti-B Lymphocyte Stimulator Monoclonal Antibody

B Lymphocyte Stimulator (BLys) is a member of the tumour necrosis factor ligand superfamily and a human monoclonal antibody against it has been shown to modulate B cell immune responses by a reduction of apoptosis and interference in B cell development and differentiation. A phase I open study using anti-BLys monoclonal antibody demonstrated a reduction in anti-dsDNA antibody titres and immunoglobulins (Furie 2003). Belimumab, the lead in a series of human monoclonal antibodies against the human protein BLyS (Human Genome Sciences, Cambridge Antibody Technology and GlaxoSmithKline), has completed phase II clinical trials in RA and SLE. The double blind placebo controlled trial with belimumab $(1,4$ or $10\,\mathrm{mg\,kg^{-1}}$ or placebo at 0,14 and 28 days followed by every 4 weeks for 24 weeks) in 283 patients with RA demonstrated drug tolerability and efficacy (McKay et al. 2005). There were significant improvements in ACR20 at 24 weeks compared to placebo, although sub-analysis revealed none of the sero-negative patients had an ACR20 response at 24 weeks. Overall, the clinical effect was negligible and may not be clinically significant, thus necessitating further studies. A phase III clinical trial of belimumab for patients with SLE is scheduled to begin in late 2006.

5 Conclusion

In studies to date, rituximab appears to be an efficacious and a generally well tolerated treatment option for patients with RA and SLE poorly or partially responsive to more conventional therapies. Definitive confirmation, however, of its role in SLE awaits the outcome of randomised controlled trials. In both RA and SLE there may be variability in the degree of B cell depletion achieved with rituximab, and also in the association between B cell depletion, levels of circulating antibodies and patient response (Edwards and Cambridge 2001; Specks et al. 2001; Anolik et al. 2004). Further studies to address these questions are necessary and future clinical trials will also continue to evaluate important long term safety data, as well as further exploring the role of rituximab in rheumatoid factor negative RA, whether rituximab therapy triggers or exacerbates other autoimmune diseases and whether it prevents disease progression or even induces long term remission. There is also a need to establish clinical and serological profiles of those patients with RA and SLE who are more, or less, likely to respond well to B cell depletion. The next few years promise to continue as exciting times as B cell targeted therapies in RA and SLE patients develop and we benefit from increasing understanding of autoimmune disease pathogenesis.

References

Albert DA, Khan SR, Stansberry JS, Tsai D, Kamoun M et al. (2003) A phase I trial of rituximab (anti-CD20) for treatment of systemic lupus. Arthritis Rheum 48:S3659
Anolik JH (2002) B lymphocyte depletion in the treatment of systemic lupus erythematosus. Arthritis Rheum 46:S717

Anolik JH, Campbell D, Felgar R et al. (2003) The relationship of FcgammaRIIIA genotype to degree of B cell depletion by rituximab in the treatment for systemic lupus erythematosus. Arthritis Rheum 48:455–459

Anolik JH, Barnard J, Cappione A, Pugh-Bernard AE, Felgar RE, Looney RJ, Sanz I (2004) Rituximab improves peripheral B cell abnormalities in human systemic lupus erythematosus. Arthritis Rheum 50:3580–3590

Buyon JP, Clancy RM (2003) Neonatal lupus: Review of proposed pathogenesis and clinical data from the US-based research registry for neonatal lupus. Autoimmunity 36:41–50

Cambridge G, Leandro MJ, Edwards JCW, Ehrenstein MR, Salden M, Bodman-Smith M, Webster ADB (2003) Serologic changes following B lymphocyte depletion therapy for rheumatoid arthritis. Arthritis Rheum 48:2146–2154

Chan OT, Hannum LG, Haberman AM, Madaio MP, Shlomchik MJ (1999) A novel mouse with B cells but lacking serum antibody reveals an antibody-independent role for B cells in murine lupus. J Exp Med 189:1639–1648

Chan OT, Madaio MP, Shlomchik MJ (1999) The central and multiple roles of B cells in lupus pathogenesis. Immunol Rev 169:107–121

Cohen SB, Emery P, Greenwald MW, Dougados M, Furie RA, Genovese MC, Keystone EC, Loveless JE, Burmester GR, Cravets MW, Hessey EW, Shaw T, Totoritis MC (2006) Rituximab for rheumatoid arthritis refractory to anti-tumor necrosis factor therapy: Results of a multicenter, randomized, double-blind, placebo-controlled, phase III trial evaluating primary efficacy and safety at twenty-four weeks. Arthritis Rheum 54:2793–2806

Davas EM, Tsirogianni A, Kappou I, Karamitsos D, Economidou I, Dantis PC (1999) Serum IL-6, TNFalpha, p55 srTNFalpha, p75srTNFalpha, srIL-2alpha levels and disease activity in systemic lupus erythematosus. Clin Rheumatol 18:17–22

De Vita S, Zaja F, Sacco S et al. (2002) Efficacy of selelctive B cell blockade in the treatment of rheumatoid arthritis: evidence for a pathogenic role of B cells. Arthritis Rheum 46:2029–2033

Dorner T, Kaufmann J, Wegener WA, Teoh N, Goldenberg DM, Burmester GR (2006) Initial clinical trial of epratuzumab (humanized anti-CD22 antibody) for immunotherapy of systemic lupus erythematosus. Arthritis Res Ther 8:R76

Edwards JCW, Cambridge G, Abrahams VM (1999) Do self-perpetuating B lymphocytes drive human autoimmune disease? Immunology 97:1868–1896

Edwards JCW, Cambridge G (2001) Sustained improvement in rheumatoid arthritis following a protocol designed to deplete B lymphocytes. Rheumatology 40:205–211

Edwards JCW, Szczepanski L, Szechinski J, Filipowicz-Sosnowska A, Emery P, Close DR, Stevens RM, Shaw T (2004) Efficacy of B-Cell-targeted therapy with rituximab in patients with rheumatoid arthritis. NEJM 350:2572–2581

Edwards JCW, Leandro MJ, Cambridge G (2005) Repeated B lymphocyte depletion therapy in rheumatoid arthritis. Arthritis Rheum 52:S13S

Emery P, Fleischmann R, Filipowicz-Sosnowska A, Schechtman J, Szczepanski L, Kavanaugh AM, Racewicz AJ, van Vollenhoven RF, Li NF, Agarwal S, Hessey EW, Shaw TM (2006) The efficacy and safety of rituximab in patients with active rheumatoid arthritis despite methotrexate treatment. Arthritis Rheum 54:1390–1400

Emilie D, Mariette X (2001) Interleukin 10: A new therapeutic target in systemic lupus erythematosus? Joint Bone Spine 68:4–5

Felson DT, Anderson JJ, Boers M, Bombardier C, Furst D, Goldsmith C, Katz LM, Lightfoot RJ, Paulus H, Strand V et al. (1995) Preliminary definition of improvement in rheumatoid arthritis. Arthritis Rheum 38:727–735

Furie R (2003) Safety, pharmacokinetic and pharmacodynamic results of a phase I single and double dose-escalation study of LymphoStat-B (human monoclonal antibody to BLyS) in SLE patients. Arthritis Rheum 48:S377

Hagelberg S, Lee Y, Bargman J et al. (2002) Longterm followup of childhood lupus nephritis. J Rheumatol 29:2635–2642

Hay EM, Bacon PA, Gordon C et al. (1993) The BILAG index: A reliable and valid instrument for measuring clinical disease activity in systemic lupus erythematosus. Q J Med 86:447–458

Herrmann M, Voll RE, Zoller OM, Hagenhofer M, Ponner BB, Kalden JR (1998) Impaired phagocytosis of apoptotic cell material by monocyte-derived macrophages from patients with systemic lupus erythematosus. Arthritis Rheum 41:1241–1250

Houssiau FA, Lefebvre C, Van den Berghe M, Lambert M, Devogelaer JP, Renauld JC (1995)
Serum interleukin 10 titers in systemic lupus erythematosus reflect disease activity. Lupus
4:393–395

Keystone EC (2005) B cells in rheumatoid arthritis: From hypothesis to the clinic. Rheumatology
44:ii8–ii12

Kneitz C, Wilhelm M, Tony HP (2004) Improvement of refractory rheumatoid arthritis after depletion of B cells. Scand J Rheumatol 33:82–86

Leandro MJ, Edwards JCW, Cambridge G (2002a) Clinical outcome in 22 patients with rheumatoid
arthritis treated with B lymphocte depletion. Ann Rheum Dis 61:883–888

Leandro MJ, Edwards JCW, Cambridge G, Ehrenstein MR, Isenberg DA (2002b) An open study
of B lymphocyte depletion in systemic lupus erythematosus. Arthritis Rheum 46:2673–2677

Leandro MJ, Ehrenstein MR, Edwards JC, Manson J, Cambridge G, Isenberg DA (2003) Treatment
of refractory lupus nephritis with B lymphocyte depletion. Arthritis Rheum 48:S924

Leandro MJ, Cambridge G, Edwards JCW, Ehrenstein MR, Isenberg DA (2005) B-cell depletion
in the treatment of patients with systemic lupus erythematosus: A longitudinal analysis of 24
patients. Rheumatology 44:1542–1545

Leandro MJ, Cambridge G, Ehrenstein MR, Edwards JCW (2006) Reconstitution of peripheral
blood B cells after depletion with rituximab in patients with rheumatoid arthritis. Arthritis
Rheum 54:613–620

Liu TF, Jones BM (1998) Impaired production of IL-12 in systemic lupus erythematosus. I. Excessive production of IL-10 suppresses production of IL-12 by monocytes. Cytokine 10:140–147

Looney RJ, Anolik JH, Campbell D, Felgar RE, Young F, Arend LJ, Sloand JA, Rosenblatt J,
Sanz I (2004) B cell depletion as a novel treatment for systemic lupus erythematosus. Arthritis
Rheum 50:2580–2589

Maloney DG, Smith B, Rose A (2002) Rituximab: Mechanism of action and resistance. Semin
Oncol 29:2–9

Mannik M, Nardella FA (1985) IgG rheumatoid factors and self-association of these antibodies.
Clin Rheum Dis 11:551–572

McKay J, Chwalinska-Sadowska H, Boling E et al. (2005) Belimumab (BmAb), a fully human
monoclonal antibody to B-lymphocyte stimulator (BLys), combined with standard of care
reduces the signs and symptoms of rheumatoid arthritis in a heterogenous subject population.
Arthritis Rheum 52:S710

Min DJ, Cho ML, Cho CS et al. (2001) Decreased production of interleukin-12 and interferon-
gamma is associated with renal involvement in systemic lupus erythematosus. Scand J Rheumatol 30:159–163

Ng KP, Leandro MJ, Edwards JCW, Ehrenstein MR, Cambridge G, Isenberg DA (2006) Repeated
B cell depletion in treatment of refractory systemic lupus erythematosus. Ann Rheum Dis
65:942–945

Panayi GS (2005) B cells: A fundamental role in the pathogenesis of rheumatoid arthritis? Rheumatology 44:ii3–ii7

Press OW, Appelbaum F, Ledbetter JA et al. (1987) Monoclonal antibody 1F5 (anti-CD20)
serotherapy of human B cell lymphomas. Blood 69:584–591

Prevoo ML, van't Hof MA, Kuper HH, van Leeuwen MA, van de Putte LB, van Riel PL (1995)
Modified disease activity scores that include twenty-eight-joint counts. Development and validation in a prospective longitudinal study of patients with rheumatoid arthritis. Arthritis Rheum
38:44–48

Rahman A, Giles I, Haley J, Isenberg D (2002) Systematic analysis of sequences of anti-DNA
antibodies – relevance to theories of origin and pathogenicity. Lupus 11:807–823

Sfikakis PP, Boletis JN, Lionaki S, Vigklis V, Fragiadaki KG, Iniotaki A et al. (2005) Remission of
proliferative lupus nephritis following B cell depletion therapy is preceded by down-regulation

of the T cell costimulatory molecule CD40ligans: An open label trial. Arthritis Rheum 52: 501–513

Specks U, Fervenza FC, McDonald TJ, Hogan MC (2001) Response of Wegener's granulomatosis to anti-CD20 chimeric monoclonal antibody therapy. Arthritis Rheum 44:2836–2840

Stasi R, Pagano A, Stipa E, Amadori S (2001) Rituximab chimeric anti-CD20 monoclonal antibody treatment for adults with chronic idiopathic thrombocytopaenic purpura. Blood 98:952–957

Tahir H, Rohrer J, Bhatia A, Wegener WA, Isenberg DA (2005) Humanized anti-CD20 monoclonal antibody in the treatment of severe resistant systemic lupus erythematosus in a patient with antibodies against rituximab. Rheumatology 44:561–562

Takemura S, Klimiuk PA, Braun A, Goronzy JJ, Weyand CM (2001) T cell activation in rheumatoid synovium is B cell dependent. J Immunol 167:4710–4718

Taylor PR, Carugati A, Fadok VA, Cook HT, Andrews M, Carroll MC, Savill JS, Henson PM, Botto M, Walport MJ (2000) A hierarchical role for classical pathway complement proteins in the clearance of apoptotic cells in vivo. J Exp Med 192:359–366

Tokano Y, Morimoto S, Kaneko H et al. (1999) Levels of IL-12 in the sera of patients with systemic lupus erythematosus (SLE) – relation to Th1- and Th2-derived cytokines. Clin Exp Immunol 16:169–173

Tokunaga M, Fujii K, Saito K, Nakayamada S, Tsujimura S, Nawata M et al. (2005) Down-regulation of CD40 and CD80 on B cells in patients with life-threatening systemic lupus erythematosus after successful treatment with rituximab. Rheumatology 44:176–182

Vigna-Perez M, Hernandez-Castro B, Paredes-Saharopulos O, Portales-Perez D, Baranda L, Abud-Mendoza C, Gonzalez-Amaro R (2006) Clinical and immunological effects of Rituximab in patients with lupus nephritis refractory to conventional therapy: A pilot study. Arthritis Res Ther 8:R83

Weng WK, Levy R (2003) Two immunoglobulin G fragment C receptor polymorphisms independently predict response to rituximab in patients with follicular lymphoma. J Clin Onc 21:3940–3947

Herceptin

H.M. Shepard(✉), P. Jin, D.J. Slamon, Z. Pirot, and D.C. Maneval

1   Magic Bullets and Monoclonal Antibodies.. 184
2   The Discovery and Development of HER Therapeutics 185
   2.1   Setting the Stage 185
   2.2   The Development of a Preclinical Rationale 186
   2.3   A Perversion of Nature 186
   2.4   Biologic Effects of Amplified HER2 Expression 189
   2.5   Proof of Concept for Antagonists of p185^{HER2} 190
   2.6   In Vivo Proof of Concept with MuMAb4D5 193
3   Proof of Concept for Therapeutic Antibodies in Solid Cancer 194
   3.1   The Controversy About Making a Successful Monoclonal Antibody Therapeutic
        vs. Solid Cancer 194
   3.2   MuMAb4D5 Therapy for Breast Cancer 195
   3.3   Phase I Investigation with MuMAb4D5.................................... 197
4   Development of Herceptin 197
   4.1   Humanized Versions of MuMAb4D5..................................... 197
   4.2   Characterization of Herceptin In Vivo 198
   4.3   Summary of the History of Clinical Trials with Herceptin..................... 201
   4.4   Current Status and Significance of Herceptin 203
5   Alternative Therapies Targeting p185^{HER2} 205
   5.1   Radiolabeled Herceptin 205
   5.2   Active Specific Immunotherapy (ASI) 206
6   New Approaches to the Human EGFR Family...................................... 207
   6.1   Current Status of the Human EGFR Family 207
   6.2   Pan-HER Ligand Traps 207
   6.3   Inhibition of Ligand-Induced Receptor Phosphorylation by Hermodulins.......... 209
   6.4   Hermodulins Inhibit Tumor Cell Proliferation In Vivo......................... 211
7   Summary and Conclusions: What We Have Learned
       and What to Do Next... 211
References 212

H.M. Shepard

Receptor BioLogix, Inc., 3350 W. Bayshore Rd., Suite 150, Palo Alto, CA 94303, USA

e-mail: hms@rblx.com

Y. Chernajovsky, A. Nissim (eds.) *Therapeutic Antibodies. Handbook of Experimental Pharmacology 181.*
© Springer-Verlag Berlin Heidelberg 2008

Abstract The biology of the human epidermal growth factor (EGF) receptor-2 (HER2) has been reviewed numerous times and provides an excellent example for developing a targeted cancer therapeutic. Herceptin, the FDA-approved therapeutic monoclonal antibody against HER2, has been used to treat over 150,000 women with breast cancer. However, the developmental history of Herceptin, the key events within the program that created pivotal decision points, and the reasons why decisions were made to pursue the monoclonal antibody approach have never been adequately described. The history of Herceptin is reviewed in a way which allows the experience to be shared for the purposes of understanding the drug discovery and development process. It is the objective of this review to describe the pivotal events and explain why critical decisions were made that resulted in the first therapeutic to successfully target tyrosine kinases in cancer. New approaches and future prospects for therapeutics targeting the HER family are also discussed.

1 Magic Bullets and Monoclonal Antibodies

The specific targeting of disease-causing organisms, or diseased cells, was first articulated by Ehrlich, who reasoned that because it is possible to differentially stain cancer and normal cells, it should be possible to specifically target cancer (perspective by Witkop 1999). Based upon this work, many successful chemotherapeutics have been created. However, because diseased and normal cells share biochemical pathways, and are much more similar than they are different, targeting disease processes by interrupting cellular metabolism without toxicity to the host has remained a problem in drug discovery.

Subtle differences between normal and tumor cells include a greater dependence of cancer cells on glucose metabolism instead of the citric acid cycle for the generation of adenosine triphosphate (the "Warburg Effect"; Ashrafian 2006), and a greater use of uracil to support their growth ("uracil flux"), leading to the discovery of fluorouracil as a chemotherapeutic (Heidelberger et al. 1957). These targets for therapy share the inherent problem that the differences are a matter of degree. While the fluorouracils are clearly effective, with a role to play in the treatment of many cancers (Dorr and Von Hoff 1994), their efficacy is more a result of the relative leakiness of blood vessels in tumors (leading to drug localization) than it is to the specific targeting of cancer cell metabolism. In fact, thymidylate synthase, the enzyme inhibited by the fluorouracils, is predictably expressed to a higher degree in tumor cells than it is in normal cells. As a result, normal cells (with lower thymidylate synthase, like gut epithelium, skin fibroblasts, and hematopoeitic cells) are generally more sensitive to the cytotoxic effects of fluorouracils than are tumor cells, which have a higher intracellular concentration of the enzyme (Lackey et al. 2001; Li et al. 2001). The goal of the modern era of cancer treatment is to create drugs that preferentially damage tumor cells based upon their specific biochemical properties, and leave normal cells relatively free from injury: the realization of Ehrlich's "magic bullet" hypothesis.

The enablement of this goal in cancer treatment required several important advances in drug discovery. Key discoveries include identifying cancer-specific antigens (e.g., tyrosine kinases and other enzymes), understanding disease pathways, and developing a means for specifically targeting diseased cells. The discovery of viral oncogenes which encode tyrosine kinases, and subsequently the finding that mutations in some normal cellular tyrosine kinases can cause them to become oncogenic, resulting in cellular transformation (immortality, anchorage independent growth, and the ability to form tumors in immune-deficient mice), reviewed by Bishop (1989) and Varmus (1989), provided the basis for targeting the human epidermal growth factor receptor 2 (HER2) protooncogene with a monoclonal antibody. Since the approval of Herceptin in 1998, the tyrosine kinases have become the archetypical example of a validated target in cancer, and monoclonal antibodies have become an accepted biopharmaceutical to target cell surface receptors.

Especially relevant to Herceptin, the early enabling oncogene discovery was the finding that the v-erb-B oncogene, derived from chicken erythroblastosis virus, shared significant homology with the human epidermal growth factor receptor (EGFR or HER1), thereby giving rise to the hypothesis that under conditions of constitutive activation, EGFR might be implicated in human cancer (Kris et al. 1985). Further work proved this hypothesis and motivated the discovery of HER2, also known as human NEU, erb-B2, or NGL (Coussens et al. 1985; King et al. 1985; Schechter et al. 1985; Semba et al. 1985; Yarden and Ullrich 1988). The focus of this chapter is the discovery and pharmacological studies that led to the approval of Herceptin, a humanized monoclonal antibody targeting the receptor extracellular domain encoded by HER2 ($p185^{HER2}$). At the time when Investigational New Drug (IND)-enabling efforts began for Herceptin, only EGFR and HER2 had been described (Yarden and Ullrich 1988). The field has made tremendous advances since this time, powered in large part by the commercial success of Herceptin. Herceptin provided the first "magic bullet" targeted at tyrosine kinases to treat cancer. A discussion later in the chapter will outline newer approaches to targeting the Human EGFR (HER) family.

2 The Discovery and Development of HER Therapeutics

2.1 Setting the Stage

Direct causal relationships between oncogene amplification and/or overexpression and certain types of cancer were less well defined in the 1980s (during the initial development efforts for Herceptin) than they are now. One of the most critical events in the research leading to Herceptin was reported by Weinberg and colleagues (Schechter et al. 1984). This involved the discovery of the first oncogenic receptor tyrosine kinase oncogene, NEU. It was discovered by gene transfection/transformation of fragmented DNA from a series of rat neuroblastomas into NIH 3T3 cells (the focus-forming assay; Shih et al. 1981).

The product of the HER2 protooncogene (p185^{HER2}) is a transmembrane Type 1 receptor tyrosine kinase with extensive homology to the EGFR (Coussens et al. 1985; Schechter et al. 1985; Yarden and Ullrich 1988) and now known to have similar homology with HER3 and HER4 (Katoh et al. 1993; Zhou and Carpenter 2002). HER2 can be distinguished from HER1, 3, and 4 by differences in chromosomal location, transcript size, molecular mass, ligand activation of the associated tyrosine kinase, and antigenicity, as determined by interaction with specific monoclonal antibodies (Citri and Yarden 2006; Kumar and Pegram 2006; Prenzel et al. 2001).

We will review the science behind Herceptin development from a historical perspective. It is our goal to provide a roadmap that can be generally applied to the assembly of the rationale for the development of other successful therapeutics. We will describe the progression of the science beginning with the discovery of the HER2 protooncogene through the demonstration that overexpression leads to cellular transformation, tumor cell resistance to elements of the host immune system, and other characteristics that create a disease-specific signaling pathway in cancer cells. This pathway was the focus of efforts that resulted in the development of Herceptin, the first biopharmaceutical to demonstrate clinical proof of concept and the value of targeting tyrosine kinases in cancer.

2.2 The Development of a Preclinical Rationale

A striking convergence of basic science, clinical research, and translational medicine occurred within a short interval that resulted in the enablement of HER2 as a therapeutic target (Fig. 1).

2.3 A Perversion of Nature

2.3.1 Growth Factor Activation of Tumor Cell Tyrosine Kinases Mediate Resistance to Immune Effector Molecules

The discovery that activation of growth factor receptors can limit the ability of tumor necrosis factor-alpha (TNF-α) to inhibit tumor growth was a key finding in the history of the development of Herceptin (Fig. 2).

These results suggested that tumor cells may be able to secrete growth factors, not only to promote their own proliferation, as suggested by the autocrine growth factor model (Sporn and Todaro 1980), but also as a protective mechanism against host immune surveillance (Fig. 4).

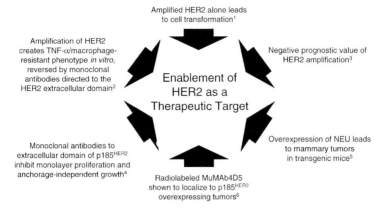

Fig. 1 Decision to develop Herceptin. Several of the most important events and data are summarized in this figure, with each step referenced by number. References: (1) Hudziak et al. (1987); (2) Hudziak et al. (1988, 1989); (3) Slamon et al. (1987, 1989); (4) Lewis et al. (1993); (5) Muller et al. (1988); (6) Maneval et al. (1991b)

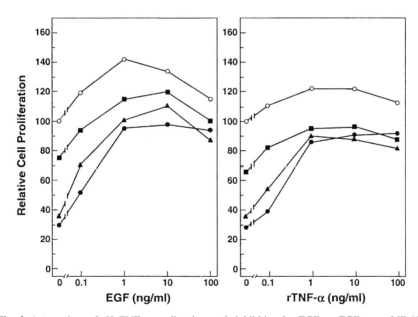

Fig. 2 Antagonism of rHuTNF-α-mediated growth inhibition by EGF or TGF-α on ME-180 cervical carcinoma cells. *Open circles*: growth factor alone; *boxes*: 50 u ml^{-1} TNF-α; *triangles*: 500 u ml^{-1}; *closed circles*: 5,000 u ml^{-1}. The left axis (0) represents the effect of rHuTNF-α alone (Sugarman et al. 1987)

2.3.2 Activation of Receptor Tyrosine Kinases is Associated with Tumor Cell Resistance to Macrophages and TNF-α

To further establish the link between tyrosine kinase activation in tumor cells and immune cell resistance, two approaches were taken. First, NIH 3T3 fibroblasts were transfected with expression plasmids encoding p185^{HER2} and cell lines were isolated as controls, or which express control plasmids and high levels of p185^{HER2}. Second, spontaneous transformants of NIH 3T3 fibroblasts, which are often associated with amplification of the c-Met protooncogene (Giordano et al. 1989), were examined for associated resistance to TNF-α. These are two independent methods and very different examples of receptor tyrosine kinases.

When cells selected for increased p185^{HER2} expression were tested for sensitivity to macrophage-mediated cytotoxicity, it was found that high levels of p185^{HER2} expression were associated with resistance to "effector" cells (Fig. 3a, Hudziak et al. 1988). Similarly, when spontaneous transformants of NIH 3T3 fibroblasts were characterized for increased c-Met gene copy number, it was found that amplified c-Met was associated with increased resistance to TNF-α (Fig. 3b).

These results support the concept that activation of tyrosine kinases by added growth factors, spontaneous gene amplification or gene transfection, are associated with resistance to immunosurveillance by macrophages/TNF-α.

a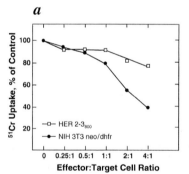

b

Cell Line	Relative Copy number	Relative expression	IC$_{50}$ (TNF-α) (units/ml)
NIH 3T3 (parent)	1.0	1.0	20
ST6	0.5	0.7	9
RST9	1.5	1.2	60
RST1	2.0	2.6	700
RST6	6.0	4.5	7000

Fig. 3 Oncogene amplification and resistance to macrophage- or TNF-α-mediated cytotoxicity. (**a**) Macrophages are known to have a key role in eliminating incipient tumors (Urban and Schreiber 1988), but the frequency of tumor cell resistance ($\sim 10^{-4}$ for some cell lines; Lewis et al. 1987) means that escape from this single mechanism is common. Macrophage effector molecules, especially TNF-α, can then act to stimulate tumor cell proliferation (Hudziak et al. 1988, Lewis et al. 1987) and angiogenesis (Leibovich et al. 1987). (**b**) The c-Met protooncogene is often amplified in spontaneous transformants of NIH 3T3 fibroblasts. In this experiment, spontaneous transformants were subcloned, then tested for sensitivity to TNF-α. The results showed decreasing sensitivity correlates with increased c-Met gene copy number (Hudziak et al. 1990)

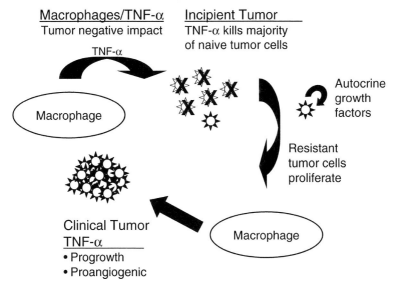

Fig. 4 Tumor cells characterized by autocrine stimulation of receptor tyrosine kinase activity are selected via activated macrophages to form a clinical tumor

2.3.3 Macrophage-mediated Antitumor Effects are Converted to Protumorigenic During In Vivo Tumor Progression

While the macrophage may be instrumental in the initial detection and destruction of tumor cells (Urban et al. 1986), its effects, if unsuccessful in the first instance, may potentiate tumor cell growth and malignancy (Lewis et al. 1987, Fig. 4, see "Clinical Tumor"). Mechanisms that modulate tumor cell sensitivity to the host immune system play an important role in the growth of an incipient tumor, and the continued presence of activated macrophages within a resistant tumor may help to establish a protumorigenic environment. Our work established that antireceptor agents can reverse oncogene-associated immune resistance, and provided a critical element in building a rationale for the use of tyrosine kinase antagonists in the treatment of cancer.

2.4 Biologic Effects of Amplified HER2 Expression

Following the first molecular description of the sequence encoding $p185^{HER2}$, its extensive homology with the rat NEU protooncogene was quickly established (Coussens et al. 1985; Yarden and Ullrich 1988). Further work distinguished NEU and HER2 by showing that a mutation in the transmembrane domain of $p185^{NEU}$ was sufficient to enable transforming activity (Weiner et al. 1989), while amplified expression of the wild-type HER2 protooncogene was sufficient to transform fibroblasts in culture (Hudziak et al. 1987). Very rapidly, Slamon and colleagues at the University of California (Los Angeles) and Ullrich (Genentech, Inc.) initiated a collaboration that provided a critical link between amplified expression of HER2 and aggressive breast and ovarian cancer (Slamon et al. 1989, 1987). In this work, it was demonstrated that threefold to fivefold overexpression of tumor-associated p185^{HER2} predicted a dramatically shortened survival in breast and ovarian cancer patients. A direct connection between HER2/NEU and breast cancer was further supported when transgenic mice overexpressing the NEU oncogene specifically developed mammary adenocarcinoma (Muller et al. 1988). Completing the cause and effect relationship between overexpression of p185^{HER2} and cellular malignancy, Hudziak et al. (1988, 1989) demonstrated that the earlier described resistance to macrophage killing that characterized growth factor activated tumor cells (Sugarman et al. 1987) also occurred in tumor cells which overexpress p185^{HER2} (Fig. 3a) or which are characterized by amplification of the c-Met protooncogene.

Many explanations have been offered for the connection between HER2 overexpression and disease progression. It is likely that HER2 overexpression leads to enhanced signaling with other members of the HER family (EGF formation; Pinkas-Kramarski et al. 1996), and potentially to coupling with other receptor tyrosine kinases, like the IGF-1 receptor (Nahta et al. 2005). This strong coupling is supported by in vitro proliferation data which show that cells overexpressing p185^{HER2} can be much more sensitive to antibodies directed to the extracellular domain of p185^{HER2} (see Sect. 2.5.2).

In summary, overexpression of p185^{HER2} transforms cells (enabling growth in soft agar and in nude mice) induces tumor cell resistance to the cytotoxic effects of macrophages, and is correlated with an aggressive form of breast and ovarian cancer.

2.5 Proof of Concept for Antagonists of p185^{HER2}

2.5.1 In Vitro Proof of Concept

No growth factor has yet been found which directly activates either p185^{NEU} or p185^{HER2} (Hynes and Lane 2005). For this reason, p185^{HER2} is a noncanonical receptor and mechanisms which may be able to modulate it were not obvious. The most similar system is the human EGFR/HER1, for which Mendelsohn and colleagues had reported successful antibody-mediated inhibition (Gill et al. 1984). Similarly, the oncogenic version of rat p185^{NEU} was found to be downregulated by monoclonal antibodies directed to its extracellular domain (Drebin et al. 1985).

Fendly et al. (1990b) prepared a large array of monoclonal antibodies directed against the extracellular domain of p185^{HER2}. These monoclonal antibodies were screened in proliferation assays against normal and tumor cells which expressed a spectrum of p185^{HER2} levels (Lewis et al. 1993; Park et al. 1992; Shepard et al. 1991). Some of these data are shown in Table 1. Multiple monoclonal

Table 1 Effect of anti-p185[HER2] monoclonal antibodies on the growth of human tumor cell lines[a]

Cell Line	Relative P185[HER] Expression[b]	Relative Cell Proliferation (% of control)					
		4D5	3H4	2C4	7F3	7C2	6E9
184	1.0	116	114	109	116	117	103
184A1	0.3	129	110	103	106	104	110
184B5	0.8	108	107	105	108	108	106
HBL-100	1.0	104	102	103	96	104	105
MCF7	1.2	101	113	100	111	112	105
MDA-MB-231	1.2	91	100	93	98	104	013
ZR-75-1	3.3	102	105	99	97	108	97
MDA-MB-436	3.3	97	91	98	93	92	101
MDA-MB-175	4.5	62	77	29	48	87	96
MDA-MB-453	16.7	61	65	88	80	70	101
MDA-MB-361	16.7	63	67	64	76	105	99
BT474	25.0	27	29	60	21	78	91
SK-BR-3	33.0	33	40	73	51	82	89
SK-OV-3	16.7	77	85	87	91	97	99
MKN7	16.7	99	102	103	111	106	108
KATO III	5.0	91	102	101	98	107	99
COLO201	8.3	107	132	123	125	122	110
SW1417	6.7	98	97	99	100	98	96

[a] Cells were seeded in 96-well microtiter plates and allowed to adhere before the addition of different anti-p185[HER2] monoclonal antibodies at a final concentration of $10\,\mu g\,ml^{-1}$. Monolayers were stained with crystal violet dye after 5 days for determination of relative cell proliferation. Each group consisted of 8–16 replicates, with the coefficient of variation for each group always less than 12%

[b] Levels of anti-p185[HER2] expression were measured by fluorescence-activated cell sorting, relative to the 184 mammary epithelial cell

antibodies were active in monolayer proliferation assays. The monoclonals induced both inhibitory and stimulatory effects on cell proliferation, and response data were dependent on the cell line. For instance, the monoclonal 7F3 had the greatest antiproliferative effect of all antibodies tested vs. the HER2-overexpressing BT474 breast tumor cell line in monolayer proliferation assays. However, 7F3 also stimulated growth of some tumor cell lines (e.g., COLO201). The cell lines shown in the box in Table 1 had high levels of expression of p185[HER2], but were less sensitive than expected. The explanation for this difference of activity between cell lines and among antibodies is not known (see Sect. 6.1). Most of the antibodies with an antiproliferative effect on HER2-overexpressing tumor cells were found to stimulate growth of nontumorigenic fibroblasts (Table 1). Overall, the best correlation between p185[HER2] expression and growth inhibitory activity in vitro (in these experiments, and in soft agar assays) was with the monoclonal 4D5 (muMAb4D5). Based upon this correlation, and animal xenograft studies (Park et al. 1992), future work, including humanization of antibody, focused on muMAb4D5. Follow-on preclinical studies have also been conducted with the 2C4 monoclonal antibody (muMAb2C4). The rationale for clinical testing of the humanized muMAb2C4 (Pertuzumab) is based upon its ability to bind to the dimerization domain of p185[HER2] and prevent

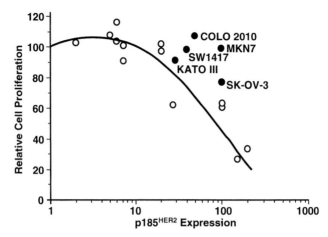

Fig. 5 Relationship between p185^{HER2} expression and growth inhibition mediated by muMAb4D5 on human breast cell lines, normal and tumor (*open circles*), and other types of tumor cells over-expressing p185^{HER2} (*filled circles,* Lewis et al. 1993)

receptor multimerization (Adams et al. 2005). Successful preliminary data with Pertuzumab in combination with chemotherapy in a subset of ovarian cancer patients have recently been reported (Makhija et al. 2007).

The data shown in Table 1 show that overall muMAb4D5 has the best activity vs. tumor cells which overexpress p185^{HER2}.

Figure 5 shows the nonlinear relationship between response to muMAb4D5 and p185^{HER2}.

There are two aspects of this nonlinear relationship which are particularly noteable: (1) the inflection point of the curve (3–5 × overexpression) is very similar to the level of expression that predicts more aggressive breast and ovarian cancer (Slamon et al. 1989, 1987); and (2) there are a number of cell types which fall above the best-fit regression line. These cells are "inherently resistant" to the growth inhibitory effects of muMAb4D5. Several theories have been advanced to help explain the inherent resistance. Probably the most common of these mechanisms is tumor cell co-expression of the human EGFR (HER) family members (Sergina et al. 2007).

2.5.2 Overcoming Tyrosine Kinase Inhibition of Macrophage (TNF-α)-Mediated Tumor Cell Cytotoxicity

The clear relationship between tyrosine kinase activation and resistance to TNF-α (Sect. 2.5.1) predicted that downregulation of tyrosine kinase activity could enhance the antitumor effect of TNF-α. To test this we treated breast tumor cells in culture with muMAb4D5 in the presence or absence of rHuTNF-α (Fig. 6).

In most HER2-overexpressing cell types, the combination of rHuTNF-α and muMAb4D5 results in an additive antiproliferative effect, and in others the effect

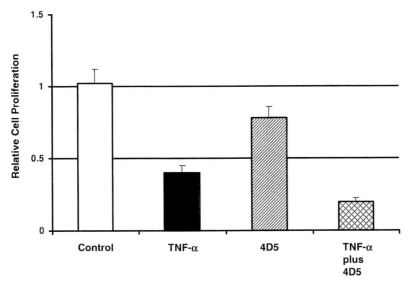

Fig. 6 MuMAb4D5 treatment sensitizes p185[HER2] breast cancer cells to the cytotoxic effects of rHuTNF-α. Monoclonal antibody 4D5 sensitizes breast tumor cells to the cytotoxic effects of TNF-α. Cells were plated in 96-well microdilution plates (4×10^4 cells per well) and allowed to adhere for 2 h. MuMAb 4D5 ($5\,\mu g\,ml^{-1}$) or antihepatitis B surface antigen monoclonal antibody 40.1.H1 ($5\,\mu g\,ml^{-1}$) was then added for a 4-h incubation prior to the addition of TNF-α to a final concentration of 10^4 units ml^{-1}. After 72 h, the monolayers were washed twice with PBS and stained with crystal violet dye for determination of relative cell proliferation. In addition, some cell monolayers were stained with crystal violet following adherence in order to determine the initial cell density for comparison with cell densities measured after 72 h (Hudziak et al. 1989)

is more pronounced. In any case, it is likely that part of the in vivo activity of Herceptin stems from the renewed ability of macrophages to inhibit the growth of HER2-overexpressing cancers.

2.6 In Vivo Proof of Concept with MuMAb4D5

2.6.1 Tumor Xenograft Studies with MuMAb4D5

Initial studies of the in vivo antitumor activity of muMAb4D5 were performed in nude mice bearing human tumor xenografts. Human breast or ovarian tumors that overexpressed p185[HER2] were implanted into the subrenal capsule, and tumors were permitted to form. Mice were then treated intravenously with muMAb4D5 or an irrelevant isotype-matched control monoclonal antibody, muMAb5B6. Tumors were excised and weighed to evaluate effects on growth. Experimental results in models of ovarian (see Table 2) and breast cancer (see Park et al. 1992) demonstrated both target-specific and dose-dependent antitumor effects of muMAb4D5.

Table 2 MuMAb4D5 inhibits growth of human ovarian tumor xenografts in mice

Material	Total dose $(mg\,kg^{-1})^a$	Tumor weight $(mg)^b$
PBS	–	$1,288 \pm 865$
Control IgG (MuMAb5B6)	90.9	$1,416 \pm 483$
MuMAb4D5	1.5	$1,187 \pm 825$
MuMAb4D5	3.0	$1,026 \pm 330$
MuMAb4D5	7.5	$1,287 \pm 919$
MuMAb4D5	15.0	812 ± 669
MuMAb4D5	36.4	715 ± 529
MuMAb4D5	90.9	698 ± 174

[a] Human ovarian tumors were implanted in the subrenal capsule of athymic mice. Monoclonal antibodies were administered as equally divided doses on days 12, 15, and 18 post tumor implantation
[b] Tumors were excised on day 22 and weighed wet. Data are mean $\pm$ SD ($n = 8$/group; Maneval, Pegram, Shepard, and Slamon, unpublished data)

The subrenal capsule nude mouse model was also used to characterize the biodistribution of muMAb4D5. ^{125}I-labeled muMAb4D5 was injected intravenously to tumor-bearing mice, and mice were sacrificed at 5 min, 3 h, 24 h, 3 or 7 days. As a control, a separate cohort of tumor-bearing mice received ^{125}I-muMAb5B6, and mice were sacrificed at 24 h or 7 days.

Whole body sagittal sections were exposed to film together with ^{125}I standards to generate autoradiograms (Fig. 7). Tumor accumulation was negligible 5 min after dosing of ^{125}I-muMAb4D5, but continually increased over the initial 24-h interval (see arrows in Fig. 7). Tumor-to-blood ratios increased throughout the 7-day study. In contrast to ^{125}I-muMAb4D5, tumor accumulation of ^{125}I was not evident after administration of the radiolabeled control antibody. These results demonstrated the in vivo localization of muMAb4D5 to tumors overexpressing p185^{HER2}. Further studies with the radiolabeled, humanized version of muMAb4D5 demonstrated that tremendous efficacy is achievable in these tumor models by combining the preferential localization and internalization by antibody with the cytotoxic effects of radioimmunotherapy.

These initial experiments with muMAb4D5 led to more comprehensive studies demonstrating the antitumor effects of therapy directed at p185^{HER2}.

3 Proof of Concept for Therapeutic Antibodies in Solid Cancer

3.1 The Controversy About Making a Successful Monoclonal Antibody Therapeutic vs. Solid Cancer

By early 1990, a number of clinical studies had been performed with murine monoclonal antibodies (muMAb), yet only one agent was approved for clinical use

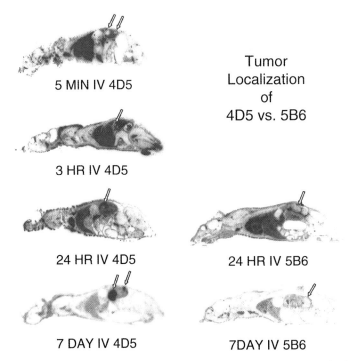

Fig. 7 Tumor localization of muMAb4D5. Athymic mice bearing human tumors in the subrenal capsule received a single intravenous (IV) dose of ^{125}I-muMAb4D5 (4D5) or control antibody ^{125}I-muMAb5B6 (5B6). Autoradiograms were generated by exposing sagittal 20 μm sections to film (nose at *left* in each panel). Radioactivity was evident in well-perfused tissues (e.g., heart, liver) at 5 min and 3 h post dosing. Tumor (T →) uptake of ^{125}I was evident by 24 h and 7 days. In contrast, no specific localization of radioactivity was detected in the tumor of mice that received ^{125}I-muMAb5B6 control (Maneval et al. 1991b)

(OKT-3). Despite more than a decade of intense research, no antibody-based drug had yet been approved for use in oncology. However, a wealth of information on the clinical use of murine antibodies, and the factors influencing effective antibody delivery to tumors was available (for perspective see Blumenthal et al. 1990; Goldenberg 1991). The development of an anti-p185^{HER2} antibody (Herceptin) required an effective strategy to address key challenges including: (1) the neutralizing effect of human antimouse antibodies (HAMA) on the serum pharmacokinetics of active antibody; (2) the inefficient in vivo delivery of macromolecules to solid tumors; and (3) the potential for adverse events due to the specific binding of nontumor tissues in humans.

3.2 MuMAb4D5 Therapy for Breast Cancer

The initial in vitro and in vivo studies described above for muMAb4D5 indicated the potential therapeutic utility of this antibody for the treatment of breast cancer. More extensive preclinical investigation at UCLA and Genentech provided additional support for muMAb4D5 therapy. Engineered cell lines were generated with differential expression of p185[HER2] (Chazin et al. 1992). Subcutaneous xenografts with these cells provided an in vivo model to demonstrate the activity of muMAb4D5 and the potential synergy when added to chemotherapy (Pietras et al. 1994). Receptor-mediated uptake and concentration of radiolabeled muMAb4D5 supported the potential for radioimmunotherapy (DeSantes et al. 1992; Maneval et al. 1992)

A series of preclinical studies was also completed in nontumor bearing animals to characterize the pharmacokinetics and biodistribution of muMAb4D5. These studies provided a dosing rationale for subsequent investigation of efficacy and safety. Consistent with expectations for murine monoclonal antibodies, muMAb4D5 was cleared slowly from the blood of all species tested (mice, rats, rabbits, and cynomolgus monkeys; Maneval et al. 1991c). Average terminal half-life ranged from 85 h in monkeys to 459 h in mice. Peak circulating concentrations of muMAb4D5 indicated an initial volume of distribution approximately equal to the plasma volume. A monkey antimouse antibody (MAMA) response was detected within 3 weeks of dosing in a majority of monkeys treated with muMAb4D5 (Fig. 8). The MAMA response occurred as early as 12 days after single intravenous injection and corresponded to a rapid decline in measurable plasma concentrations of muMAb4D5.

Efficacy studies with muMAb4D5 indicated the need for sustained concentrations of anti-p185[HER2] antibody for therapeutic benefit. However, primate studies

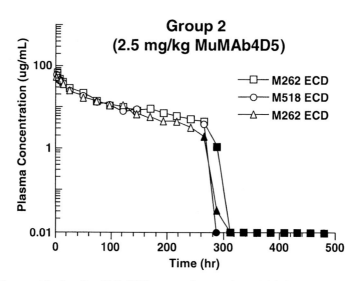

Fig. 8 Pharmacokinetics of muMAb4D5 in cynomolgus monkeys. Adult female cynomolgus monkeys received a single intravenous injection of muMAb4D5 ($2.5\,mg\,kg^{-1}$), and blood samples were collected over a 21-day interval. Plasma concentrations of muMAb4D5 were measured by ELISA, and data from individual monkeys ($N = 3$) were plotted vs. time (represented by *squares, triangles*, and *circles*). Monkey antimurine antibodies (MAMA) were detected in the plasma as early as day 12 (indicated by *solid symbols*). The MAMA response corresponded to a precipitous decline in the measurable plasma concentrations of muMAb4D5 (Maneval et al. 1991a)

with muMAb4D5 indicated a HAMA response was very likely to neutralize the therapeutic activity of the murine antibody. Consequently, humanization of muMAb4D5 was considered essential to develop an antibody therapeutic directed at p185^{HER2}, and efforts to engineer Herceptin began in 1990 (Carter et al. 2000, 1992).

The availability of muMAb4D5 for clinical studies provided the opportunity for parallel testing of other critical hypotheses for development of antibodies to p185^{HER2}. Would binding the HER2 receptor using pharmacological doses of muMAb4D5 result in unanticipated toxicity in humans? Would muMAb4D5 target tumors in patients? Could evidence for antitumor activity be detected in cancer patients treated with muMAb4D5? Clinical investigation with muMAb4D5 was also expected to establish methodologies for patient selection, tissue sampling, serum analysis, and dose optimization. Consequently, a Phase I trial with muMAb4D5 was conducted under the direction of Dr. Dennis Slamon at UCLA.

3.3 Phase I Investigation with MuMAb4D5

Seeking answers to the questions described above, a Phase I clinical study to evaluate the safety, pharmacokinetics, and tumor localization of an anti-p185^{HER2} antibody was initiated with muMAb4D5. Twelve breast and ovarian cancer patients that overexpressed p185^{HER2} were enrolled in an open-label dose-escalation study. Patients received a single intravenous administration of muMAb4D5 at doses ranging from 3 to 500 mg kg^{-1}. Prior to dosing, muMAb4D5 was mixed with 1–5 mCi ^{131}I-muMAb4D5 to enable external gamma scintigraphy and evaluation of tumor localization.

MuMAb4D5 was well tolerated at all doses tested. Gamma camera imaging provided evidence for tumor localization. Pharmacokinetic analyses indicated a small initial volume of distribution, dose dependent clearance, and a long terminal half-life. Consistent with observations from preclinical studies in primates, a HAMA response was encountered, confirming a limitation of muMAb4D5 as an effective biopharmaceutical. Results from this pivotal Phase I study provided the foundation for creation and development of a humanized version of muMAb4D5, which became Herceptin.

4 Development of Herceptin

4.1 Humanized Versions of MuMAb4D5

Humanized versions of muMAb4D5 were engineered to retain the binding specificity of the parent antibody and also to encode human-like residues even in the hypervariable complementarity determining regions (CDRs). Some variants had higher affinity than others and binding affinity varied from 0.3 to 25 nM (Carter et al. 1992). There was a general correlation between lower Kd and growth inhibitory activity until an affinity of 1 nM was reached. The antibody chosen for further study and development was designated rhuMab4D5 (later renamed Herceptin/Trastuzumab). As a result of humanization, Herceptin is an IgG1 isotype and was demonstrated to mediate antibody-dependent cellular cytotoxicity (ADCC). Human peripheral blood mononuclear cells were isolated in the initial studies of ADCC and the results showed 30–40% cytotoxicity utilizing SK-BR-3 tumor cells (up to 25:1 effector to target cell ratio), as opposed to a maximum cytotoxicity of about 10% utilizing WI-38 fibroblasts as target cells (Carter et al. 1992). These results were promising and meant that both direct antiproliferative activity and ADCC could be important for discriminating between normal cells and tumor cells. It is not known whether ADCC is an important component for the general efficacy of Herceptin, although there is evidence that it may have a role in at least some patients (Arnould et al. 2006).

4.2 Characterization of Herceptin In Vivo

Study designs for the in vivo characterization of Herceptin were similar to the preclinical studies performed with muMAb4D5. Tumor localization was demonstrated using radiolabeled Herceptin (see Fig. 9), and dose–response studies resulted in antitumor effects in nude mice bearing human tumor xenografts overexpressing $p185^{HER2}$. Herceptin was compared to control human immunoglobulin to demonstrate target-specific activity. Comparisons of Herceptin with muMAb4D5 resulted in similar but somewhat diminished antitumor activity in immunodeficient mouse models of human cancer (Pietras et al. 1998). Subsequent investigation in other mouse models of human cancer confirmed these observations (Baselga et al. 1998; Pietras et al. 1998; Tokuda et al. 1996).

The novel mechanism of action of Herceptin encouraged investigation of the effects of anti-$p185^{HER2}$ antibodies when combined with chemotherapeutic agents commonly used in cancer therapy (Baselga et al. 1998; Pegram et al. 1999; Pietras et al. 1998). The observation that an antibody directed against EGFR (HER1) significantly enhanced the antitumor activity of cisplatin provided a basis for experimental investigation (Aboud-Pirak et al. 1988). Initial studies combining muMAb4D5 with cisplatin or carboplatin resulted in synergistic effects in human breast and ovarian cancer cells that overexpressed $p185^{HER2}$ (Pietras et al. 1994). Synergism was not demonstrated in cells that expressed a low level of the receptor. The mechanism of action of Herceptin when combined with cisplatin or doxorubicin was further investigated in a series of in vitro and in vivo studies. In vitro studies demonstrated that Herceptin interfered with drug-induced DNA repair and unscheduled DNA synthesis. Dose-ranging studies evaluated the relative timing of administration, and results indicated receptor-enhanced chemosensitivity when the two agents were given in close temporal proximity. These preclinical data provided the basis

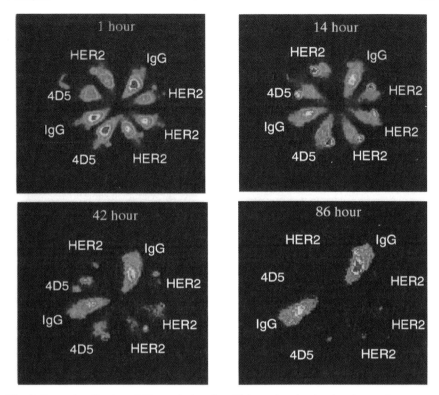

Fig. 9 Tumor localization of Herceptin in mice. Eight nude mice bearing large subcutaneous tumors ($>1\,cm^3$) on the right flank received a single intravenous injection of ^{186}Re-muMAb4D5 (4D5), ^{186}Re-Herceptin (HER2), or ^{186}Re-human IgG (IgG). Mice were anesthetized and arranged (nose facing image center) on the face of a gamma camera equipped with a parallel-hole collimator. A 5-min acquisition was performed 1h post injection, and mice were returned to their cages. Radioactivity was localized to tumors only in mice treated with 4D5 or HER2 (Maneval et al. 1993)

for dosing schedules for subsequent clinical investigation of Herceptin with DNA-reactive drugs (Pietras et al. 1998).

Investigators at UCLA also performed an extensive series of preclinical studies to characterize the effects of anti-p185^{HER2} antibodies when combined with other chemotherapeutic agents. In vitro experiments were completed that used eight drugs from seven different classes of cytotoxic agents. These drugs were individually combined with Herceptin, and the effects on breast cancer cells that overexpressed p185^{HER2} were quantitatively assessed using a statistically robust index for drug interactions. Synergy was demonstrated when Herceptin was combined with cisplatin, thiotepa, or etoposide. Additive effects were observed when the antibody was combined with doxorubicin, paclitaxel, methotrexate, and vinblastine. Interestingly, the quantitative analysis resulted in a less-than-additive effect when Herceptin was combined with 5-fluorouracil. A series of in vivo studies combining Herceptin with these cytotoxic agents was also performed using mice bearing human tumor xenografts. Although quantitative assessment of synergy in vivo was not feasible, the combination therapy resulted in enhanced antitumor effects that were consistent with the in vitro observations (Pegram et al. 1999). These results provided a solid preclinical rationale for combinations of Herceptin and chemotherapeutic drugs in the treatment of breast cancer (Pegram et al. 1997, 2004).

A series of preclinical studies evaluating the pharmacokinetics and toxicology of Herceptin was completed to support the submission of an IND and permit Phase I clinical trials. Serum pharmacokinetics was characterized in mice and monkeys. Similar to muMAb4D5, Herceptin was cleared slowly from the blood after intravenous administration. Whole body autoradiography also indicated a similar pattern of tissue distribution of the two anti-p185^{HER2} antibodies in nude mice bearing human tumors. In contrast to the HAMA response detected within 3 weeks of dosing of muMAb4D5 (see Fig. 8), no evidence for anti-Herceptin antibody was detected in the sera of cynomolgus monkeys dosed with single or multiple intravenous injections of Herceptin. Consequently, Herceptin serum concentrations were detected for >2 months in the primate model (see Fig. 10). These data supported the assumption

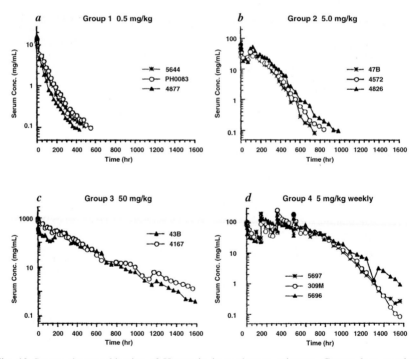

Fig. 10 Serum pharmacokinetics of Herceptin in nonhuman primates. Cynomolgus monkeys received a single or four weekly intravenous injections of Herceptin and blood samples were collected over a 2-month interval. Serum concentrations of Herceptin were analyzed by ELISA and are plotted vs. time after dosing. Symbols represent concentrations from individual monkeys (unpublished)

that Herceptin was likely to be less immunogenic than the parent murine antibody, and serum concentrations were expected to be maintained for extended periods in patients.

Measurements of the extracellular domain of immunoreactive $p185^{HER2}$ in the serum (i.e., shed antigen) were shown to correlate with tumor size in tumor-bearing nude mouse models. Whole body clearance of radiolabeled Herceptin increased in animals with larger tumors (Fig. 9). Taken together, these data supported the hypothesis that shed antigen can affect the pharmacokinetics of Herceptin and suggested that measurement of shed antigen may be important in clinical studies (Pegram et al. 1998). Shed antigen/receptor continues to be important in the evaluation of antibody therapeutics and "ligand trap"-based biologics – for different reasons. If the level of shed receptor is high, then higher doses of antireceptor monoclonal antibody may be required, at least in the loading doses. Also, the presence of shed receptor in the serum can interfere in analysis of the pharmacokinetics of therapeutic monoclonal antibody (Maple et al. 2004).

4.3 Summary of the History of Clinical Trials with Herceptin

Phase I investigation with Herceptin was initiated in 1992. Studies were designed to evaluate safety, characterize serum pharmacokinetics, and test for evidence of clinical activity of Herceptin in cancer patients that overexpressed $p185^{HER2}$. The initial single-dose open-label dose escalation (10–500 mg per patient) study in cancer patients was followed by two additional studies designed to test weekly dosing and combination with cisplatin (50 or $100 \, mg \, m^{-2}$, Shak 1999). Results from Phase I investigation indicated that Herceptin was well tolerated at all doses tested. A maximum tolerated dose was not achieved. Analysis of serum concentrations demonstrated that Herceptin pharmacokinetics were well-predicted from clinical experience with muMAb4D5 and preclinical studies with Herceptin in nonhuman primates. Objective responses were reported in 4 of 15 patients that received the combination therapy (Pegram et al. 1998), and co-administration of cisplatin had no measurable effect on Herceptin pharmacokinetics. Importantly, no evidence for an anti-Herceptin antibody response was detected after single or multiple dosing (Baselga 2001; Leyland-Jones 2001; Yeon and Pegram 2005).

Pharmacokinetic modeling of Phase I data provided a rationale basis for the design of the Phase II dosing strategies. In nonhuman primates, Herceptin exhibited nonlinear pharmacokinetics, with an extended terminal half-life and slower serum clearance at higher doses of the drug (see Fig. 10). Similar observations were made in the Phase I studies (see Table 1, Leyland-Jones 2001). These results were consistent with a model that involves saturation of the clearance mechanisms and provided the basis for a "loading dose" that was incorporated into subsequent clinical investigation.

In vitro studies with anti-p185^{HER2} antibodies demonstrated maximum inhibition of cell proliferation that varied with cell line and ranged from 1–10 µg ml^{-1} (Carter et al. 1992; Chazin et al. 1992; Lewis et al. 1993; Pegram et al. 1999; Pietras et al. 1994). Tumor growth inhibition in vivo was typically observed with tumor xenografts models at Herceptin doses that ranged from 1 to 10 mg kg^{-1}, with interstudy variations due to tumor type, level of p185^{HER2} expression, tumor vascularity, tumor size, and the presence of serum ECD (Baselga et al. 1998; Pegram et al. 1999; Pietras et al. 1998; Tokuda et al. 1996). Based on these preclinical findings, a target trough serum concentration of >10 µg ml^{-1} was set for Phase II clinical studies with Herceptin (Pegram et al. 1999). Although measurable antitumor activity could have been anticipated by maintaining a lower target trough serum concentration, the absence of adverse events in Phase I supported the conservative notion of proceeding to pivotal Phase II investigation with a relatively high dose of Herceptin. Phase II study designs included a 250 mg loading dose followed by 100 mg weekly dosing, a schedule that ensured >90% of patients would exceed the target (10 µg ml^{-1}) trough concentration.

Two Phase II studies were initiated in 1993–1994 to determine the overall response rate of Herceptin therapy. Both studies enrolled patients with metastatic breast cancers that overexpressed p185^{HER2}. The objectives of these studies included further investigation of the safety and pharmacokinetics of Herceptin as a single agent and in combination with cisplatin (Shak 1999).

In the first study, 10 weekly doses of Herceptin were administered to 46 patients that had received extensive prior therapy. Objective responses were reported in five patients, including one complete remission. Herceptin was well tolerated and detailed blood sampling indicated that serum concentrations were maintained above 10 µg ml^{-1} in >90% of patients. Serum pharmacokinetics were shown to be influenced by the presence of circulating ECD. Anti-Herceptin antibodies were not detected in any patient (Baselga et al. 1996).

Pegram and colleagues conducted a Phase II study that expanded on preclinical and Phase I data combining Herceptin with cisplatin. Thirty-nine extensively treated advanced breast cancer patients received 10 weekly doses of Herceptin in combination with cisplatin on days 1, 29, and 57. Nearly half of patients treated achieved a partial or minor response to therapy. The toxicity profile was consistent with expectations for cisplatin alone, and serum pharmacokinetics of Herceptin were not affected by the addition of chemotherapy. A significant inverse correlation was demonstrated between circulating ECD and trough serum concentrations of Herceptin. Although serum ECD was not considered a predictor of clinical response in this trial, ECD had a measurable effect on serum pharmacokinetics and may be a source of significant interpatient variability associated with Herceptin therapy (Pegram et al. 1998).

Successful results from Phase II investigation led to the design of Phase III studies with Herceptin alone or in combination with chemotherapy. Based on results from Phase II investigation, patient dosing was modified to normalize for body weight (4 mg kg^{-1} loading dose; 2 mg kg^{-1} weekly dosing). Herceptin treatment as a single agent resulted in an objective response rate of 15% in a study of 222 women with HER2-overexpressing breast cancer that had progressed after chemotherapy (Cobleigh et al. 1999). Serum concentrations were maintained above $20\,\mu g\,ml^{-1}$ in >90% of patients. Mean trough concentrations were reported to be higher in complete $(70.3\,\mu g\,ml^{-1})$ and partial $(58.4\,\mu g\,ml^{-1})$ responders than in nonresponders $(44.3\,\mu g\,ml^{-1}; P < 0.001)$. A single patient was shown to have detectable antibodies directed against the Fab region of Herceptin. Although peak serum concentrations were lower in this individual, no clinical signs of allergy were observed.

Clear evidence of clinical benefit of Herceptin therapy was reported by Slamon and colleagues in 2001 (Slamon et al. 2001). Four hundred sixty-nine patients were enrolled in a study and randomly assigned to receive standard chemotherapy alone or in combination with Herceptin. Combination therapy resulted in an increased objective response rate, a longer time to disease progression, a longer duration of response, longer survival, and a 20% reduction in the risk of death. Importantly, Herceptin significantly increased the cardiac dysfunction associated of anthracycline therapy, an observation not anticipated from preclinical or early clinical studies. Although cardiotoxicity was severe in some cases, symptoms were effectively treated with standard medical management. Data from the clinical trials summarized above provided the basis for United States Food and Drug Administration approval of Herceptin in September 1998, eight years after the molecular engineering of the humanized antibody.

Recent results from a series of ongoing trials indicate that Herceptin is also effective in the adjuvant setting. Four large-scale international clinical trials involving >13,000 patients with early-stage breast cancer positive for p185[HER2] overexpression have demonstrated a survival benefit for patients treated with Herceptin (reviewed in Baselga et al. 2006). Notwithstanding differences in patient populations, types and regimens of chemotherapy, randomization methods, and follow up times, adjuvant therapy with Herceptin reduced the risk of disease recurrence in early breast cancer patients by approximately 50% (see Table 3).

These extended trials have further demonstrated that Herceptin-related adverse cardiac events remained at a clinically acceptable number, and no new or unexpected toxicities were reported. However, longer follow-up is needed to make conclusive statements regarding cardiac safety. Further clinical investigation is also required to determine duration of dosing and optimal dosing regimens, relative timing of administration with chemotherapy, and to compare combinations with anthracycline or nonanthracycline-based chemotherapy. Overall, these international trials support one year of adjuvant Herceptin treatment for women with early breast cancer that overexpress p185[HER2] (Baselga et al. 2006).

4.4 Current Status and Significance of Herceptin

Currently, more than 150,000 women have been treated with Herceptin (Genentech, Inc.). Additional clinical studies are underway to further investigate the therapeutic potential of Herceptin in breast cancer patients that overexpress p185[HER2], with

Table 3 Clinical efficacy data with Herceptin as single agent and in combination with chemotherapy in breast cancer patients

Therapy	# Patients	Response rate[a]	Hazard ratio[b]	Reference
Herceptin	46	11.6%		(Baselga et al. 1996)
Herceptin + cisplatin	39	24.3%		(Pegram et al. 1998)
Herceptin	222	15%		(Cobleigh et al. 1999)
Herceptin	114	26%		(Vogel et al. 2002)
Herceptin + AC[c]	143	56%		(Slamon and
Herceptin + paclitaxel	92	38%		Pegram 2001)
Herceptin + paclitaxel	98	36%	0.66 PFS[d]	(Robert et al. 2006)
Herceptin + paclitaxel + carboplatin	98	52%	0.90 OS[e]	
docetaxel	94	34%		(Marty et al. 2005)
Herceptin + docetaxel	92	61%		
doxorubicin, cyclophosphamide, paclitaxel	1,679		0.48 DFS[f] 0.67 OS	(Romond et al. 2005)
Herceptin + doxorubicin, cyclophosphamide, paclitaxel	1,672			
Herceptin	1,694		0.54 DFS	(Piccart-Gebhart
Observation	1,693			et al. 2005)
FEC[g], docetaxel or vinorelbine	116		0.42 RFS[h]	(Joensuu et al. 2006)
Herceptin + FEC, docetaxel, or vinorelbine	115		0.41 OS	

[a] Response rate includes complete responders and partial responders
[b] The hazard ratio is calculated from time to event data for the individual studies and reflects the beneficial effect of Herceptin vs. control. A hazard ratio of 1.0 indicates no effect
[c] Anthracycline (doxorubicin or epirubicin) plus cyclophosphamide
[d] Progression-free survival
[e] Overall survival
[f] Disease-free survival
[g] Fluorouracil, epirubicin, cyclophosphamide
[h] Survival free of recurrence

additional work focused on the possibility of targeting breast and other malignancies with lower levels of HER2 expression. The latter work is quite important since high overexpressing HER2 patients make up no more than 25% of all breast cancer.

The Herceptin project has also provided guidance for other therapeutic advances, including the first proof for the role of tyrosine kinase in cancer, methods for measuring and standardizing target expression, and a model for development of novel antireceptor therapeutics.

5 Alternative Therapies Targeting p185^{HER2}

5.1 Radiolabeled Herceptin

Arming antibodies with cytotoxic drugs or radionuclides provides a conceptual strategy to increase antitumor activity, consistent with Ehrlich's fundamental hypothesis. Radionuclides have been conjugated to monoclonal antibodies to enhance tumor imaging (radioimmunodiagnosis, RAID) or tumor therapy (radioimmunotherapy, RAIT). The recent FDA approvals of Zevalin and Bexxar demonstrated the potential for therapeutic development of RAIT for cancer. Determinants that influence successful RAIT and RAID include antibody size (full length vs. fragment), antibody affinity, protein dose and antibody pharmacokinetics, tumor size, location, vascularity, and levels of target expression in vivo. The selection of an appropriate radionuclide is also dependent on physical half-life, the nature of physical decay (α, β, or γ emission), available radiochemistry techniques for conjugation, and whether the intended use includes imaging, therapy, or both. The interplay of numerous factors can affect the development of a radiolabeled monoclonal antibody for clinical use (for reviews, see Blumenthal et al. 1990; Brechbiel and Waldmann 2000; Goldenberg and Sharkey 2006).

Phase I investigation with radiolabeled ^{131}I-muMAb4D5 was designed to characterize the in vivo distribution of the antibody and evaluate tumor localization. ^{131}I was chosen because of the ease of iodination of monoclonal antibodies and the wealth of experience with this radionuclide in clinical nuclear medicine. Preclinical studies to view the distribution of Herceptin have also used ^{186}Re to improve the quality of gamma scintigraphy (Kotts et al. 1996). Recently, a clinical study that included 17 patients treated with ^{111}In-Herceptin was reported. The primary objective of the study was to assess whether ^{111}In-scintigraphy could predict Herceptin-based cardiotoxicity. Although gamma camera images did not correlate with cardiac dysfunction, new tumor lesions were detected in 13 of 15 patients evaluated, suggesting that radiolabeled Herceptin may have clinical utility in the management of breast cancer (Perik et al. 2006).

Because of the long circulating residence times of full-length antibodies, truncated versions of anti-p185^{HER2} antibodies have been evaluated to maximize tumor-to-blood ratios and optimize p185^{HER2} radionuclide imaging. Olafsen and colleagues (2005) evaluated Fab fragments, single chain Fv fragments, and Herceptin-derived diabodies using ^{111}In and ^{64}Cu to optimize tumor targeting in mouse xenografts. Other investigators have used ^{68}Ga to label an F(ab$'$)$_2$ fragment of Herceptin to characterize p185^{HER2} expression in animal models. Using positron-emission tomography, these investigators were able to demonstrate a noninvasive strategy to evaluate the pharmacodynamics of drug action in vivo (Smith-Jones et al. 2004). RAID techniques may complement current biopsy-based methods to identify and select patients for Herceptin therapy.

Specific delivery of radionuclides to the tumor cell provides the opportunity to enhance the antitumor activity of Herceptin. DeSantes et al. (1992), first demonstrated an antitumor effect using ^{131}I-muMAb4D5 in the mouse subcutaneous tumor model. Although radioiodine has been used extensively in the clinic, alternative radionuclides that deposit energy over a shorter range may prove superior for RAIT (for review, see Brechbiel and Waldmann 2000). Preclinical studies with beta emitters such as ^{90}Y (Crow et al. 2005) and ^{177}Lu (Persson et al. 2005) have been completed and may improve anti-p185^{HER2} antibody therapy. Radionuclides that emit alpha particles provide another strategy for RAIT with Herceptin. Preclinical studies have been reported using Herceptin radiolabeled with ^{225}Ac (Ballangrud et al. 2004), ^{213}Bi (Milenic et al. 2004), ^{211}At (Persson et al. 2006), and ^{212}Pb (Milenic et al. 2005). Although in vivo delivery can be influenced by a number of factors, RAIT provides an attractive target to increase the anticancer activity of Herceptin.

The pursuit of this approach was not considered viable at the time of initial development of Herceptin. There were a few reasons for this. First, it was a big step for a biotechnology company to commit itself to the development of a humanized antibody against a solid tumor, and against the extracellular domain of a receptor tyrosine kinase – neither of which were proven therapeutic targets at the time. Second, it was not clear how to package and deliver such a drug. In the face of the success of Herceptin and Erbitux (targeting the EGFR/HER1), and the success of Bexxar and Zevalin (radiolabeled anti-CD 20 antibodies), it is possible that this approach should be pursued. Furthermore, resistance to Herceptin (innate or acquired) does not require loss of HER2 expression, but rather the acquisition of other tumor cell characteristics (discussed in Sect. 6). This latter observation suggests that, similarly to the use of Bexxar in the case of Rituxan failures (Horning et al. 2005), the radiolabeled version of Herceptin could be used successfully in Herceptin nonresponders, or patients who have developed resistance to Herceptin.

5.2 Active Specific Immunotherapy (ASI)

Active specific immunotherapy is the vaccination of a patient with antigen(s) characteristic of an ongoing malignancy. Usually such antigens are weakly immunogenic (Aloysius et al. 2006). This approach has been most rigorously championed by Mitchell (Mitchell 2003; Sosman and Sondak 2003). The initial therapeutic approach to p185^{HER2} was to develop a successful vaccination of breast cancer patients with the extracellular domain of HER2 (ECD; Fendly et al. 1990a). This concept was successfully used in a primate model in which it was shown that immunized animals developed a cellular immune response as monitored by delayed-type hypersensitivity to ECD, and antigen-specific cellular cytotoxicity. Antisera derived from successfully immunized animals specifically inhibited the in vitro proliferation of HER2-overexpressing tumor cells. Despite these encouraging preclinical results, the development of ASI was not pursued in 1990 primarily for two reasons: (1) the uncertainties surrounding breaking tolerance with self-antigen (HER2 ECD); and (2) the relative pharmacologic intractability of successful immunization vs. the "known" pharmacologic properties of passive immunotherapy. There are currently a number of ASI protocols ongoing which target p185^{HER2}, as well as other malignancies. One of the most promising ASIs in development is antigastrin vaccination for gastric cancer (Ajani et al. 2006; Aloysius et al. 2006). There are advantages to the development of a humoral response to disease-related ligands and receptors. In the case of p185^{HER2} the best evidence to this effect is that multiple monoclonal antibodies targeting distinct epitopes are much more effective in mediating downregulation and degradation of receptors than single monoclonal antibody administration (Friedman et al. 2005).

6 New Approaches to the Human EGFR Family

6.1 Current Status of the Human EGFR Family

From the time clinical work was begun for Herceptin, a great deal has been learned about the human EGFR (HER) family of receptors. There are now four recognized members of the family, all of which have been crystallized, and at least 11 ligands (Fig. 11; Yarden and Sliwkowski 2001).

Both homodimerization and heterodimerization occur among these receptors, mediated by a dimerization domain (Burgess et al. 2003) located in subdomain II of the ECD. Further diversity is added by the multiplicity of ligands, greater or lesser signaling based upon the composition of the heterodimer, and other issues. For instance, the EGFR/HER1 is stimulated in response to ligand; HER2 has no canonical ligand; HER3 has no tyrosine kinase activity; and HER4, while retaining both ligand-initiated signaling and tyrosine kinase activity, may assert its activity primarily after the intracellular region is cleaved and relocalized to the nucleus (Muraoka-Cook et al. 2006; Vidal et al. 2005).

6.2 Pan-HER Ligand Traps

Sensitivity of cells to Herceptin or its murine parent, muMAb4D5 is related to the level of p185^{HER2} expression but not in a linear manner (Lewis et al. 1993; Shepard et al. 1991). These studies demonstrated a marked increase in sensitivity when the tumor cell expresses approximately threefold to fivefold the level of receptor expressed by normal fibroblasts, coinciding remarkably with the level of

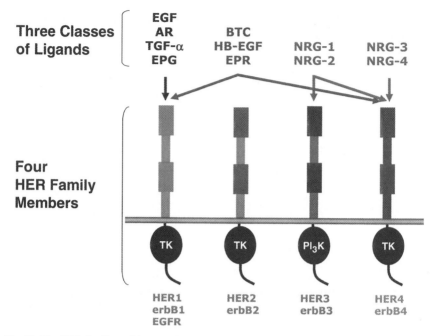

Fig. 11 The HER family and its canonical ligands. There are four members of the human EGFR family. Subdomains I and III contribute to ligand binding. Subdomain II contains the dimerization domain which is important for both homo- and heterodimerization. Subdomain IV contains a "tether" domain that can interact and stabilize the "closed" form of the receptor in the absence of ligand, except in the case of HER2 which most data indicate is constitutively in an open "ready to dimerize" configuration

overexpression required to predict shorter survival in patients who have tumors characterized by HER2 overexpression (Slamon et al. 1989; 1987). However, some tumor cells with quite high expression of HER2 do not respond as predicted by regression analysis (see boxed cell lines in Table 2). Similarly, about 25–50% of patients predicted to respond to Herceptin, based upon HER2 gene amplification or immunohistochemistry, do not respond to treatment (Joensuu et al. 2006; Piccart-Gebhart et al. 2005; Robert et al. 2006; Romond et al. 2005).

Mechanisms of inherent or adaptive resistance to Herceptin include alterations in the expression or mutations in p27[kip1], PTEN, survivin, p95[HER2], and IGF-1 receptor (Nahta et al. 2006). Not surprisingly, altered expression of unrelated cell surface proteins like MUC1, CD44, and hyaluronic acid, all of which may impact the ability of HER2 to cluster on the cell membrane, may also play a role in the activity of Herceptin (Ghatak et al. 2005; Hommelgaard et al. 2004). However, perhaps the most common and best documented factor associated with inherent resistance of tumor cells to Herceptin, and disease progression, is the co-expression of other HER family members (Bianchi et al. 2006; Robinson et al. 2006; Wiseman et al. 2005). While most of this work has been done with cohorts of breast cancer patients, similar data are available in a wide range of malignancies (Bladder, Chow et al. 2001;

Hepatocellular, Ito et al. 2001; Non small cell lung, Onn et al. 2004; Ovarian, Wang et al. 2005). It would be a great mistake to infer from this review that the human EGFR and its ligands are only associated with cancer. Data associated dysfunctional expression of Heregulin/Neuregulin, initially fully characterized as activators of the HER system by Holmes et al. (1992), have now shown that the HER family and its ligands participate in cardiac development, neuronal differentiation, schizophrenia, and Alzheimer's disease (Hahn et al. 2006; Meeks et al. 2006; Rohrbach et al. 2005; Vidal et al. 2005).

There is a clear need for therapeutic approaches that address multiple HER family members simultaneously. One approach has been to develop an antibody (muMAb2C4, Table 1) that binds the dimerization domain of p185^{HER2}, thereby preventing its heterodimerization with other HER family members (Adams et al. 2005). A second approach has been the development of Lapatinib, a small molecule tyrosine kinase inhibitor with apparent efficacy against Herceptin-resistant breast cancers, perhaps because it simultaneously inhibits both the HER2 and EGFR/HER1 tyrosine kinases (Konecny et al. 2006; Nelson and Dolder 2006). Other approaches to address this latter mechanism are principally aimed at inhibiting receptor multi-merization. This concept was first introduced by Greene and colleagues (Berezov et al. 2003; Qian et al. 1996). It has been extended to natural splice variants of the HER2 ECD acting as dominant negative ligands (Doherty et al. 1999) as well as several other approaches (Kumar and Pegram 2006). Our laboratory has chosen to focus on an alternative approach, which uses molecularly engineered heterodimers of the HER1 and HER3 extracellular domains to create receptor decoys that bind a wide range of HER family ligands. Because these proteins have the ability to broadly regulate juxtacrine and paracrine activation of the HER family, they are called Her-modulins. One example of a Hermodulin (RB200h) is shown in Fig. 12a,b.

These molecules are able to bind most of the ligands which normally activate HER1, 3, and 4. Because ligand overexpression promotes cellular transformation, resistance to tyrosine kinase inhibitors, and pathologies in addition to cancer, there is considerable interest in such reagents.

The concept of the Hermodulins is supported by Enbrel (a homodimeric TNF-α ligand trap), which is effective in the treatment of autoimmune disease (Nash and Florin 2005), and a homodimeric VEGF trap (Ferrara 2004) aimed at angiogenic diseases. In addition, cell biological experiments have demonstrated that receptor cooperativity and ligand stimulation are required for maximum transforming activity (Cohen et al. 1996; Zhang et al. 1996), providing further support that Hermod-ulins should be active anticancer agents.

6.3 Inhibition of Ligand-Induced Receptor Phosphorylation by Hermodulins

Early experiments with RB200h were intended to compare the breadth of its activity with the proposed pan-HER activity of Pertuzumab (reported by Adams et al. 2005)

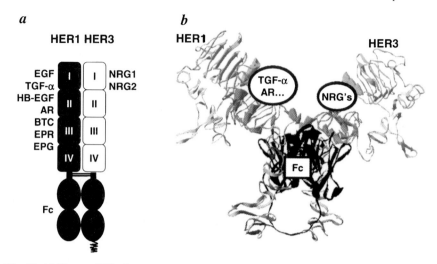

Fig. 12 (**a**) The pan-HER ligand trap. Shown are subdomains I–IV of both the EGFR/HER1 and HER 3, dimerized via IgG1 Fc domains. The canonical ligands bound by each member of the heterodimer are also listed. (**b**) The predicted solution structure of RB200h in a high affinity conformation and a schematic of TGF-α/Amphiregulin bound to subdomains I and III of HER1; and the neuregulins bound to subdomains I and III of HER3

and with Herceptin. The results of these experiments are shown in Table 4. The data are summarized as a "Pan-HER Index" which is a measure of the maximum inhibition of ligand-stimulated receptor phosphorylation achieved by the three agents. Inhibition of $p185^{HER2}$ phosphorylation is likely indirect, and secondary to inhibition of ligand binding mediated by RB200h.

These data clearly suggest that "trapping" is a more effective means of inhibiting ligand-associated receptor activation than direct antibody-mediated receptor binding. The result is that muMAb2C4 seems to stimulate NRG-mediated receptor phosphorylation.

Table 4 Pan-HER antagonist activity of muMab2C4 (parent of Pertuzumab), Herceptin, and RB200h[a]

Molecule	EGFR/HER1		HER2		HER3		Pan-HER Index[b]
	EGF	NRG	EGF	NRG	EGF	NRG	
MuMAb2C4	15	−75	20	−200	62	59	−19.8
Herceptin	5	10	90	70	45	3	37.2
RB200h	90	50	65	15	60	60	56.7

Phosphorylation of HER receptors in the presence of growth factors or antagonists (2C4, Herceptin, or RB200h) was assessed in an ELISA-based receptor phosphorylation assay

[a] Values given are percent control stimulated with 3 nM EGF or 5 nM NRG1-β1. Standard deviations are less than 20%

[b] Pan-HER Index is the average inhibition of receptor phosphorylation for EGFR/HER1, HER2, and HER 3. A negative number indicates stimulation of phosphorylation

Table 5 Growth inhibition by RB200h is distinct from growth inhibition by Herceptin

Cell line	IC_{50}^{a}	Max inhibition[b]	
	(nM)	RB200h (%)	Herceptin(%)
SK-BR-3 (breast)	1	60	69
A549 (NSCLC)	1	30	<10
ZR-75-1 (breast)	2	22	<10

[a] Inhibition of tumor cell proliferation by RB200h was measured at 72 h using alamar blue as described by the vendor (Biotium, Inc.; www.biotium.com). The IC_{50} values shown reflect half-maximum growth inhibition for RB200h
[b] Maximum inhibition of tumor cell growth at the highest doses tested

6.4 Hermodulins Inhibit Tumor Cell Proliferation In Vivo

The spectrum of growth inhibitory activity of Hermodulins is distinct from Herceptin. RB200h and its related protein, RB210h, were tested for their ability to inhibit the proliferation of tumor cells in monolayer culture. To test whether RB200h/210h inhibited tumor cell line proliferation in vitro, monolayer growth assays were performed (Table 5).

The receptor phosphorylation and cell growth inhibition data show that RB200 has biological activities which are distinct from Herceptin and muMAb2C4 (the parent of Pertuzumab).

7 Summary and Conclusions: What We Have Learned and What to Do Next

Herceptin has helped many women with breast cancer. More than 150,000 patients have been treated with Herceptin, and there is about 50% success rate in patients whose malignancy is characterized by a high level of $p185^{HER2}$ expression, or gene amplification. This is, however, less than 25% of all breast cancer. The utility of Herceptin outside of this discrete population has been difficult to demonstrate. Attempts at optimizing administration using different schedules and combinations with chemotherapy may improve this situation. In particular, combinations of Herceptin with tyrosine kinase inhibitors like Lapatinib, or other monoclonal antibodies which target either distinct epitopes on the ECD of $p185^{HER2}$, or other members of the HER family, are likely to improve the overall percentage of patients that can be helped, perhaps even outside of breast cancer. Because HER family members cooperate to promote malignancy, it is necessary that we develop approaches, such as the pan-HER Ligand Trap, which can specifically target several members of the family simultaneously. Other antibody-based approaches to the treatment of HER-driven diseases need further examination. For instance, radioimmunotherapy using Herceptin conjugated with the appropriate radioisotope would likely be effective in $HER2^{+++}$ patients, even when they co-express multiple other receptors, because its efficacy depends only upon the enhanced internalization which occurs with HER2 overexpression. Finally, increased understanding of the HER system and its ligands has led to "unrelated" potential applications of reagents such as Hermodulins. As an example, it is now known that dysregulation of the neuregulins may be involved in diseases as disparate as autommune diseases, cardiac myopathy, and neurodegenerative diseases (Garratt 2006; Hall et al. 2004; Nawa and Takei 2006; Zanazzi et al. 2001). What has been learned from the application of α-HER agents in cancer is likely to eventually benefit patients with other chronic and life-threatening diseases.

References

Aboud-Pirak E, Hurwitz E, Pirak ME, Bellot F, Schlessinger J, Sela M (1988) Efficacy of antibodies to epidermal growth factor receptor against KB carcinoma in vitro and in nude mice. J Natl Cancer Inst 80:1605–1611

Adams CW, Allison DE, Flagella K, Presta L, Clarke J, Dybdal N, McKeever K, Sliwkowski MX (2005) Humanization of a recombinant monoclonal antibody to produce a therapeutic HER dimerization inhibitor, pertuzumab. Cancer Immunol Immunother 55:717–727

Ajani JA, Randolph HJ, Ho L, Baker J, Oortgiesen M, Eduljee A, Michaeli D (2006) An open-label, multinational, multicenter study of G17DT vaccination combined with cisplatin and 5-fluorouracil in patients with untreated, advanced gastric or gastroesophageal cancer: the GC4 study. Cancer 106:1908–1916

Aloysius MM, Robins RA, Eremin JM, Eremin O (2006) Vaccination therapy in malignant disease. Surgeon 4:309–320

Arnould L, Gelly M, Penault-Llorca F, Benoit L, Bonnetain F, Migeon C, Cabaret V, Fermeaux V, Bertheau P, Garnier J, Jeannin JF, Coudert B (2006) Trastuzumab-based treatment of HER2-positive breast cancer: an antibody-dependent cellular cytotoxicity mechanism? Br J Cancer 94:259–267

Ashrafian H (2006) Cancer's sweet tooth: the Janus effect of glucose metabolism in tumorigenesis. Lancet 367:618–621

Ballangrud AM, Yang WH, Palm S, Enmon R, Borchardt PE, Pellegrini VA, McDevitt MR, Scheinberg DA, Sgouros G (2004) Alpha-particle emitting atomic generator (Actinium-225)-labeled trastuzumab (herceptin) targeting of breast cancer spheroids: efficacy versus HER2/neu expression. Clin Cancer Res 10:4489–4497

Baselga J (2001) Clinical trials of Herceptin(R) (trastuzumab). Eur J Cancer 37 Suppl 1:18–24

Baselga J, Norton L, Albanell J, Kim YM, Mendelsohn J (1998) Recombinant humanized anti-HER2 antibody (Herceptin) enhances the antitumor activity of paclitaxel and doxorubicin against HER2/neu overexpressing human breast cancer xenografts. Cancer Res 58:2825–2831

Baselga J, Perez EA, Pienkowski T, Bell R (2006) Adjuvant trastuzumab: a milestone in the treatment of HER-2-positive early breast cancer. Oncologist 11 Suppl 1:4–12

Baselga J, Tripathy D, Mendelsohn J, Baughman S, Benz CC, Dantis L, Sklarin NT, Seidman AD, Hudis CA, Moore J, Rosen PP, Twaddell T, Henderson IC, Norton L (1996) Phase II study of weekly intravenous recombinant humanized anti-p185HER2 monoclonal antibody in patients with HER2/neu-overexpressing metastatic breast cancer. J Clin Oncol 14:737–744

Berezov A, Greene MI, Murali R (2003) Structure-based approaches to inhibition of erbB receptors with peptide mimetics. Immunol Res 27:303–308

Bianchi S, Palli D, Falchetti M, Saieva C, Masala G, Mancini B, Lupi R, Noviello C, Omerovic J, Paglierani M, Vezzosi V, Alimandi M, Mariani-Costantini R, Ottini L (2006) ErbB-receptors expression and survival in breast carcinoma: a 15-year follow-up study. J Cell Physiol 206: 702–708

Bishop JM (1989) Nobel Prize Lecture: Retroviruses and Oncogenes II

Blumenthal RD, Sharkey RM, Goldenberg DM (1990) Current perspectives and challenges in the use of monoclonal antibodies as imaging and theraputic agents. Adv Drug Deliv Rev 4:279–318

Brechbiel MW, Waldmann TA (2000) Anti-HER2 radioimmunotherapy. Breast Dis 11:125–132

Burgess AW, Cho HS, Eigenbrot C, Ferguson KM, Garrett TP, Leahy DJ, Lemmon MA, Sliwkowski MX, Ward CW, Yokoyama S (2003) An open-and-shut case? Recent insights into the activation of EGF/ErbB receptors. Mol Cell 12:541–552

Carter P, Fendly BM, Lewis GD, Sliwkowski MX (2000) Development of herceptin. Breast Dis 11:103–111

Carter P, Presta L, Gorman CM, Ridgway JB, Henner D, Wong WL, Rowland AM, Kotts C, Carver ME, Shepard HM (1992) Humanization of an anti-p185HER2 antibody for human cancer therapy. Proc Natl Acad Sci USA 89:4285–4289

Chazin VR, Kaleko M, Miller AD, Slamon DJ (1992) Transformation mediated by the human HER-2 gene independent of the epidermal growth factor receptor. Oncogene 7:1859–1866

Chow NH, Chan SH, Tzai TS, Ho CL, Liu HS (2001) Expression profiles of ErbB family receptors and prognosis in primary transitional cell carcinoma of the urinary bladder. Clin Cancer Res 7:1957–1962

Citri A, Yarden Y (2006) EGF-ERBB signalling: towards the systems level. Nat Rev Mol Cell Biol 7:505–516

Cobleigh MA, Vogel CL, Tripathy D, Robert NJ, Scholl S, Fehrenbacher L, Wolter JM, Paton V, Shak S, Lieberman G, Slamon DJ (1999) Multinational study of the efficacy and safety of humanized anti-HER2 monoclonal antibody in women who have HER2-overexpressing metastatic breast cancer that has progressed after chemotherapy for metastatic disease. J Clin Oncol 17:2639–2648

Cohen BD, Kiener PA, Green JM, Foy L, Fell HP, Zhang K (1996) The relationship between human epidermal growth-like factor receptor expression and cellular transformation in NIH3T3 cells. J Biol Chem 271:30897–30903

Coussens L, Yang-Feng TL, Liao YC, Chen E, Gray A, McGrath J, Seeburg PH, Libermann TA, Schlessinger J, Francke U (1985) Tyrosine kinase receptor with extensive homology to EGF receptor shares chromosomal location with neu oncogene. Science 230:1132–1139

Crow DM, Williams L, Colcher D, Wong JY, Raubitschek A, Shively JE (2005) Combined radioimmunotherapy and chemotherapy of breast tumors with Y-90-labeled anti-Her2 and anti-CEA antibodies with taxol. Bioconjug Chem 16:1117–1125

De Santes K, Slamon D, Anderson SK, Shepard M, Fendly B, Maneval D, Press O (1992) Radio labeled antibody targeting of the HER-2/neu oncoprotein. Cancer Res 52:1916–1923

Doherty JK, Bond C, Jardim A, Adelman JP, Clinton GM (1999) The HER-2/neu receptor tyrosine kinase gene encodes a secreted autoinhibitor. Proc Natl Acad Sci USA 96:10869–10874

Dorr RT, Von Hoff DD (1994) Cancer Chemotherapy Handbook., 2nd edn. Appleton and Lange, Norwalk, pp 500–515

Drebin JA, Link VC, Stern DF, Weinberg RA, Greene MI (1985) Down-modulation of an oncogene protein product and reversion of the transformed phenotype by monoclonal antibodies. Cell 41:697–706

Fendly BM, Kotts C, Vetterlein D, Lewis GD, Winget M, Carver ME, Watson SR, Sarup J, Saks S, Ullrich A (1990a) The extracellular domain of HER2/neu is a potential immunogen for active specific immunotherapy of breast cancer. J Biol Response Mod 9:449–455

Fendly BM, Winget M, Hudziak RM, Lipari MT, Napier MA, Ullrich A (1990b) Characterization of murine monoclonal antibodies reactive to either the human epidermal growth factor receptor or HER2/neu gene product. Cancer Res 50:1550–1558

Ferrara N (2004) Vascular endothelial growth factor: basic science and clinical progress. Endocr Rev 25:581–611

Friedman LM, Rinon A, Schechter B, Lyass L, Lavi S, Bacus SS, Sela M, Yarden Y (2005) Synergistic down-regulation of receptor tyrosine kinases by combinations of mAbs: implications for cancer immunotherapy. Proc Natl Acad Sci USA 102:1915–1920

Garratt AN (2006) "To erb-B or not to erb-B…" Neuregulin-1/ErbB signaling in heart development and function. J Mol Cell Cardiol 41:215–218

Ghatak S, Misra S, Toole BP (2005) Hyaluronan constitutively regulates ErbB2 phosphorylation and signaling complex formation in carcinoma cells. J Biol Chem 280:8875–8883

Gill GN, Kawamoto T, Cochet C, Le A, Sato JD, Masui H, McLeod C, Mendelsohn J (1984) Monoclonal anti-epidermal growth factor receptor antibodies which are inhibitors of epidermal growth factor binding and antagonists of epidermal growth factor binding and antagonists of epidermal growth factor-stimulated tyrosine protein kinase activity. J Biol Chem 259: 7755–7760

Giordano S, Ponzetto C, Di Renzo MF, Cooper CS, Comoglio PM (1989) Tyrosine kinase receptor indistinguishable from the c-met protein. Nature 339:155–156

Goldenberg DM (1991) Challenges to the therapy of cancer with monoclonal antibodies. J Natl Cancer Inst 83:78–79

Goldenberg DM, Sharkey RM (2006) Advances in cancer therapy with radiolabeled monoclonal antibodies. Q J Nucl Med Mol Imag 50:248–264

Hahn CG, Wang HY, Cho DS, Talbot K, Gur RE, Berrettini WH, Bakshi K, Kamins J, Borgmann-Winter KE, Siegel SJ, Gallop RJ, Arnold SE (2006) Altered neuregulin 1-erbB4 signaling contributes to NMDA receptor hypofunction in schizophrenia. Nat Med 12:824–828

Hall D, Gogos JA, Karayiorgou M (2004) The contribution of three strong candidate schizophrenia susceptibility genes in demographically distinct populations. Genes Brain Behav 3:240–248

Heidelberger C, Chaudhuri Nk, Danneberg P, Mooren D, Griesbach L, Duschinsky R, Schnitzer Rj, Pleven E, Scheiner J (1957) Fluorinated pyrimidines, a new class of tumour-inhibitory compounds. Nature 179:663–666

Holmes WE, Sliwkowski MX, Akita RW, Henzel WJ, Lee J, Park JW, Yansura D, Abadi N, Raab H, Lewis GD (1992) Identification of heregulin, a specific activator of p185erbB2. Science 256:1205–1210

Hommelgaard AM, Lerdrup M, van DB (2004) Association with membrane protrusions makes ErbB2 an internalization-resistant receptor. Mol Biol Cell 15:1557–1567

Horning SJ, Younes A, Jain V, Kroll S, Lucas J, Podoloff D, Goris M (2005) Efficacy and safety of tositumomab and iodine-131 tositumomab (Bexxar) in B-cell lymphoma, progressive after rituximab. J Clin Oncol 23:712–719

Hudziak RM, Lewis GD, Holmes WE, Ullrich A, Shepard HM (1990) Selection for transformation and met protooncogene amplification in NIH 3T3 fibroblasts using tumor necrosis factor alpha. Cell Growth Differ 1:129–134

Hudziak RM, Lewis GD, Shalaby MR, Eessalu TE, Aggarwal BB, Ullrich A, Shepard HM (1988) Amplified expression of the HER2/ERBB2 oncogene induces resistance to tumor necrosis factor alpha in NIH 3T3 cells. Proc Natl Acad Sci USA 85:5102–5106

Hudziak RM, Lewis GD, Winget M, Fendly BM, Shepard HM, Ullrich A (1989) p185HER2 monoclonal antibody has antiproliferative effects in vitro and sensitizes human breast tumor cells to tumor necrosis factor. Mol Cell Biol 9:1165–1172

Hudziak RM, Schlessinger J, Ullrich A (1987) Increased expression of the putative growth factor receptor p185HER2 causes transformation and tumorigenesis of NIH 3T3 cells. Proc Natl Acad Sci USA 84:7159–7163

Hynes NE, Lane HA (2005) ERBB receptors and cancer: the complexity of targeted inhibitors. Nat Rev Cancer 5:341–354

Ito Y, Takeda T, Sakon M, Tsujimoto M, Higashiyama S, Noda K, Miyoshi E, Monden M, Matsuura N (2001) Expression and clinical significance of erb-B receptor family in hepatocellular carcinoma. Br J Cancer 84:1377–1383

Joensuu H, Kellokumpu-Lehtinen PL, Bono P, Alanko T, Kataja V, Asola R, Utriainen T, Kokko R, Hemminki A, Tarkkanen M, Turpeenniemi-Hujanen T, Jyrkkio S, Flander M, Helle L, Ingalsuo S, Johansson K, Jaaskelainen AS, Pajunen M, Rauhala M, Kaleva-Kerola J, Salminen T, Leinonen M, Elomaa I, Isola J (2006) Adjuvant docetaxel or vinorelbine with or without trastuzumab for breast cancer. N Engl J Med 354:809–820

Katoh M, Yazaki Y, Sugimura T, Terada M (1993) c-erbB3 gene encodes secreted as well as trans-membrane receptor tyrosine kinase. Biochem Biophys Res Commun 192:1189–1197

King CR, Kraus MH, Aaronson SA (1985) Amplification of a novel v-erbB-related gene in a human mammary carcinoma. Science 229:974–976

Konecny GE, Pegram MD, Venkatesan N, Finn R, Yang G, Rahmeh M, Untch M, Rusnak DW, Spehar G, Mullin RJ, Keith BR, Gilmer TM, Berger M, Podratz KC, Slamon DJ (2006) Activity of the dual kinase inhibitor lapatinib (GW572016) against HER-2-overexpressing and trastuzumab-treated breast cancer cells. Cancer Res 66:1630–1639

Kotts CE, Su FM, Leddy C, Dodd T, Scates S, Shalaby MR, Wirth CM, Giltinan D, Schroff RW, Fritzberg AR, Shepard HM, Slamon DJ, Hutchins BM (1996) 186Re-labeled antibodies to p185HER2 as HER2-targeted radioimmunopharmaceutical agents: comparison of physical and biological characteristics with 125I and 131I-labeled counterparts. Cancer Biother Radiopharm 11:133–144

Kris RM, Lax I, Gullick W, Waterfield MD, Ullrich A, Fridkin M, Schlessinger J (1985) Antibodies against a synthetic peptide as a probe for the kinase activity of the avian EGF receptor and v-erbB protein. Cell 40:619–625

Kumar PS, Pegram M (2006) Targeting HER2 Epitopes. Semin Oncol 33:386–391

Lackey DB, Groziak MP, Sergeeva M, Beryt M, Boyer C, Stroud RM, Sayre P, Park JW, Johnston P, Slamon D, Shepard HM, Pegram M (2001) Enzyme-catalyzed therapeutic agent (ECTA) design: activation of the antitumor ECTA compound NB1011 by thymidylate synthase. Biochem Pharmacol 61:179–189

Leibovich SJ, Polverini PJ, Shepard HM, Wiseman DM, Shively V, Nuseir N (1987) Macrophage-induced angiogenesis is mediated by tumour necrosis factor-alpha. Nature 329:630–632

Lewis GD, Aggarwal BB, Eessalu TE, Sugarman BJ, Shepard HM (1987) Modulation of the growth of transformed cells by human tumor necrosis factor-alpha and interferon-gamma. Cancer Res 47:5382–5385

Lewis GD, Figari I, Fendly B, Wong WL, Carter P, Gorman C, Shepard HM (1993) Differential responses of human tumor cell lines to anti-p185HER2 monoclonal antibodies. Cancer Immunol Immunother 37:255–263

Leyland-Jones B (2001) Dose scheduling–Herceptin. Oncology 61 Suppl 2:31–36

Li Q, Boyer C, Lee JY, Shepard HM (2001) A novel approach to thymidylate synthase as a target for cancer chemotherapy. Mol Pharmacol 59:446–452

Makhija, Glenn D, Ueland F, Gold M, Dizon D, Paton V, Birkner M, Lin C, Derynck M, Matulonis U (2007) Results from a phase II randomized, placebo-controlled, double-blind trial suggest improved PFS with the addition of pertuzumab to gemcitabine in patients with platinum-resistant ovarian, fallopian tube, or primary peritoneal cancer. J Clin Oncol 25:5507

Maneval DC, Baughman S, Hutchins B, Mordenti J (1991a) Pharmacokinetics of MuMab4D5 in cynomolgus monkeys. Pharm Res 8:54

Maneval DC, Hutchins B, Osaka G, Leddy C, Kotts C, Mohler M, Lewis D, Hansen S, Terrell T, Dodd T, Beaumier P, Giltinan D, Shalaby R, Stagg R, Mordenti J, Green J, Fritzberg A, Su FM (1993) Studies with a radiolabeled humanized anti-p185HER2 monoclonal antibody (rhuMab HER2) in tumor-bearing mice. Antibody Immunoconjugates and Radiopharmaceuticals 6:80

Maneval DC, Hutchins B, Osaka G, Leddy C, Kotts C, Vetterlein D, Dodd T, Axworthy D, Beaumeier P, Vanderheyden JL, Shalaby R, Shepard HM, Mordenti J, Fritzberg A, Su FM (1992) Comparative evaluation of I-125 and Re-186 labeled murine anti-p185HER2 antibody (muMAb 4D5) in an animal tumor model. J Nucl Med 33:934

Maneval DC, Mordenti J, Hutchins B, Scates S, Hansen S, Keith D, Kotts C, Fletcher B, Fendly B, Blank G, Vetterlein D, Slamon D, Shepard HM, Green JD (1991b) Pharmacokinetics and whole body autoradiography of I-125 muMAb 4D5 in mice. J Nucl Med 32:1837

Maneval DC, Thomas D, Mordenti J, Green J (1991c) Utilization of interspecies scaling techniques to support dose selection in the development of a monoclonal antibody in GN 1445. The Toxicologist 11:235

Maple L, Lathrop R, Bozich S, Harman W, Tacey R, Kelley M, nilkovitch-Miagkova A (2004) Development and validation of ELISA for herceptin detection in human serum. J Immunol Methods 295:169–182

Marty M, Cognetti F, Maraninchi D, Snyder R, Mauriac L, Tubiana-Hulin M, Chan S, Grimes D, Anton A, Lluch A, Kennedy J, O'Byrne K, Conte P, Green M, Ward C, Mayne K, Extra JM (2005) Randomized phase II trial of the efficacy and safety of trastuzumab combined with docetaxel in patients with human epidermal growth factor receptor 2-positive metastatic breast cancer administered as first-line treatment: the M77001 study group. J Clin Oncol 23: 4265–4274

Meeks TW, Ropacki SA, Jeste DV (2006) The neurobiology of neuropsychiatric syndromes in dementia. Curr Opin Psychiat 19:581–586

Milenic DE, Garmestani K, Brady ED, Albert PS, Ma D, Abdulla A, Brechbiel MW (2005) Alpha-particle radioimmunotherapy of disseminated peritoneal disease using a (212)Pb-labeled radioimmunoconjugate targeting HER2. Cancer Biother Radiopharm 20:557–568

Milenic DE, Garmestani K, Brady ED, Albert PS, Ma D, Abdulla A, Brechbiel MW (2004) Targeting of HER2 antigen for the treatment of disseminated peritoneal disease. Clin Cancer Res 10:7834–7841

Mitchell MS (2003) Combinations of anticancer drugs and immunotherapy. Cancer Immunol Immunother 52:686–692

Muller WJ, Sinn E, Pattengale PK, Wallace R, Leder P (1988) Single-step induction of mammary adenocarcinoma in transgenic mice bearing the activated c-neu oncogene. Cell 54:105–115

Muraoka-Cook RS, Sandahl M, Husted C, Hunter D, Miraglia L, Feng SM, Elenius K, Earp HS, III (2006) The intracellular domain of ErbB4 induces differentiation of mammary epithelial cells. Mol Biol Cell 17:4118–4129

Nahta R, Yu D, Hung MC, Hortobagyi GN, Esteva FJ (2006) Mechanisms of Disease: under-standing resistance to HER2-targeted therapy in human breast cancer. Nat Clin Pract Oncol 3:269–280

Nahta R, Yuan LX, Zhang B, Kobayashi R, Esteva FJ (2005) Insulin-like growth factor-I recep-tor/human epidermal growth factor receptor 2 heterodimerization contributes to trastuzumab resistance of breast cancer cells. Cancer Res 65:11118–11128

Nash PT, Florin TH (2005) Tumour necrosis factor inhibitors. Med J Aust 183:205–208

Nawa H, Takei N (2006) Recent progress in animal modeling of immune inflammatory processes in schizophrenia: implication of specific cytokines. Neurosci Res 56:2–13

Nelson MH, Dolder CR (2006) Lapatinib: a novel dual tyrosine kinase inhibitor with activity in solid tumors. Ann Pharmacother 40:261–269

Olafsen T, Kenanova VE, Sundaresan G, Anderson AL, Crow D, Yazaki PJ, Li L, Press MF, Gambhir SS, Williams LE, Wong JY, Raubitschek AA, Shively JE, Wu AM (2005) Optimizing radiolabeled engineered anti-p185HER2 antibody fragments for in vivo imaging. Cancer Res 65:5907–5916

Onn A, Correa AM, Gilcrease M, Isobe T, Massarelli E, Bucana CD, O'Reilly MS, Hong WK, Fidler IJ, Putnam JB, Herbst RS (2004) Synchronous overexpression of epidermal growth factor receptor and HER2-neu protein is a predictor of poor outcome in patients with stage I non-small cell lung cancer. Clin Cancer Res 10:136–143

Park JW, Stagg R, Lewis GD, Carter P, Maneval D, Slamon DJ, Jaffe H, Shepard HM (1992) Anti-p185HER2 monoclonal antibodies: biological properties and potential for immunother-apy. Cancer Treat Res 61:193–211

Pegram MD, Finn RS, Arzoo K, Beryt M, Pietras RJ, Slamon DJ (1997) The effect of HER-2/neu overexpression on chemotherapeutic drug sensitivity in human breast and ovarian cancer cells. Oncogene 15:537–547

Pegram MD, Hsu S, Lewis G, Pietras R, Beryt M, Sliwkowski M, Coombs D, Baly D, Kabbinavar F, Slamon D (1999) Inhibitory effects of combinations of HER-2/neu antibody and chemotherapeutic agents used for treatment of human breast cancers. Oncogene 18:2241–2251

Pegram MD, Konecny GE, O'Callaghan C, Beryt M, Pietras R, Slamon DJ (2004) Rational combinations of trastuzumab with chemotherapeutic drugs used in the treatment of breast cancer. J Natl Cancer Inst 96:739–749

Pegram MD, Lipton A, Hayes DF, Weber BL, Baselga JM, Tripathy D, Baly D, Baughman SA, Twaddell T, Glaspy JA, Slamon DJ (1998) Phase II study of receptor-enhanced chemosensitivity using recombinant humanized anti-p185HER2/neu monoclonal antibody plus cisplatin in patients with HER2/neu-overexpressing metastatic breast cancer refractory to chemotherapy treatment. J Clin Oncol 16:2659–2671

Perik PJ, Lub-De Hooge MN, Gietema JA, Van der Graaf WT, de Korte MA, Jonkman S, Kosterink JG, Van Veldhuisen DJ, Sleijfer DT, Jager PL, De Vries EG (2006) Indium-111-labeled trastuzumab scintigraphy in patients with human epidermal growth factor receptor 2-positive metastatic breast cancer. J Clin Oncol 24:2276–2282

Persson MI, Gedda L, Jensen HJ, Lundqvist H, Malmstrom PU, Tolmachev V (2006) Astatinated trastuzumab, a putative agent for radionuclide immunotherapy of ErbB2-expressing tumours. Oncol Rep 15:673–680

Persson MI, Tolmachev V, Andersson K, Gedda L, Sandstrom M, Carlsson J (2005) [(177)Lu]pertuzumab: experimental studies on targeting of HER-2 positive tumour cells. Eur J Nucl Med Mol Imaging 32:1457–1462

Piccart-Gebhart MJ, Procter M, Leyland-Jones B, Goldhirsch A, Untch M, Smith I, Gianni L, Baselga J, Bell R, Jackisch C, Cameron D, Dowsett M, Barrios CH, Steger G, Huang CS, Andersson M, Inbar M, Lichinitser M, Lang I, Nitz U, Iwata H, Thomssen C, Lohrisch C, Suter TM, Ruschoff J, Suto T, Greatorex V, Ward C, Straehle C, McFadden E, Dolci MS, Gelber RD (2005) Trastuzumab after adjuvant chemotherapy in HER2-positive breast cancer. N Engl J Med 353:1659–1672

Pietras RJ, Fendly BM, Chazin VR, Pegram MD, Howell SB, Slamon DJ (1994) Antibody to HER-2/neu receptor blocks DNA repair after cisplatin in human breast and ovarian cancer cells. Oncogene 9:1829–1838

Pietras RJ, Pegram MD, Finn RS, Maneval DA, Slamon DJ (1998) Remission of human breast cancer xenografts on therapy with humanized monoclonal antibody to HER-2 receptor and DNA-reactive drugs. Oncogene 17:2235–2249

Pinkas-Kramarski R, Soussan L, Waterman H, Levkowitz G, Alroy I, Klapper L, Lavi S, Seger R, Ratzkin BJ, Sela M, Yarden Y (1996) Diversification of Neu differentiation factor and epidermal growth factor signaling by combinatorial receptor interactions. EMBO J 15:2452–2467

Prenzel N, Fischer OM, Streit S, Hart S, Ullrich A (2001) The epidermal growth factor receptor family as a central element for cellular signal transduction and diversification. Endocr Relat Cancer 8:11–31

Qian X, O'Rourke DM, Zhao H, Greene MI (1996) Inhibition of p185neu kinase activity and cellular transformation by co-expression of a truncated neu protein. Oncogene 13:2149–2157

Robert N, Leyland-Jones B, Asmar L, Belt R, Ilegbodu D, Loesch D, Raju R, Valentine E, Sayre R, Cobleigh M, Albain K, McCullough C, Fuchs L, Slamon D (2006) Randomized phase III study of trastuzumab, paclitaxel, and carboplatin compared with trastuzumab and paclitaxel in women with HER-2-overexpressing metastatic breast cancer. J Clin Oncol 24:2786–2792

Robinson AG, Turbin D, Thomson T, Yorida E, Ellard S, Bajdik C, Huntsman D, Gelmon K (2006) Molecular predictive factors in patients receiving trastuzumab-based chemotherapy for metastatic disease. Clin Breast Cancer 7:254–261

Rohrbach S, Niemann B, Silber RE, Holtz J (2005) Neuregulin receptors erbB2 and erbB4 in failing human myocardium – depressed expression and attenuated activation. Basic Res Cardiol 100:240–249

Romond EH, Perez EA, Bryant J, Suman VJ, Geyer CE, Jr., Davidson NE, Tan-Chiu E, Martino S, Paik S, Kaufman PA, Swain SM, Pisansky TM, Fehrenbacher L, Kutteh LA, Vogel VG, Visscher DW, Yothers G, Jenkins RB, Brown AM, Dakhil SR, Mamounas EP, Lingle WL, Klein PM, Ingle JN, Wolmark N (2005) Trastuzumab plus adjuvant chemotherapy for operable HER2-positive breast cancer. N Engl J Med 353:1673–1684

Schechter AL, Hung MC, Vaidyanathan L, Weinberg RA, Yang-Feng TL, Francke U, Ullrich A, Coussens L (1985) The neu gene: an erbB-homologous gene distinct from and unlinked to the gene encoding the EGF receptor. Science 229:976–978

Schechter AL, Stern DF, Vaidyanathan L, Decker SJ, Drebin JA, Greene MI, Weinberg RA (1984) The neu oncogene: an erb-B-related gene encoding a 185,000-Mr tumour antigen. Nature 312:513–516

Semba K, Kamata N, Toyoshima K, Yamamoto T (1985) A v-erbB-related protooncogene, c-erbB-2, is distinct from the c-erbB-1/epidermal growth factor-receptor gene and is amplified in a human salivary gland adenocarcinoma. Proc Natl Acad Sci USA 82:6497–6501

Sergina NV, Rausch M, Wang D, Blair J, Hann B, Shokat KM, Moasser MM (2007) Escape from HER-family tyrosine kinase inhibitor therapy by the kinase-inactive HER3. Nature 445: 437–441

Shak S (1999) Overview of the trastuzumab (Herceptin) anti-HER2 monoclonal antibody clinical program in HER2-overexpressing metastatic breast cancer. Herceptin Multinational Investigator Study Group. Semin Oncol 26:71–77

Shepard HM, Lewis GD, Sarup JC, Fendly BM, Maneval D, Mordenti J, Figari I, Kotts CE, Palladino MA, Jr., Ullrich A (1991) Monoclonal antibody therapy of human cancer: taking the HER2 protooncogene to the clinic. J Clin Immunol 11:117–127

Shih C, Padhy LC, Murray M, Weinberg RA (1981) Transforming genes of carcinomas and neuroblastomas introduced into mouse fibroblasts. Nature 290:261–264

Slamon D, Pegram M (2001) Rationale for trastuzumab (Herceptin) in adjuvant breast cancer trials. Semin Oncol 28:13–19

Slamon DJ, Clark GM, Wong SG, Levin WJ, Ullrich A, McGuire WL (1987) Human breast cancer: correlation of relapse and survival with amplification of the HER-2/neu oncogene. Science 235:177–182

Slamon DJ, Godolphin W, Jones LA, Holt JA, Wong SG, Keith DE, Levin WJ, Stuart SG, Udove J, Ullrich A (1989) Studies of the HER-2/neu proto-oncogene in human breast and ovarian cancer. Science 244:707–712

Slamon DJ, Leyland-Jones B, Shak S, Fuchs H, Paton V, Bajamonde A, Fleming T, Eiermann W, Wolter J, Pegram M, Baselga J, Norton L (2001) Use of chemotherapy plus a monoclonal antibody against HER2 for metastatic breast cancer that overexpresses HER2. N Engl J Med 344:783–792

Smith-Jones PM, Solit DB, Akhurst T, Afroze F, Rosen N, Larson SM (2004) Imaging the pharmacodynamics of HER2 degradation in response to Hsp90 inhibitors. Nat Biotechnol 22:701–706

Sosman JA, Sondak VK (2003) Melacine: an allogeneic melanoma tumor cell lysate vaccine. Expert Rev Vaccines 2:353–368

Sporn MB, Todaro GJ (1980) Autocrine secretion and malignant transformation of cells. N Engl J Med 303:878–880

Sugarman BJ, Lewis GD, Eessalu TE, Aggarwal BB, Shepard HM (1987) Effects of growth factors on the antiproliferative activity of tumor necrosis factors. Cancer Res 47:780–786

Tokuda Y, Ohnishi Y, Shimamura K, Iwasawa M, Yoshimura M, Ueyama Y, Tamaoki N, Tajima T, Mitomi T (1996) In vitro and in vivo anti-tumour effects of a humanised monoclonal antibody against c-erbB-2 product. Br J Cancer 73:1362–1365

Urban JL, Schreiber H (1988) Host-tumor interactions in immunosurveillance against cancer. Prog Exp Tumor Res 32:17–68

Urban JL, Shepard HM, Rothstein JL, Sugarman BJ, Schreiber H (1986) Tumor necrosis factor: a potent effector molecule for tumor cell killing by activated macrophages. Proc Natl Acad Sci USA 83:5233–5237

Varmus HE (1989) Nobel Prize Lecture: Retroviruses and Oncogenes I.

Vidal GA, Naresh A, Marrero L, Jones FE (2005) Presenilin-dependent gamma-secretase processing regulates multiple ERBB4/HER4 activities. J Biol Chem 280:19777–19783

Vogel CL, Cobleigh MA, Tripathy D, Gutheil JC, Harris LN, Fehrenbacher L, Slamon DJ, Murphy M, Novotny WF, Burchmore M, Shak S, Stewart SJ, Press M (2002) Efficacy and safety of trastuzumab as a single agent in first-line treatment of HER2-overexpressing metastatic breast cancer. J Clin Oncol 20:719–726

Wang Y, Kristensen GB, Helland A, Nesland JM, Borresen-Dale AL, Holm R (2005) Protein expression and prognostic value of genes in the erb-b signaling pathway in advanced ovarian carcinomas. Am J Clin Pathol 124:392–401

Weiner DB, Liu J, Cohen JA, Williams WV, Greene MI (1989) A point mutation in the neu onco-gene mimics ligand induction of receptor aggregation. Nature 339:230–231

Wiseman SM, Makretsov N, Nielsen TO, Gilks B, Yorida E, Cheang M, Turbin D, Gelmon K, Huntsman DG (2005) Coexpression of the type 1 growth factor receptor family members HER-1, HER-2, and HER-3 has a synergistic negative prognostic effect on breast carcinoma survival. Cancer 103:1770–1777

Witkop B (1999) Paul Ehrlich and his Magic bullets–revisited. Proc Am Philos Soc 143:540–557

Yarden Y, Sliwkowski MX (2001) Untangling the ErbB signalling network. Nat Rev Mol Cell Biol 2:127–137

Yarden Y, Ullrich A (1988) Growth factor receptor tyrosine kinases. Annu Rev Biochem 57: 443–478

Yeon CH, Pegram MD (2005) Anti-erbB-2 antibody trastuzumab in the treatment of HER2-amplified breast cancer. Invest New Drugs 23:391–409

Zanazzi G, Einheber S, Westreich R, Hannocks MJ, Bedell-Hogan D, Marchionni MA, Salzer JL (2001) Glial growth factor/neuregulin inhibits Schwann cell myelination and induces demyeli-nation. J Cell Biol 152:1289–1299

Zhang K, Sun J, Liu N, Wen D, Chang D, Thomason A, Yoshinaga SK (1996) Transformation of NIH 3T3 cells by HER3 or HER4 receptors requires the presence of HER1 or HER2. J Biol Chem 271:3884–3890

Zhou W, Carpenter G (2002) ErbB-4: a receptor tyrosine kinase. Inflamm Res 51:91–101

The Use of CD3-Specific Antibodies in Autoimmune Diabetes: A Step Toward the Induction of Immune Tolerance in the Clinic

L. Chatenoud

1 Introduction 221
2 The Physiopathology of Autoimmune Insulin-Dependent Diabetes 222
3 The Use of CD3-Specific Antibodies in Experimental Models 225
4 Immunopharmacology of CD3-Specific Antibodies (Fig. 1) 228
5 Clinical Use of CD3-Specific Antibodies in Type 1 Diabetes........................ 229
6 Conclusions 230
References 231

Abstract CD3-specific monoclonal antibodies were the first rodent monoclonals introduced in clinical practice in the mid 1980s as approved immunosuppressants to prevent and treat organ allograft rejection. Since then compelling evidence has been accumulated to suggest that in addition to their immunosuppressive properties, CD3-specific antibodies can also afford inducing immune tolerance especially in the context of ongoing immune responses. Thus, they are highly effective at restoring self-tolerance in overt autoimmunity, a capacity first demonstrated in the experimental setting, which was recently transferred to the clinic with success.

1 Introduction

OKT3, a mouse IgG2a (Kung et al. 1979), was the first monoclonal antibody (MAb) introduced in clinical practice in 1981 to treat and prevent renal allograft rejection (Cosimi et al. 1981a, b; Vigeral et al. 1986; Debure et al. 1988). Amazingly, this

Lucienne Chatenoud

Université Paris Descartes, 75015 Paris, France; Institut National de la Santé et de la Recherche Médicale, Unité 580, 75015 Paris, France; Hôpital Necker-Enfants Malades, 161 rue de Sèvres 75743 Paris Cedex 15, France

e-mail: chatenoud@necker.fr

Y. Chernajovsky, A. Nissim (eds.) *Therapeutic Antibodies. Handbook of Experimental Pharmacology 181.*
© Springer-Verlag Berlin Heidelberg 2008

occurred about 4 years before the complexities of its target molecule, CD3 were discovered (Clevers et al. 1988; Davis and Chien 1999). In addition, due to the tight species-specificity of anti-human CD3 antibodies, which only cross-react with chimpanzees T cells and not those from more commonly used nonhuman primates (i.e., *Rhesus* or *Cynomolgus*), conventional in vivo preclinical toxicology data were not available when the first patients were treated with OKT3. In this particular case this was fortunate since the risk was high for this antibody to be excluded because of its T cell mitogenic potential leading to the well described cytokine-mediated "flu-like" syndrome. Several controlled trials were conducted demonstrating the very efficient immunosuppressive properties of OKT3 both to reverse and prevent acute organ allograft rejection episodes (Cosimi et al. 1981a, b; Ortho 1985; Debure et al. 1988), thus explaining that the MAb was licensed both in the USA and Europe for use in transplantation.

Over the last 10 years, as other immunosuppressants developed, the use of OKT3 was almost completely abandoned, essentially because of the aforementioned cytokine releasing potential (Chatenoud et al. 1986, 1989, 1990; Cosimi 1987; Abramowicz et al. 1989; Eason and Cosimi 1999; Chatenoud 2003). In parallel, however, second generation CD3-specific MAbs have been produced by molecular engineering that are humanized (Bolt et al. 1993; Alegre et al. 1994), or even fully human, and Fc mutated. Because of the Fc mutation these antibodies are well tolerated since they express a significantly decreased cytokine releasing potential. In addition, the experimental work conducted in different autoimmunity and transplant models have demonstrated that far beyond their immunosuppressive potential, CD3 MAbs are also unique tools to promote immune tolerance in naïve hosts (Hayward and Shreiber 1989; Nicolls et al. 1993; Plain et al. 1999) and, perhaps more impressively and more important in terms of clinical translation, to reestablish self-tolerance in established autoimmunity (Chatenoud et al. 1994, 1997; Belghith et al. 2003; Chatenoud 2003).

It is on this basis that in the early 2000, CD3-specific MAbs were back in the clinic in the context of challenging protocols that mostly aim at testing whether one may translate into patients the tolerogenic potential observed in preclinical models. It is the aim of this review to gather the data showing the reader that this may indeed be the case. Since the most compelling clinical evidence in support of such conclusion presently derives from the experience with CD3-specific MAbs in an autoimmune disease that is insulin-dependent diabetes, it appears important to start with a brief description of the physiopathology of this condition.

2 The Physiopathology of Autoimmune Insulin-Dependent Diabetes

Diabetes mellitus is a clinical syndrome characterized by chronic hyperglycemia. It became apparent by the 70s that this definition included two major physiopathological entities namely, Type 1 (T1D) and Type 2 (T2D) diabetes. Type I diabetes is an autoimmune disease causing the progressive and selective destruction of insulin secreting β cells of the islets of Langerhans. Thus patients with overt T1D, also termed insulin-dependent diabetes, rely on the chronic administration of exogenous insulin to maintain an adequate metabolic control. In non insulin-dependent diabetes in T2D, when compared with T1D, the abnormal glucose control is not due to deficient insulin production by β cells but to an aberrant sensitivity of peripheral tissues to the effect of the hormone, thus impairing their capacity to handle glucose (i.e., insulin resistance). The two diseases are genetically controlled and are polygenic. Interestingly, 5–15% of patients diagnosed as T2D present in fact slow progressing autoimmune T1D. They are now defined as LADA patients for late autoimmune diabetes of the adult.

In humans the autoimmune origin of T1D was initially suspected from data showing that patients' sera contained antibodies that stained islet cells from normal human pancreas tissue sections (ICAs or islet cell autoantibodies) (Bottazzo et al. 1974). The obvious difficulties of having access to the target organ greatly hampered a more in depth analysis of the disease. This explains that spontaneous animal models of T1D in rodents, such as the bio-breeding (BB) rat and the nonobese diabetic (NOD) mouse, constituted invaluable tools to address not only the physiopathology and the genetics of the disease but also to test for immunointervention strategies aimed at both preventing and reversing established T1D (Bach 1994).

The BB rat was derived from outbred Wistar rats (Nakhooda et al. 1977). This model was the one which provided the first robust evidence that autoimmune T1D was a T cell-mediated disease (Crisa et al. 1992). BB-diabetes prone (DP) rats express the $RT1^u$ MHC haplotype and diabetes develops in 90% of males and females between 2 and 4 months of age. Overt disease is preceded by an infiltration of the islets of Langerhans of the pancreas by mononuclear cells, i.e., insulitis that starts 2–3 weeks prior to the advent of overt hyperglycemia and glycosuria and is present also in the few BB–DP rats that never develop full blown disease. Although very useful, one major problem of BB rats as a model for human T1D is that they are lymphopenic, which is not the case in T1D patients. This in part explains that since they were characterized in Japan almost 30 years ago but now the NOD mouse model is more extensively used (Makino et al. 1980). A wide number of NOD colonies were rapidly developed in various laboratories that, quite interestingly, showed a high variability in disease incidence. The initial interpretation of genetic variations among substrains was invalidated by reports showing that the pathogen environment plays a major role in disease development; high disease incidence is only observed under very "clean" specific pathogen-free (SPF) conditions (Ohsugi and Kurosawa 1994; Bach 2002). Under SPF conditions, disease incidence is higher in females when compared with males (90–95% vs. 40–50% by 45 weeks of age).

Aside to T1D, NOD mice present other autoimmune manifestations: they often exhibit thyroiditis and sialitis (Garchon et al. 1991; 1995; Many et al. 1996), they may develop autoimmune haemolytic anemia (Baxter and Mandel 1991), they produce antinuclear antibodies Humphreys Beher et al. 1993, and are prone to lupus-like syndrome following particular treatments (Baxter et al. 1994). It is interesting to note that in the clinic about 10% of T1D patients also present with multiple endocrinopathies (in particular thyroiditis); these patients are essentially young/middle aged women.

In NOD mice, overt T1D appears by 3 months of age and is preceded by progressive infiltration with mononuclear cells (i.e., insulitis). Insulitis first appears by 3–4 weeks of age and up to 8–10 weeks of age it is a benign process, often defined as prediabetes, with cells remaining confined to the periphery of the islets (Fujino-kurihara et al. 1985; Katz et al. 1993). By 10–14 weeks of age the insulatis becomes invasive and active β cell destruction progresses until overt disease appears characterized as in humans by hyperglycemia, glycosuria.

Disease is caused by pathogenic $CD4^+$ and $CD8^+$ T lymphocytes. This was clearly demonstrated by the capacity of "diabetogenic" T cells from the spleen of diabetic NOD mice to transfer disease into syngeneic immunoincompetent recipients (NOD neonates, adult irradiated NOD mice, NOD SCID mice) (Wicker et al. 1986; Bendelac et al. 1987; Christianson et al. 1993; Rohane et al. 1995). Pathogenic T cells recognize various β cell antigens including insulin (Wegmann et al. 1994; Daniel et al. 1995; Wegmann 1996), proinsulin (French et al. 1997; Harrison et al. 1997), glutamic acid decarboxylase (GAD) (Baekkeskov et al. 1990; Honeyman et al. 1993; Tisch et al. 1994; Panina-bordignon et al. 1995), a β cell-specific protein phosphatase I-A2 (Hawkes et al. 1996; Lampasona et al. 1996; Trembleau et al. 1997; Dotta et al. 1999), a peptide (p277) of heat shock protein 60 (hsp60) (Elias et al. 1991; Elias and Cohen 1994; Elias et al. 1997), and the islet-specific glucose-6-phosphatase catalytic subunit-related protein (IGRP) (Lieberman et al. 2003). This latter antigen was characterized as being a preferential target of a significant proportion of pathogenic $CD8^+$ T cells from infiltrated NOD islets Utsugi et al. 1996.

Islet cell reactive autoantibodies are also found in NOD mice, albeit in lower amounts when compared with T1D patients, but they are not pathogenic. Interestingly, however, disease development is B cell-dependent as B cell-less NOD mice are disease free (Serreze et al. 1996). The interpretation is that B lymphocytes are in T1D as in many other autoimmune diseases' key autoantigen presenting cells (Akashi et al. 1997; Noorchashm et al. 1997; Serreze and Silveira 2003).

There is very compelling evidence to show that T1D progression (to overt disease) is tightly controlled by T cell-mediated immunoregulatory circuits. T cell depletion that follows thymectomy at 3 weeks of age (i.e., weaning) or cyclophosphamide treatment accelerates disease onset (Yasunami and Bach 1988; Charlton et al. 1989; Dardenne et al. 1989; Yasunami et al. 1990; Mahiou et al. 2001). More direct evidence came from adoptive transfer models showing that diabetes transfer by pathogenic cells is prevented by coinjection of $CD4^+$ suppressor or regulatory T cells (Tregs) from the spleen or the thymus of young prediabetic mice (Boitard et al. 1989; Herbelin et al. 1998). Spleen cells mediating effective protection from diabetes transfer include not only thymic-derived "natural suppressive" $CD4^+CD25^+FoxP3^+$ T cells (Nishizuka and Sakakura 1969; Asano et al. 1996; Sakaguchi 2005), but also a $CD4^+FoxP3^+$ T cell subset expressing variable levels of CD25, which appear to be cytokine dependent (i.e., TGF-dependent) thus responding to the definition of "adaptive regulatory cells" differentiating at the periphery from CD4$^+$CD25$^-$ precursors (Bach and Chatenoud 2001; Bluestone and Abbas 2003; You et al. 2006, 2007). CD62-L (L-selectin) is also expressed by some of the Tregs involved in control of T1D (Herbelin et al. 1998; Lepault and Gagnerault 2000; You et al. 2005).

Importantly, at the time of overt T1D both in experimental models and in patients, β cells are not all destroyed, a finding that is highly relevant for our following discussion on immunointervention strategies. In fact, at such quite late disease stage, the residual β cell mass may still represent about 30% of normal values (Sreenan et al. 1999). This is so because the physical destruction of β cells is preceded by a phase of functional impairment (which translates into incapacity to release insulin in response to conventional stimulations) due to the immune-mediated inflammation. Infiltrated pancreatic islets from nondiabetic 13-week-old female NOD do not secrete insulin in response to glucose stimulation if examined immediately after the isolation. However, this inhibition is fully reversed upon clearing of insulitis following a few days of in vitro culture (Strandell et al. 1990). The same is observed in vivo. In NOD mice, the administration of agents that clear insulitis within the first days of overt hyperglycemia, such as polyclonal anti-T cell antibodies (Maki et al. 1992) or monoclonal antibodies to the constant portion of the T cell receptor (TCR) (Sempe et al. 1991) or to CD3 (Chatenoud et al. 1994) (as we shall discuss in more detail), promote immediate return to normal glycemia. In T1D patients, the same is observed when effective T cell directed immunointervention is applied as assessed by a preservation of the endogenous insulin secreting capacity (i.e., release of C-peptide after stimulation) and a decrease in insulin needs (Feutren et al. 1986; Herold et al. 2002, 2005; Keymeulen et al. 2005).

3 The Use of CD3-Specific Antibodies in Experimental Models

The capacity of CD3-specific MAbs to promote immune tolerance in naïve hosts were first reported by the group of B. Hall in a rat transplant model (Nicolls et al. 1993; Plain et al. 1999). The authors demonstrated that a short course of a non-mitogenic anti-rat CD3 MAb induced permanent engraftment of fully mismatched vascularized heart allografts. Interestingly, the establishment of alloantigen-specific tolerance was proven in this model since CD3-specific MAb-treated recipients accepted secondary donor-matched skin grafts while third party skin allografts were rejected (Nicolls et al. 1993; Plain et al. 1999).

Without diminishing the relevance of these findings, it is fair, however, to stress first that similar results had been obtained with several other MAbs or fusion proteins targeting key T cell signalling pathways and in particular CD4, alone or in combination with CD8 and costimulatory pathway receptors (Wood et al. 1971; Cobbold et al. 1992; Maki et al. 1992; Cobbold et al. 1996; Waldmann and Cobbold 1998; Adler and Turka 2002; Wekerle et al. 2002; Quezada et al. 2004). Second, when one comes to clinical translation the obvious problem is that both in the auto-immunity setting, and now more and more frequently also in transplantation, one deals with presensitized hosts, a situation that is far more complex. It is thus highly relevant to our discussion that indeed in the context of an established autoimmune disease CD3-specific MAbs still expressed their tolerogenic ability, a quite unique capacity.

Data from our laboratory were the first to show that in NOD mice CD3-specific MAb could reverse recent onset disease and restore tolerance to β cell antigens (Chatenoud et al. 1994, 1997; Chatenoud 2003). In NOD mice presenting with full-blown diabetes, as assessed by hyperglycemia (values $\geq$ 3–3.5 g l^{-1}) and glyco-suria, a five consecutive day treatment with low doses (5–20 μg) of the hamster CD3-specific MAb 145 2C11 (Leo et al. 1987) or of its F(ab')2 fragments (i.e., that are nonmitogenic when compared with the intact antibody) induces within 2–4 weeks complete remission of disease manifested by progressive return to normal glycemia in the absence of insulin treatment. The remission is durable (follow-up was pro-tracted for up to 8–10 months) and not related to long standing immunosuppression since, by 8 weeks from the last injection, treated mice regain full immunocompe-tence: they normally reject histoincompatible skin grafts (Chatenoud et al. 1994, 1997; Chatenoud 2003). The effect is antigen specific since syngeneic islet grafts implanted in CD3-specific MAb-treated mice are not destroyed, at variance with what is regularly observed in untreated diabetic NOD females in which relapse of the autoimmune aggression rapidly destroys autologous islet implants (Chatenoud et al. 1994, 1997; Chatenoud 2003). Our data also indicated that to be effective at fully reversing established disease and allowing complete and durable metabolic reconstitution, the treatment had to be started within 7 days from the detection of the first signs of overt diabetes (Chatenoud et al. 1994, 1997, Chatenoud 2003). In fact, if treatment is started too late the β cell mass left is insufficient to guarantee the return to a normal metabolic balance. Yet immunological self-tolerance is restored, which explains that if a syngeneic islet graft is performed, providing again a suffi-cient source of insulin-secreting β cells, mice enter long-standing disease remission (Chatenoud et al. 1994).

Similar data, namely, of restoration of self tolerance in overtly diabetic NOD mice have also been reported by Maki et al., using polyclonal antilymphocyte serum (Maki et al. 1992). However, at variance with CD3 antibody, profound and quite prolonged T cell depletion was induced.

Contrasting with its potent therapeutic effect when applied at disease onset, CD3-specific MAb treatment was without any effect as a preventive treatment applied to young prediabetic NOD mice (4–8 weeks of age) (Chatenoud et al. 1997). This is another distinctive feature between CD3-specific MAbs and various other poten-tially tolerogenic biological agents that in NOD mice showed great effectiveness at disease prevention but did not act on the ongoing destructive disease (Shoda et al. 2005). Interestingly, these particular features of CD3-specific MAbs, which are of utmost importance for potential clinical translation, were recently extended to a model in SJL mice of induced autoimmunity namely, proteolipid protein (PLP)-induced relapsing experimental allergic encephalomyelitis (EAE) (Kohm et al. 2005). Also in this situation, CD3-specific MAbs are effective at treating ongoing PLP-triggered disease while no effect is obtained when the MAb is administered at the same time the triggering autoantigen is injected. Treatment is still active if started when disease activity peaks; disease remission is induced and further relapses of this chronic relapsing/remitting form of EAE are prevented (Kohm et al. 2005).

It is also important to mention here that the data reported by the group of W. Strober showing that a single injection of CD3-specific MAb fully inhibited the development of experimental inflammatory bowel disease (i.e., colitis) induced following administration of TNP-KLH (2,4,6-trinitrophenol-conjugated keyhole limpet hemocyanin) (Ludviksson et al. 1997).

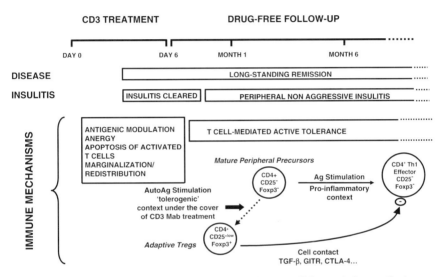

Fig. 1 The mode of action of CD3-specific MAbs in autoimmune diabetes. A short antibody treatment induces durable remission of established disease. The immune mechanisms that mediate this remarkable therapeutic activity of CD3 MAbs may be distinguished into two clearly distinct phases. The first one is coincident with CD3 MAb administration. The insulitis is completely cleared due to various mechanisms that include CD3/TCR antigenic modulation followed by recirculation/marginalization of T cells and some degree of T cell apoptosis that preferential involves activated T cells. This phase is short lasting and cannot on its own account for the long-lasting restoration of self-tolerance that is induced by the antibody. The hallmark of this second phase of the antibody action is the resetting of peripheral tolerance mechanisms, which are mediated by TGF-β dependent Treg cells that are mostly of the adaptive type namely, they are induced from mature CD4+ T lymphocytes at the periphery. A still pending fundamental issue is to better define the initial cellular and molecular mechanisms triggering the preferential expansion of these adaptive Tregs following CD3 MAb treatment.

4 Immunopharmacology of CD3-Specific Antibodies (Fig. 1)

CD3-specific MAb used in experimental models and the ones recognizing human CD3 are all directed to the ε chain of the CD3 complex that is tightly associated to TCR. CD3-specific MAb in both their Fc receptor binding and nonbinding forms cross-link CD3/TCR complexes, a key step in the unique spectrum of biological activities they elicit among which are antigenic modulation, redirected T cell lysis, apoptosis mainly of activated T cells, and anergy. One key property of CD3-specific MAb is that they do not promote massive T cell depletion; transient lymphopenia is observed following treatment but T cell counts return to baseline levels within a few days after the MAb is cleared from the circulation (Chatenoud et al. 1982, 1986; Decochez et al. 2000). This lymphopenia ensues from partial apoptosis, from the redistribution of cells within the various lymphocyte compartments, and also from an increased adhesiveness of endothelial cells favoring lymphocyte marginalization that is secondary to their activation triggered by CD3-specific MAbs released cytokines, even in the case of non Fc-receptor binding antibodies (see later). In mice treated with non Fc-receptor binding CD3-specific MAbs only 20–30% of $CD3^+$ cells disappear, because of physical destruction and/or redistribution, from the spleen and lymph nodes (Hirsch et al. 1990, Chatenoud 2003; Chatenoud et al. 1997). In the particular case of non Fc binding, CD3-specific MAbs depletion was shown to be mediated by redirected T cell lysis (i.e., bridging of cytotoxic T cells to the target) (Wong and Colvin 1991) and the induction of apoptosis to which, once again, activated T cells appear the most sensitive (Wesselborg et al. 1993).

T lymphocytes that are not destroyed following CD3-specific MAb binding will experience antigenic modulation of CD3/TCR (Chatenoud et al. 1982, 1984). $CD3^+$ T cells will transiently loose CD3/TCR expression and become unresponsive to various antigen-mediated or mitogenic stimuli (Chatenoud et al. 1982). It is important at this point to mention the interesting data showing that non-Fc-receptor binding CD3-specific Mab triggers partial signalling and promotes T cell anergy in vitro (Smith et al. 1997, 1998). T cell signalling is central to the in vivo tolerogenic effect of non Fc-receptor binding CD3-specific MAb in NOD mice since the therapeutic effect is lost when the well known calcineurin inhibitor cyclosporine is given in association with CD3-specific Mab (Chatenoud et al. 1997). In the NOD mouse, the short antibody administration promotes a rapid, complete clearing of insulitis, which correlates with the return to normoglycemia. Transient polarization toward a Th2-type phenotype, i.e., increased production of IL-4 by stimulated T cells from CD3-specific MAb-treated mice is also observed. This is, however, irrelevant for the long-term tolerogenic effect since remission of disease following CD3-specific MAb treatment is also seen in NOD mice whose IL-4 gene was invalidated (NOD $IL - 4^{-/-}$) (Belghith et al. 2003; Chatenoud 2003). Over long term, the antigen-specific therapeutic effect is best explained by the up-regulation of T cell-mediated "active" tolerance mediated by specialized subsets of Tregs including $CD4^+CD25^+$ and $CD4^+CD62L^+$ T cells that control the pathogenic potential of diabetogenic effector T cells. The numbers of Tregs increase in pancreatic and mesenteric lymph nodes, but not in the spleen of treated tolerant mice; in adoptive transfer experiments, Tregs effectively block disease induced by diabeto-genic T cells (Belghith et al. 2003). Our most recent data demonstrate that an impor-tant proportion of the CD3-specific MAb-induced Tregs are from the adaptive type that derive from peripheral CD4$^+$CD25$^-$ precursors (Belghith et al. 2003; You et al. 2006, 2007). One direct proof of this conclusion is that diabetes remission was also induced following CD3-specific MAb treatment in NOD mice deficient for the cos-timulation molecule CD28 (NOD CD28$^{-/-}$), which are devoid of thymic natural suppressor CD4$^+$CD25$^+$ cells (Salomon et al. 2000; Belghith et al. 2003). These adaptive Tregs are TGF-β-dependent: the in vivo neutralization of TGF-β, following injection of specific monoclonal antibodies, fully prevents CD3-specific antibody-induced remission (Belghith et al. 2003). It remains to be determined whether in this setting TGF-β acts as a growth and/or differentiation factor for Tregs or is also a mediator of their regulatory effect.

5 Clinical Use of CD3-Specific Antibodies in Type 1 Diabetes

On the basis of the preclinical data we just described clinical trials were established using humanized CD3-specific Fc mutated MAbs to decrease their ability to bind Fc receptors. In fact, there was quite compelling data in the literature to show that the mitogenic activity of rodent CD3-specific MAbs and thus their cytokine-releasing ability is monocyte-dependent, linked to their capacity to interact with Fc recep-tors on monocyte/macrophages thus enhancing cross-linking. Thus, the mitogenic response varies with the murine antibody isotype (IgG2a >> IgG1 >> IgG2b >> IgA), and CD3-specific F(ab′)2 fragments, lacking the Fc portion, are nonmito-genic (Van Lier et al. 1987; Hirsch et al. 1990; Chatenoud et al. 1994; Parlevliet et al. 1994; Chatenoud et al. 1997).

We are going to restrict our discussion to the two humanized complementarity determining region (CDR)-grafted nonmitogenic CD3-specific MAbs, which were so far the most extensively used and which in particular were tested in patients with T1D. One of these antibodies is hOKT3γ1 Ala-Ala, the humanized version of OKT3, with two mutations in the Fc portion (Alegre et al. 1994). The other antibody is ChAglyCD3, derived from the rat YTH 12.5 antibody, with a single mutation that prevents glycosylation of its γ1 Fc portion (Bolt et al. 1993).

Phase I trials were first carried out in renal allograft recipients presenting acute rejection episodes and to confirm their good tolerance (Friend et al. 1999; Woodle et al. 1999). Although they are termed "nonmitogenic" both of the antibodies still elicit some cytokine release, which is, however, minimal when compared with what usually observed with OKT3 (Friend et al. 1999; Woodle et al. 1999; Herold et al. 2002, 2005; Keymeulen et al. 2005). Although the number of patients included in these trials was small, a favorable trend was observed concerning their capacity to reverse rejection very similar to what reported in the very first studies using OKT3 (Cosimi et al. 1981).

The real question was whether, given the encouraging safety profile, these humanized CD3-specific MAbs could be used in settings other than transplantation and, if possible, within protocols aiming at more than simple immunosuppression similar to the strategy discussed above in NOD mice. Two trials were started in 2000. hOKT3γ1 Ala-Ala alone was used in a Phase I/II trial where patients with recent onset T1D were treated for two consecutive weeks (Herold et al. 2002, 2005). Results showed that the treatment stopped disease progression over 1 year and even at 36 months as assessed by C-peptide production and insulin usage when compared with the control group (Herold et al. 2002, 2005).

In parallel, a randomized double blind multicenter Phase II placebo-controlled study was started by an European consortium recruiting patients in Belgium and Germany. The trial included 80 patients who received 8 mg of ChAglyCD3 (40 patients) or placebo (40 patients) daily for six consecutive days. The treatment very efficiently preserved β cell function, maintaining significantly higher levels of endogenous insulin secretion when compared with those observed in placebo-treated patients at 6, 12, and even 18 months (Keymeulen et al. 2005). In addition, up to 18 months after treatment a significant decrease in the insulin needs was observed, which was more obvious in the subset of patients who showed a higher β cell mass at the time of treatment (Keymeulen et al. 2005). Seventy-five percent of these patients if treated with ChAglyCD3 received insulin doses $\leq 0.25 \, U \, kg^{-1} \, day^{-1}$ that are compatible with clinical insulin independency (Keymeulen et al. 2005).

As previously mentioned, in the two trials some degree of T cell activation is still observed leading to limited cytokine release and consequent minor acute side effects mainly including moderate fever, headaches, and self-limiting gastrointestinal manifestations, which were all responsive to palliative treatment (Herold et al. 2002; Keymeulen et al. 2005).

Transient reactivation of Epstein Barr virus (EBV) was also observed as assessed by an increase in numbers of EBV copies measured in peripheral blood mononuclear cells using quantitative PCR by 10–20 days after the first injection. Within 1–3 weeks in all patients the number of EBV copies returned to normal baseline pretreatment levels. Concomitantly, an efficient humoral and cellular immune response specific to EBV developed. This effective anti-EBV response is for obvious reasons very important in terms of safety. In addition, it suggests that, as we observed in NOD mice, the effect of ChAglyCD3 in patients is antigen-specific i.e., the antibody treatment affects the autoimmune reaction but does not refrain immune responses to unrelated exogenous antigens.

6 Conclusions

In developed countries, autoimmune diseases represent the third cause of morbidity and mortality after cardiovascular diseases and cancer and their frequency has been steadily increasing over the last 3 decades. Thus autoimmune diseases represent a major therapeutic challenge. Present treatments are substitutive, antiinflammatory, or immunosuppressive without any specificity for the pathogenic mechanisms of the disease. Therefore, much interest is devoted to modern technologies that have made new biological agents available such as anti-TNF antibodies in rheumatoid arthritis or anti-VLA4 in multiple sclerosis. However, even in these cases, which represented a major step forward, continuous treatment is needed to maintain efficacy thus still confronting patients to the risk of increased infections due to over-immunosuppression such as mycobacterial infections with TNF antagonists (Keane et al. 2001; Gomez-Reino et al. 2003) or JC virus infection with anti-VLA4 (natalizumab) treatment (Langer-Gould et al. 2005; Van Assche et al. 2005).

At variance with these therapies, CD3-specific MAbs afford long term effects following a short administration. At least in the experimental setting, the capacity to trigger TGF-β-dependent Tregs mediating long-standing active suppression appears as a central mechanism explaining their unique tolerogenic properties.

From the pharmacological point of view, one major challenge is now to better dissect the molecular mechanisms underlying this effect to optimize the use of CD3-specific MAbs. In addition, gaining further insights into specific signalling pathways mediating the effect will pave the way toward the identification of small molecules endowed with less side effects and sharing identical tolerogenic properties.

From a more practical point of view and in the short term, the clinical challenge is to build on the available results to establish the use of CD3-specific MAbs in T1D, possibly in well-selected subsets of patients, and to extend it to the treatment to other autoimmune diseases. Last but not least, organ transplantation is for obvious reasons another potential clinical indication.

References

Abramowicz D, Schandene L et al. (1989) Release of tumor necrosis factor, interleukin-2, and gamma-interferon in serum after injection of OKT3 monoclonal antibody in kidney transplant recipients. Transplantation 47(4):606–608

Adler SH, Turka LA (2002) Immunotherapy as a means to induce transplantation tolerance. Curr Opin Immunol 14(5):660–665

Akashi T, Nagafuchi S et al. (1997) Direct evidence for the contribution of B cells to the progression of insulitis and the development of diabetes in non-obese diabetic mice. Int Immunol 9(8):1159–1164

Alegre ML, Peterson LJ et al. (1994) A non-activating "humanized" anti-CD3 monoclonal antibody retains immunosuppressive properties in vivo. Transplantation 57(11):1537–1543

Asano M, Toda M et al. (1996) Autoimmune disease as a consequence of developmental abnormality of a T cell subpopulation. J Exp Med 184(2):387–396

Bach JF (1994) Insulin-dependent diabetes mellitus as an autoimmune disease. Endocrine Rev 15(4):516–542

Bach JF (2002) The effect of infections on susceptibility to autoimmune and allergic diseases. N Engl J Med 347(12):911–920

Bach JF, Chatenoud L (2001) Tolerance to islet autoantigens and type I diabetes. Annu Rev Immunol 19:131–161

Baekkeskov S, Aanstoot HJ et al. (1990) Identification of the 64K autoantigen in insulin-dependent diabetes as the GABA-synthesizing enzyme glutamic acid decarboxylase. Nature 347(6289):151–156

Baxter AG, Horsfall AC et al. (1994) Mycobacteria precipitate an SLE-like syndrome in diabetes-prone NOD mice. Immunology 83(2):227–231

Baxter AG, Mandel TE (1991) Hemolytic anemia in non-obese diabetic mice. Eur J Immunol 21(9):2051–2055

Belghith M, Bluestone JA et al. (2003) TGF-beta-dependent mechanisms mediate restoration of self-tolerance induced by antibodies to CD3 in overt autoimmune diabetes. Nat Med 9(9):1202–1208

Bendelac A, Carnaud C et al. (1987) Syngeneic transfer of autoimmune diabetes from diabetic NOD mice to healthy neonates. Requirement for both L3T4+ and Lyt-2+ T cells. J Exp Med 166(4):823–832

Bluestone JA, Abbas AK (2003) Natural versus adaptive regulatory T cells. Nat Rev Immunol 3(3):253–257

Boitard C, Yasunami R et al. (1989) T cell-mediated inhibition of the transfer of autoimmune diabetes in NOD mice. J Exp Med 169(5):1669–1680

Bolt S, Routledge E et al. (1993) The generation of a humanized, non-mitogenic CD3 monoclonal antibody which retains in vitro immunosuppressive properties. Eur J Immunol 23(2):403–411

Bottazzo GF, Florin-christensen A et al. (1974) Islet-cell antibodies in diabetes mellitus with autoimmune polyendocrine deficiencies. Lancet 2(7892):1279–1283

Charlton B, Bacelj A et al. (1989) Cyclophosphamide-induced diabetes in NOD/WEHI mice. Evidence for suppression in spontaneous autoimmune diabetes mellitus. Diabetes 38(4):441–447

Chatenoud L (2003) CD3-specific antibody-induced active tolerance: from bench to bedside. Nat Rev Immunol 3(2):123–132

Chatenoud L, Bach JF (1984) Antigenic modulation: a major mechanism of antibody action. Immunol Today 5(1):20–25

Chatenoud L, Baudrihaye MF et al. (1986) Restriction of the human in vivo immune response against the mouse monoclonal antibody OKT3. J Immunol 137(3):830–838

Chatenoud L, Baudrihaye MF et al. (1982) Human in vivo antigenic modulation induced by the anti-T cell OKT3 monoclonal antibody. Eur J Immunol 12(11):979–982

Chatenoud L, Ferran C et al. (1990) In vivo cell activation following OKT3 administration. Systemic cytokine release and modulation by corticosteroids. Transplantation 49(4):697–702

Chatenoud L, Ferran C et al. (1989) "Systemic reaction to the anti-T-cell monoclonal antibody OKT3 in relation to serum levels of tumor necrosis factor and interferon-gamma. N Engl J Med 320(21):1420–1421

Chatenoud L, Primo J et al. (1997) CD3 antibody-induced dominant self tolerance in overtly diabetic NOD mice. J Immunol 158(6):2947–2954

Chatenoud L, Thervet E et al. (1994) Anti-CD3 antibody induces long-term remission of overt autoimmunity in nonobese diabetic mice. Proc Natl Acad Sci USA 91(1):123–127

Christianson SW, Shultz LD et al. (1993) Adoptive transfer of diabetes into immunodeficient NOD-scid/scid mice. Relative contributions of CD4+ and CD8+ T-cells from diabetic versus prediabetic NOD.NON-Thy-1a donors. Diabetes 42(1):44–55

Clevers H, Alarcon B et al. (1988) The T cell receptor/CD3 complex: a dynamic protein ensemble. Annu Rev Immunol 6(1):629–662

Cobbold SP, Adams E et al. (1996) Mechanisms of peripheral tolerance and suppression induced by monoclonal antibodies to CD4 and CD8. Immunol Rev 149:5–33

Cobbold SP, Qin S et al. (1992) Reprogramming the immune system for peripheral tolerance with CD4 and CD8 monoclonal antibodies. Immunol Rev 129:165–201

Cosimi AB (1987) Clinical development of Orthoclone OKT3. Transplant Proc 19(2 Suppl 1):7–16

Cosimi AB, Burton RC et al. (1981a) Treatment of acute renal allograft rejection with OKT3 monoclonal antibody. Transplantation 32(6):535–539

Cosimi AB, Colvin RB et al. (1981b) Use of monoclonal antibodies to T-cell subsets for immunologic monitoring and treatment in recipients of renal allografts. N Engl J Med 305(6):308–314

Crisa L, Mordes JP et al. (1992) Autoimmune diabetes mellitus in the BB rat. Diabetes Metab Rev 8(1):4–37

Daniel D, Gill RG et al. (1995) Epitope specificity, cytokine production profile and diabetogenic activity of insulin-specific T cell clones isolated from NOD mice. Eur J Immunol 25(4):1056–1062

Dardenne M, Lepault F et al. (1989) Acceleration of the onset of diabetes in NOD mice by thymectomy at weaning. Eur J Immunol 19(5):889–895

Davis MM, Chien YH (1999) T cell antigen receptors. In: Paul W (ed) Fundamental immunology. Raven, New York, pp 341–366

Debure A, Chkoff N et al. (1988) One-month prophylactic use of OKT3 in cadaver kidney transplant recipients. Transplantation 45(3):546–553

Decochez K, Keymeulen B et al. (2000) Use of an islet cell antibody assay to identify type 1 diabetic patients with rapid decrease in C-peptide levels after clinical onset. Belgian Diabetes Registry. Diabetes Care 23(8):1072–1078

Dotta F, Dionisi S et al. (1999) T-cell mediated autoimmunity to the insulinoma-associated protein 2 islet tyrosine phosphatase in type 1 diabetes mellitus. Eur J Endocrinol 141(3):272–278

Eason JD, Cosimi AB (1999) Biologic immunosuppressive agents. In: Ginns L, Cosimi A, Morris P (eds) Transplantation. Blackwell, Malden, USA, pp 196–224

Elias D, Cohen IR (1994) Peptide therapy for diabetes in NOD mice. Lancet 343(8899):704–706

Elias D, Meilin A et al. (1997) Hsp60 peptide therapy of NOD mouse diabetes induces a Th2 cytokine burst and downregulates autoimmunity to various beta-cell antigens. Diabetes 46(5):758–764

Elias D, Reshef T et al. (1991) Vaccination against autoimmune mouse diabetes with a T-cell epitope of the human 65-kDa heat shock protein. Proc Natl Acad Sci USA 88(8):3088–3091

Feutren G, Papoz L et al. (1986) Cyclosporin increases the rate and length of remissions in insulin-dependent diabetes of recent onset. Results of a multicentre double-blind trial. Lancet 2(8499):119–124

French MB, Allison J et al. (1997) Transgenic expression of mouse proinsulin II prevents diabetes in nonobese diabetic mice. Diabetes 46(1):34–39

Friend PJ, Hale G et al. (1999) Phase I study of an engineered aglycosylated humanized CD3 antibody in renal transplant rejection. Transplantation 68:1632–1637

Fujino-kurihara H, Fujita H et al. (1985) Morphological aspects on pancreatic islets of non-obese diabetic (NOD) mice. Virchows Arch B Cell Pathol Incl Mol Pathol 49(2):107–120

Garchon HJ, Bedossa P et al. (1991) Identification and mapping to chromosome 1 of a susceptibility locus for periinsulitis in non-obese diabetic mice. Nature 353(6341):260–262

Gomez-Reino JJ, Carmona L et al. (2003) Treatment of rheumatoid arthritis with tumor necrosis factor inhibitors may predispose to significant increase in tuberculosis risk: a multicenter active-surveillance report. Arthritis Rheum 48(8):2122–2127

Harrison LC, Honeyman MC et al. (1997) A peptide-binding motif for I-A(g7), the class II major histocompatibility complex (MHC) molecule of NOD and Biozzi AB/H mice. J Exp Med 185(6):1013–1021

Hawkes CJ, Wasmeier C et al. (1996) Identification of the 37-kDa antigen in IDDM as a tyrosine phosphatase-like protein (phogrin) related to IA-2. Diabetes 45(9):1187–1192

Hayward AR, Shreiber M (1989) Neonatal injection of CD3 antibody into nonobese diabetic mice reduces the incidence of insulitis and diabetes. J Immunol 143(5):1555–1559

Herbelin A, Gombert JM et al. (1998) Mature mainstream TCR alpha beta(+)CD4(+) thymocytes expressing L-selectin mediate "active tolerance" in the nonobese diabetic mouse. J Immunol 161(5):2620–2628

Herold KC, Gitelman SE et al. (2005) A single course of anti-CD3 monoclonal antibody hOKT3gamma1(Ala-Ala) results in improvement in C-peptide responses and clinical parameters for at least 2 years after onset of type 1 diabetes. Diabetes 54(6):1763–1769

Herold KC, Hagopian W et al. (2002) Anti-CD3 monoclonal antibody in new-onset type 1 diabetes mellitus. N Engl J Med 346(22):1692–1698

Hirsch R, Bluestone JA et al. (1990) Anti-CD3 F(ab')2 fragments are immunosuppressive in vivo without evoking either the strong humoral response or morbidity associated with whole mAb. Transplantation 49(6):1117–1123

Honeyman MC, Cram DS et al. (1993) Glutamic acid decarboxylase 67-reactive T cells: a marker of insulin-dependent diabetes. J Exp Med 177(2):535–540

Humphreys Beher MG, Brinkley L et al. (1993) Characterization of antinuclear autoantibodies present in the serum from nonobese diabetic (NOD) mice. Clin Immunol Immunopathol 68(3):350–356

Katz JD, Wang B et al. (1993) Following a diabetogenic T cell from genesis through pathogenesis. Cell 74(6):1089–1100

Keane J, Gershon S et al. (2001) Tuberculosis associated with infliximab, a tumor necrosis factor alpha-neutralizing agent. N Engl J Med 345(15):1098–1104

Keymeulen B, Vandemeulebroucke E et al. (2005) Insulin needs after CD3-antibody therapy in new-onset type 1 diabetes. N Engl J Med 352(25):2598–2608

Kohm AP, Williams JS et al. (2005) Treatment with nonmitogenic anti-CD3 monoclonal antibody induces CD4+ T cell unresponsiveness and functional reversal of established experimental autoimmune encephalomyelitis. J Immunol 174(8):4525–4534

Kung P, Goldstein G et al. (1979) Monoclonal antibodies defining distinctive human T cell surface antigens. Science 206(4416):347–349

Lampasona V, Bearzatto M et al. (1996) Autoantibodies in insulin-dependent diabetes recognize distinct cytoplasmic domains of the protein tyrosine phosphatase-like IA-2 autoantigen. J Immunol 157(6):2707–2711

Langer-Gould A, Atlas SW et al. (2005) Progressive multifocal leukoencephalopathy in a patient treated with natalizumab. N Engl J Med 353(4):375–381

Leo O, Foo M et al. (1987) Identification of a monoclonal antibody specific for a murine T3 polypeptide. Proc Natl Acad Sci USA 84(5):1374–1378

Lepault F, Gagnerault MC (2000) Characterization of peripheral regulatory CD4(+) T cells that prevent diabetes onset in nonobese diabetic mice. J Immunol 164(1):240–247

Lieberman SM, Evans AM et al. (2003) Identification of the beta cell antigen targeted by a prevalent population of pathogenic CD8+ T cells in autoimmune diabetes. Proc Natl Acad Sci USA 100(14):8384–8388

Ludviksson BR, Ehrhardt RO et al. (1997) TGF-beta production regulates the development of the 2,4,6-trinitrophenol-conjugated keyhole limpet hemocyanin-induced colonic inflammation in IL-2-deficient mice. J Immunol 159(7):3622–3628

Mahiou J, Walter U et al. (2001) In vivo Blockade of the Fas-Fas Ligand Pathway Inhibits Cyclophosphamide-induced Diabetes in NOD Mice. J Autoimmun 16(4):431–440

Maki T, Ichikawa T et al. (1992) Long-term abrogation of autoimmune diabetes in nonobese diabetic mice by immunotherapy with anti-lymphocyte serum. Proc Natl Acad Sci USA 89(8):3434–3438

Makino S, Kunimoto K et al. (1980) Breeding of a non-obese, diabetic strain of mice. Exp Anim 29(1):1–13

Many MC, Maniratunga S et al. (1996) The non-obese diabetic (NOD) mouse: An animal model for autoimmune thyroiditis. Exp Clin Endocrinol Diabetes 104:17–20

Many MC, Maniratunga S et al. (1995) Two-step development of Hashimoto-like thyroiditis in genetically autoimmune prone non-obese diabetic mice: effects of iodine-induced cell necrosis. J Endocrinol 147(2):311–320

Nakhooda AF, Like AA et al. (1977) The spontaneously diabetic Wistar rat. Metabolic and morphologic studies. Diabetes 26(2):100–112

Nicolls MR, Aversa GG et al. (1993) Induction of long-term specific tolerance to allografts in rats by therapy with an anti-CD3-like monoclonal antibody. Transplantation 55(3):459–468

Nishizuka Y, Sakakura T (1969) Thymus and reproduction: sex-linked dysgenesia of the gonad after neonatal thymectomy in mice. Science 166(906):753–755

Noorchashm H, Noorchashm N et al. (1997) B-cells are required for the initiation of insulitis and sialitis in nonobese diabetic mice. Diabetes 46(6):941–946

Ohsugi T, Kurosawa T (1994) Increased incidence of diabetes mellitus in specific pathogen-eliminated offspring produced by embryo transfer in NOD mice with low incidence of the disease. Lab Anim Sci 44(4):386–388

Ortho Multicenter Transplant Study Group (1985) A randomized clinical trial of OKT3 monoclonal antibody for acute rejection of cadaveric renal transplants. N Engl J Med 313(6):337–342

Panina-bordignon P, Lang R et al. (1995) Cytotoxic T cells specific for glutamic acid decarboxylase in autoimmune diabetes. J Exp Med 181(5):1923–1927

Parlevliet KJ, Ten Berge IJ et al. (1994) In vivo effects of IgA and IgG2a anti-CD3 isotype switch variants. J Clin Invest 93(6): 2519–2525

Plain KM, Chen J et al. (1999) Induction of specific tolerance to allografts in rats by therapy with non-mitogenic, non-depleting anti-CD3 monoclonal antibody: association with TH2 cytokines not anergy. Transplantation 67(4):605–613

Quezada SA, Jarvinen LZ et al. (2004) CD40/CD154 interactions at the interface of tolerance and immunity. Annu Rev Immunol 22:307–328

Rohane PW, Shimada A et al. (1995) Islet-infiltrating lymphocytes from prediabetic NOD mice rapidly transfer diabetes to NOD-scid/scid mice. Diabetes 44(5):550–554

Sakaguchi S (2005) Naturally arising Foxp3-expressing CD25 + CD4+ regulatory T cells in immunological tolerance to self and non-self. Nat Immunol 6(4):345–352

Salomon B, Lenschow DJ et al. (2000) B7/CD28 Costimulation is essential for the homeostasis of the CD4 + CD25+ immunoregulatory T cells that control autoimmune diabetes. Immunity 12:431–440

Sempe P, Bedossa P et al. (1991) Anti-alpha/beta T cell receptor monoclonal antibody provides an efficient therapy for autoimmune diabetes in nonobese diabetic (NOD) mice. Eur J Immunol 21(5):1163–1169

Serreze DV, Chapman HD et al. (1996) B lymphocytes are essential for the initiation of T cell-mediated autoimmune diabetes: Analysis of a new "speed congenic" stock of NOD.Ig mu(null) mice. J Exp Med 184(5):2049–2053

Serreze DV, Silveira PA (2003). The role of B lymphocytes as key antigen-presenting cells in the development of T cell-mediated autoimmune type 1 diabetes. Curr Dir Autoimmun 6:212–227

Shoda LK, Young DL et al. (2005) A Comprehensive Review of Interventions in the NOD Mouse and Implications for Translation. Immunity 23(2):115–126

Smith JA, Tang Q et al. (1998) Partial TCR signals delivered by FcR-nonbinding anti-CD3 monoclonal antibodies differentially regulate individual Th subsets. J Immunol 160(10):4841–4849

Smith JA, Tso JY et al. (1997) Nonmitogenic anti-CD3 monoclonal antibodies deliver a partial T cell receptor signal and induce clonal anergy. J Exp Med 185(8):1413–1422

Sreenan S, Pick AJ et al. (1999) Increased beta-cell proliferation and reduced mass before diabetes onset in the nonobese diabetic mouse. Diabetes 48(5):989–996

Strandell E, Eizirik DL et al. (1990) Reversal of beta-cell suppression in vitro in pancreatic islets isolated from nonobese diabetic mice during the phase preceding insulin-dependent diabetes mellitus. J Clin Invest 85(6):1944–1950

Tisch R, Yang XD et al. (1994) Administering glutamic acid decarboxylase to NOD mice prevents diabetes. J Autoimmun 7(6):845–850

Trembleau S, Penna G et al. (1997) Deviation of pancreas-infiltrating cells to Th2 by interleukin-12 antagonist administration inhibits autoimmune diabetes. Eur J Immunol 27(9):2330–2339

Utsugi T, Yoon JW et al. (1996) Major histocompatibility complex class I-restricted infiltration and destruction of pancreatic islets by NOD mouse-derived beta-cell cytotoxic CD8(+) T-cell clones in vivo. Diabetes 45(8):1121–1131

Van Assche G, Van Ranst M et al. (2005) Progressive multifocal leukoencephalopathy after natalizumab therapy for Crohn's disease. N Engl J Med 353(4):362–368

Van Lier RA, Boot JH et al. (1987) Induction of T cell proliferation with anti-CD3 switch-variant monoclonal antibodies: effects of heavy chain isotype in monocyte-dependent systems. Eur J Immunol 17(11):1599–1604

Vigeral P, Chkoff N et al. (1986) Prophylactic use of OKT3 monoclonal antibody in cadaver kidney recipients. Utilization of OKT3 as the sole immunosuppressive agent. Transplantation 41(6):730–733

Waldmann H, Cobbold S (1998) How do monoclonal antibodies induce tolerance? A role for infectious tolerance? Annu Rev Immunol 16:619–644

Wegmann DR (1996) The immune response to islets in experimental diabetes and insulin-dependent diabetes mellitus. Curr Opin Immunol 8(6):860–864

Wegmann DR, Norbury-glaser M et al. (1994) Insulin-specific T cells are a predominant component of islet infiltrates in pre-diabetic NOD mice. Eur J Immunol 24(8):1853–1857

Wekerle T, Kurtz J et al. (2002) Mechanisms of transplant tolerance induction using costimulatory blockade. Curr Opin Immunol 14(5):592–600

Wesselborg S, Janssen O et al. (1993) Induction of activation-driven death (apoptosis) in activated but not resting peripheral blood T cells. J Immunol 150(10):4338–4345

Wicker LS, Miller BJ et al. (1986) Transfer of autoimmune diabetes mellitus with splenocytes from nonobese diabetic (NOD) mice. Diabetes 35(8):855–860

Wong JT, Colvin RB (1991) Selective reduction and proliferation of the CD4+ and CD8+ T cell subsets with bispecific monoclonal antibodies: evidence for inter-T cell-mediated cytolysis. Clin Immunol Immunopathol 58(2):236–250

Wood ML, Monaco AP et al. (1971) Use of homozygous allogeneic bone marrow for induction of tolerance with antilymphocyte serum: dose and timing. Transplant Proc 3(1):676–679

Woodle ES, Xu D et al. (1999) Phase I trial of a humanized, Fc receptor nonbinding OKT3 antibody, huOKT3gamma1(Ala–Ala) in the treatment of acute renal allograft rejection. Transplantation 68(5):608–616

Yasunami R, Bach JF (1988) Anti-suppressor effect of cyclophosphamide on the development of spontaneous diabetes in NOD mice. Eur J Immunol 18(3):481–484

Yasunami R, Debray-sachs M et al. (1990) Ontogeny of regulatory and effector T cells in autoimmune NOD mice. In: Shafrir E (eds) Frontiers in diabetes research. Lessons from animal diabetes III. vol 19, Smith-Gordon, London pp 88–93

You S, Belghith M, et al. (2005) Autoimmune diabetes onset results from qualitative rather than quantitative age-dependent changes in pathogenic T cells. Diabetes 54:1415–1422

You S, Leforban B, et al. (2007) Adaptive TGF-{beta}-dependent regulatory T cells control autoimmune diabetes and are a privileged target of anti-CD3 antibody treatment. Proc Natl Acad Sci USA 104(15):6335–6340

You S, Thieblemont N, et al. (2006) Transforming growth factor-beta and T-cell-mediated immunoregulation in the control of autoimmune diabetes. Immunol Rev 212:185–202

Monoclonal Antibody Therapy for Prostate Cancer

A. Jakobovits

1 Overview of Prostate Cancer 238
2 Therapeutic Antibodies in Cancer Therapy 238
3 Antibody Therapy in Prostate Cancer 240
   3.1 Antibodies to Established Targets 240
   3.2 Antibodies to Emerging Targets 246
4 Conclusions 250
References 251

Abstract Early detection of prostate cancer (PCa) and advances in hormonal and chemotherapy treatments have provided great clinical benefits to patients with early stages of the disease. However, a significant proportion of patients still progress to advanced, metastatic disease, for which no effective therapies are available. Therefore, there is a critical need for new treatment modalities, ideally targeted specifically to prostate cancer cells. The recent clinical and commercial successes of monoclonal antibodies (MAbs) have made them the most rapidly expanding class of therapeutics being developed for many disease indications, including cancer. PCa is well suited for antibody-based therapy due to the size and location of recurrent and metastatic tumors, and the lack of necessity to avoid targeting the normal prostate, a nonessential organ. These properties have fostered interest in the development and clinical evaluation of therapeutic MAbs directed to both well established and newly discovered targets in PCa. MAbs directed to established targets include those approved for other solid tumors, including anti-human epidermal growth factor receptor-2 (HER2) MAb trastuzumab, anti-epidermal growth factor receptor (EGFR) MAbs cetuximab and panitumumab, and the antivascular endothelial growth factor (VEGF) MAb bevacizumab. Genomics efforts have yielded a

A. Jakobovits
Agensys, Inc., 1545 17th Street, Santa Monica, CA 90404, USA
e-mail: ajakobovits@agensys.com

Y. Chernajovsky, A. Nissim (eds.) *Therapeutic Antibodies. Handbook of Experimental Pharmacology 181.*
© Springer-Verlag Berlin Heidelberg 2008

large number of novel, clinically relevant targets in PCa with the desirable expression profiling in tumor and normal tissues, and with an implicated role in tumor growth and spread. Growing efforts are directed to the development of naked or payload-conjugated therapeutic antibodies to these targets, and a variety of MAb products are currently progressing through preclinical and various stages of clinical development. The clinical experience with some of the commercialized MAb products points out specific challenges in conducting clinical trials with targeted therapy in PCa. Encouraging results with MAbs directed to both established and emerging targets indicate a potential key role for MAb-based therapy in future treatments for different stages of PCa.

1 Overview of Prostate Cancer

Prostate cancer (PCa) is the most commonly diagnosed cancer and the second leading cause of cancer-related deaths in American males. In 2005, over 230,000 men were diagnosed with PCa and approximately 30,000 died of the disease (Jemel et al. 2005). The ability to measure prostate-specific antigen (PSA) levels in men has allowed earlier diagnosis of PCa. Although several curative therapies exist for localized disease, such as radical prostatectomy, radiation therapy, and cryotherapy, approximately one-third of treated patients will relapse with distant metastases to bone and other organs (Jemel 2005, Pound et al. 1999). Since prostate cancer cell growth is regulated by androgens, systemic androgen deprivation is the common treatment for recurrent, locally advanced and metastatic disease. Despite an initial positive response by a large percentage of patients, most will develop hormone-refractory, metastatic disease (Saad and Schulman 2004). Treatment of hormone-refractory prostate cancer (HPRC) patients with docetaxel in combination with prednisone has been shown to improve patient overall survival (OS), time to disease progression, and quality of life, and was approved by the FDA in 2004 (Tannock et al. 2004). The treatment, however, is accompanied by significant toxicity and most patients become resistant to the chemotherapy after several treatment cycles. The paucity of therapeutic options for hormone and/or chemotherapy refractory patients and the need for more effective and less toxic agents for earlier stages of the disease indicate a critical need for new therapeutic approaches. Monoclonal antibody (MAb)-based targeted therapy is emerging as one of the leading therapeutic modalities under development in PCa.

2 Therapeutic Antibodies in Cancer Therapy

The therapeutic potential of MAbs stems from their specific and high affinity binding to their targets, coupled with their diversity of effector functions. More than a quarter century after the discovery of MAbs (Kohler and Milstein 1975), their therapeutic utility is now being realized, with over 20 MAbs approved in the US for use in various clinical settings, including human malignancies. At present, with

160 MAb products under development, antibodies are the most rapidly expanding class of human therapeutics (PhRMA report 2006). The recent success in the development and commercialization of therapeutic antibodies can be attributed to the technical progress made in producing safer, more stable, and efficacious MAbs. The primary contribution to this progress has been development of technologies for generation of more human-like antibodies, allowing overcoming of the efficacy and safety issues related to immunogenicity of mouse antibodies in human patients (Jakobovits 1998, Lonberg 2005). The transition from mouse to human antibodies has progressed from chimeric antibodies with ~30% residual mouse sequences (Morrison and Oi 1975) to humanized MAbs with ~5% residual mouse sequences (Riechmann et al. 1988), to fully human antibodies derived from combinatorial libraries (Griffiths and Hooggenboom 1993) or mice engineering with the human humoral immune system (Mendez et al. 1997, Fishwild et al. 1996). This technical progress, together with better understanding of targets, therapeutic indications, and clinical designs that suit antibody therapy, has allowed for an increased rate in successful development and commercialization of therapeutic MAbs.

Utilization of antibodies to affect tumor cell growth and survival has been one of the most appealing applications for MAbs since their discovery. Of the 20 approved MAbs, 9 MAbs are being commercialized for different hematological and solid cancer indications and over 115 additional MAb products are being evaluated in clinical trials (PhRMA report 2006).

In oncology settings, MAbs can be developed either as naked agents or armed with a toxic payload such as radioisotopes or toxins (Wu and Senter 2005). Naked antibodies are directed against targets that play a role in the tumor pathogenesis and progression. Upon binding to their target, such MAbs are capable of modulating their function to inhibit tumor cell growth, survival, or spread. In addition, naked antibodies bearing the IgG1 isotype are capable of recruiting the patient's complement and immune cells to induce complement-dependent cytotoxicity (CDC) and antibody dependent cellular cytotoxicity (ADCC) (Adams and Weiner 2005). For many of the approved naked antibodies, their administration with the relevant chemotherapy has led to enhanced clinical benefit.

Armed MAbs utilize the antibody as a vehicle to deliver to target-expressing tumor cells a toxic agent, such as radioisotopes (e.g., ^{90}Y, ^{177}Lu, ^{131}I) or potent toxins (e.g., maytansinoid, auristatin) (Wu and Senter 2005). The payload approach benefits from high affinity antibodies directed to targets that are highly expressed on tumor cells and minimally on essential normal tissues. Utilization of antibody-drug conjugates (ADCs) requires their internalization into the cells to induce specific release of the active drug and subsequent cell killing (Doronina et al. 2003, Smith 2004). Among the nine FDA-approved MAbs for cancer indications, six are naked and three are conjugated to a payload. Among the naked antibodies are: (1) rituximab (Rituxan® BiogenIdec/Genentech), a mouse MAb targeting CD20 for non-Hodgkin's lymphoma; (2) alemtuzumab (Campath®, Ilex), a humanized anti-CD52 MAb for chronic lymphocytic leukemia; (3) trastuzumab (Herceptin®, Genentech), a humanized anti-HER2 MAb for breast cancer; (4) cetuximab (Erbitux®, ImClone/Bristol-Myers Squibb), a chimeric MAb targeting EGFR for colorectal and head and neck cancers; (5) bevacizumab (Avastin®, Genentech), a humanized

MAb targeting VEGF for the treatment of colorectal and lung cancers; and (6) pan-itumumab (Vectimib™, Amgen), an anti-EGFR fully human MAb for the treatment of colorectal cancer.

The three approved payload-conjugated MAbs include the anti-CD20 ibritumo-mab tiuxetan (Zevalin®, BiogenIdec) and tositumomab (Bexxar®, GlaxoSmith-Kline) mouse MAbs, conjugated to the radioisotopes ^{90}Y and ^{131}I, respectively, for non-Hodgkin's lymphoma; and gemtuzumab (Mylotarg®, Wyeth) anti-CD33 humanized MAb conjugated to the toxin calicheamicin for acute myeloid leukemia.

3 Antibody Therapy in Prostate Cancer

Different aspects of prostate cancer make it an excellent indication for antibody-based therapy: (1) normal prostate, being a nonessential organ, allows for targeting of antigens that are expressed in both normal prostate and prostate cancer cells; (2) PCa metastases predominately involve bone marrow and lymph nodes, locations that are accessible to circulating antibodies and that have shown responses to MAb therapies in other tumor types (e.g., lymphoma, breast cancer); (3) the early diag-nosis of the disease and the availability of the biomarker PSA allow for initiation of treatment when primary/recurrent tumors or metastatic lesions are small and well suited for antibody penetration; and (4) the demonstrated response of PCa to radio-therapy and chemotherapy justifies the use of naked antibodies in combination with chemotherapeutic agents and the use of payload-conjugated MAbs.

The premise of the antibody-based therapy in prostate cancer led to clinical evaluation of the four MAbs approved for solid tumor indications (cetuximab, trastuzumab, bevacizumab, and panitumumab) in different PCa settings. In paral-lel, significant academic and corporate efforts have been made toward identification of novel targets in PCa and evaluation of their suitability for a therapeutic antibody approach. This review will focus on the major clinical and preclinical developments in both areas.

3.1 Antibodies to Established Targets

3.1.1 Human Epidermal Growth Factor Receptor-2 (HER2/neu)

HER2 is a 185-kD growth factor receptor tyrosine kinase encoded by the HER2 (c-erb-2) proto-oncogene. It is one of the four members of the HER receptor tyrosine kinase family, which includes EGFR (HER1), HER3, and HER4, shown to regulate cell growth, survival, and differentiation. The ligand to HER2 has not yet been iden-tified but it appears that HER2 heterodimerization with other HER receptors leads to activation of cell signaling pathways and thus to cell proliferation (Olayioye et al. 2000; Pegram and Slamon 2000). In breast cancer, HER2 gene amplification or pro-tein overexpression occurs in 25–30% of patients and has been associated with a poor clinical prognosis (Pauletti et al. 2000; Yeon and Pegram 2005). Trastuzumab is a humanized $IgG_1\kappa$ anti-HER2 MAb that binds with high affinity ($K_d \sim 5\,nM$) to HER2 expressed on the cell surface. It received FDA approval for treatment of metastatic breast cancer based on two large clinical studies, which demonstrated that antibody treatment (initial dose of $4\,mg\,kg^{-1}$ followed by $2\,mg\,kg^{-1}$ dose, weekly) increased survival of patients whose tumors overexpressed HER2, both as a single agent in second- and third-line therapy, and in combination with chemotherapy as first-line therapy (Slamon et al. 2001). Clinical benefits were shown to correlate with HER2 overexpression leading to patient selection based on the target expression levels (Yeon and Pegram 2005). More recently, trastuzumab was approved for adjuvant treatment of women with node-positive, HER2-overexpressing breast cancer, in combination with doxorubicin, cyclophosphamide, and paclitaxel. The antibody mode of action is not fully understood, but it may combine different mechanisms, including effect on HER2 signaling, internalization, downregulation, and proteolysis, as well as MAb-induced ADCC (Yeon and Pegram 2005).

In PCa, studies of HER2 expression resulted in variable results and a consensus for target expression and its predictive value has not been achieved (Scher 2000, Solit and Angus 2001). In various studies, only low proportion of patients exhibited HER2 overexpression (Scher 2000, Koeppen et al. 2001, Lara et al. 2004). In studies where overexpression was detected, it was correlated with progression to androgen-independent and metastatic disease (Signoretti et al. 2000, Morris et al. 2002, Nishio et al. 2006). Furthermore, unlike breast cancer, HER2 amplification in PCa has been decidedly uncommon (Scher 2000, Signoretti et al. 2000). The role of HER2 expression in PCa progression is not clear. Some studies have shown that HER2 overexpression activated the androgen receptor pathway in the absence of ligand and conferred androgen-independent growth to an androgen-dependent cell line (Craft et al. 1999). In addition, HER2 transfection in prostate cell lines induced metastatic capacity in an orthotopic model (Marengo et al. 1997). These findings concur with the correlation between HER2 expression levels and progression to androgen-independent disease (Signoretti et al. 2000). These data, together with the anti-tumor activity of trastuzumab in PCa mouse xenograft models (Agus et al. 1999, Solit and Angus 2001), provided the rationale for evaluation of the MAb in patients with advanced PCa.

In phase II clinical trials with trastuzumab in HPRC patients, no objective responses, based on PSA decline or regression of measurable disease, were observed (Morris et al. 2002, Lara et al. 2004). Attempts to correlate between HER2 expression, hormone sensitivity, and trastuzumab efficacy have failed due to the low number of patients identified as HER2-positive, based on their archived primary tumor specimens (Morris et al. 2002, Lara et al. 2004).

Clinical trials in PCa were also performed with a new anti-HER2 humanized MAb, pertuzumab (Omnitag™, Genentech), selected to inhibit HER2 dimerization with other HER family members, thereby inhibiting target signaling pathways in a mechanism distinct from trastuzumab. In xenograft models, the antibody was shown to inhibit growth of HER2 non-overexpressing breast and prostate tumors (Agus et al. 2002), suggesting that pertuzumab may allow to extend HER2-directed antibody therapy to patients that do not respond to trastuzumab. In a phase I dose escalating study, one of five PCa patients, dosed at 15 mg kg^{-1} experienced a partial response (Agus et al. 2003). However, in phase II studies with pertuzumab as single agent in 41 HPRC patients that failed taxane-based therapy, no PSA or objective radiographic responses were observed (Agus et al. 2005).

The overall limited clinical efficacy in PCa observed to date with trastuzumab and pertuzumab suggests that modulation of HER2 by naked antibodies does not impact the disease, potentially due to either insufficient expression levels or the nonessential role of the target in PCa pathogenesis. Recently, phase I clinical studies have been initiated in breast cancer patients with trastuzumab conjugated to the maytansinoid derivative DM1 (trastuzumab-MCC-DM1, Genentech). Application of this ADC in PCa may provide a more efficacious HER2-directed antibody therapy.

3.1.2 Epidermal Growth Factor Receptor (EGFR)

EGFR (HER1, c-erb-1), a member of the HER receptor family, is a 150-kD transmembrane glycoprotein with an extracellular ligand-binding domain and an intracellular tyrosine kinase domain. Interaction of EGFR with its ligands (e.g., EGF and transforming growth factor-α) leads to receptor dimerization and autophosphorylation, which triggers a cascade of signaling pathways that regulate cell proliferation, survival, motility, and transformation (Mendelsohn and Baselga 2006, Citri and Yarden 2006). EGFR is expressed in epithelial cells from multiple normal tissues, including skin and liver. EGFR protein overexpression has been detected in many human epithelial carcinomas (Wujcik 2006). Increased EGFR overexpression in tumors was shown to be associated with increased production of ligands, in particular TGFα, by the tumor cells, suggesting an autocrine regulatory loop for EGFR stimulation (Di Marco et al. 1989). Due to these properties, EGFR has been considered an attractive target for MAb therapy for more than 20 years and was the first target to which antibody-mediated anti-tumor activity was demonstrated in preclinical xenograft models (Mendelsohn and Baselga 2006, Sebastian et al. 2006).

Two anti-EGFR MAbs have been approved by the US FDA: cetuximab for the treatment of colorectal cancer and squamous cell carcinoma of head and neck (SCCHN), and panitumumab for the treatment of colorectal cancer (Mendelsohn and Baselga 2006, Yang et al. 2005). Cetuximab, a chimeric IgG$_1$κ derivative of the mouse MAb 225, binds with high affinity ($K_d \sim 0.39$ nM) to the extracellular domain of EGFR expressed on cells. The antibody was shown to block ligand binding, receptor dimerization, and to inhibit activation of EGFR-mediated signal transduction pathways associated with cell growth and transformation, invasion, and angiogenesis (Baselga 2001, Mendelsohn and Baselga 2006). As a result, the antibody inhibited tumor cell proliferation, angiogenesis, and metastasis. In preclinical xenograft models, cetuximab was shown to enhance antitumor effects of different classes of chemotherapy and radiotherapy (Baselga 2001, Mendelsohn and Baselga 2006). Cetuximab was approved for treatment of patients with advanced colorectal cancer based on demonstrated higher objective response rate in patients treated with the MAb (initial dose of $400\,\mathrm{mg\,m}^{-2}$ followed by $250\,\mathrm{mg\,m}^{-2}$ weekly) in combination with irinotecan as compared to those treated with antibody alone (Cunningham et al. 2004). More recently, the antibody was approved for treatment of SCCHN based on significant benefit in disease control and OS (Bonner et al. 2004).

Panitumumab is a fully human $IgG_2\kappa$ MAb that binds to EGFR with very high affinity ($K_d \sim 0.05\,\mathrm{nM}$) (Mendez et al. 1997). The IgG_2 isotype was selected to minimize CDC- and ADCC-mediated toxicity to normal organs. The MAb was shown to inhibit ligand binding, receptor autophosphorylation, and activation of receptor associated kinases, resulting in inhibition of cell growth, induction of apoptosis, and VEGF production (Yang et al. 1999). In various xenograft mouse models, panitumumab has demonstrated significant antitumor activity, including eradication of large established tumors (Yang et al. 1999, 2001). The antibody activity was further enhanced when combined with chemotherapy or radiation. Panitumumab was approved as a single agent treatment ($6\,\mathrm{mg\,kg}^{-1}$, every 2 weeks) for patients with advanced colorectal cancer who failed one or more chemotherapy regimens. The approval was based on a demonstrated statistically significant prolongation in progression free survival (PFS) in EGFR-expressing patients receiving the MAb compared to those receiving best supportive care alone (Peeters et al. 2006, Van Cutsem et al. 2007).

EGFR is expressed in the basal/neuroendocrine compartment of the normal prostate and there is some evidence that EGF and TGFα play a role in the structural and functional integrity of the prostatic epithelium (Sherwood and Lee 1995). The role of EGFR in the development of PCa is not clear. Most studies did not detect increased EGFR expression in PCa as compared to benign prostatic tissue, and no correlation with EGFR expression and prognosis has been established. However, Di Lorenzo et al. (2002) reported that increased EGFR expression was associated with progression to androgen-independent disease. Constitutive EGFR activation has been shown in PCa cell lines and the autocrine/paracrine loop interaction of EGFR with EGF and TGFα has been implicated in PCa proliferation. Studies with cetuximab and panitumumab in various PCa xenograft models have shown inhibition of tumor growth and enhanced sensitivity to cytotoxic agents (Yang et al. 2001, Prewett et al. 1996).

In phase I/II studies in HPRC patients with cetuximab and doxorubicin, one patient out of 19 experienced a partial response (Slovin et al. 1997), a limited response as compared to the efficacy observed from combination of MAb and chemotherapy treatment in colon cancer. Similarly, in phase II clinical studies with panitumumab as a single agent in HPRC patients, no PSA or tumor responses have been observed.

3.1.3 Vascular Endothelial Growth Factor (VEGF)

VEGF is a growth factor that is essential for the regulation of both physiological and pathological angiogenesis. VEGF acts as a potent mitogen and a survival factor for vascular endothelial cells. In addition, it modulates the migration of endothelial cells to sites of angiogenesis, mediates the secretion and activation of enzymes involved with degrading extracellular matrix, and increases vascular permeability (Ferrara et al. 2003). The role of VEGF in promoting development of tumor vasculature supports a primary role for this growth factor in tumor development. VEGF expression is detected in many human cancers, with higher expression in hypoxic cells adjacent to necrotic areas. Tumor cells and their associated stroma represent the main source of VEGF. Many anti-VEGF agents, including MAbs, were shown to inhibit tumor growth in vivo. Studies also demonstrated that combining antibodies with chemotherapy or radiation results in a greater antitumor effect (Ferrara et al. 2004).

Bevacizumab is a high-affinity ($K_d \sim 0.5\,nM$) humanized IgG$_1$κ antibody that binds to human VEGF-A and prevents its interaction with its receptors, VEGFR1 and VEGFR2, on the surface of endothelial cells. The antibody prevents endothelial cell proliferation, new blood vessel formation, and inhibits the growth of various human tumor cell lines in mouse xenograft models (Ferrara et al. 2004). Bevacizumab was approved by the FDA as first- and second-line treatment with 5-fluorouracil-based chemotherapy for metastatic carcinoma of the colon or rectum. The approval was based on demonstration of a statistically significant improvement in OS, PFS, and objective response in patients receiving bevacizumab ($5\,mg\,kg^{-1}$, every 14 days) plus FOLFOX4 when compared to those receiving chemotherapy alone (Hurwitz et al. 2004). More recently, based on improvement in OS, bevacizumab in combination with carboplatin and paclitaxel was approved for first-line treatment of patients with unresectable, locally advanced, recurrent or metastatic nonsmall cell lung cancer.

Although no increased VEGF expression levels have been detected in prostate tumors, various findings suggest that VEGF may play a role in the pathogenesis and progression of the disease. In patients with metastatic prostate cancer, plasma VEGF levels are significantly higher than in patients with localized disease and high urine VEGF levels are associated with progressive HPRC (Duque et al. 1999, Bok et al. 2001). Tumor angiogenesis has been correlated with adverse outcome in PCa and increased microvascularity has been found to correlate with the pathologic stage of the disease (Weidner et al. 1993, Silberman et al. 1997). Antibodies to VEGF slowed tumor growth in androgen-independent PCa xenograft models, and the antitumor activity was augmented with the addition of chemotherapy (Kirschenbaum et al. 1997, Melynk et al. 1999, Borgstrom et al. 1998).

Evaluation of bevacizumab as a single agent ($10\,mg\,kg^{-1}$, every 14 days) in HPRC patients did not produce significant objective responses (Reese et al. 2001). Phase II studies of bevacizumab in combination with docetaxel and estramustine in metastatic HPRC patients led to objective responses, including PSA decline in 81% of the patients, and tumor responses in 53% of the patients. The observed time to progression and OS were 9.7 months and 21 months, respectively (Picus et al. 2003). These results led to the ongoing randomized phase III study in HPRC patients, comparing treatment with bevacizumab ($15\,mg\,kg^{-1}$, every 3 weeks) in combination with docetaxel and prednisone to treatment with chemotherapy and placebo. The primary endpoint is OS and the secondary endpoints are PSA response and PFS. Another planned study is aimed at evaluation of bevacizumab in combination with docetaxel as neoadjuvant treatment of high-risk patients with localized PCa undergoing prostatectomy.

3.1.4 Insulin-Like Growth Factor I Receptor (IGF-IR)

IGF-IR is a receptor tyrosine kinase (Adams et al. 2000). IGF-IR and its ligands, IGF-I and IGF-II, are implicated in the regulation of cell proliferation, survival, differentiation, and angiogenesis, as well as in the maintenance of the transformed phenotype for different cancer types (Grothey et al. 1999, Valentinis and Baserga 2001). IGF-IR has widespread expression among normal tissues and many tumors exhibit increased expression of IGF-IR (Burtscher and Christofori). Blocking the IGF-IR pathway by inhibitory peptides, soluble receptor, and antisense oligonucleotides resulted in decreased cell growth, increased cell apoptosis, and inhibition of tumor formation in animal models. IGF-IR-specific MAbs have been shown to block IGF-1 binding to its receptors, to induce receptor downregulation, and to inhibit cell proliferation in vitro. The MAbs also significantly inhibited tumor growth in various xenografts models as single agents and in combination with chemotherapy (Maloney et al. 2003, Wu et al. 2005, Burtrum et al. 2003, Cohen et al. 2005). Among the MAbs that are progressing in clinical development are: (1) CP-751,871 (Pfizer), a fully human $IgG_2\kappa$ MAb ($K_d \sim 1.5\,nM$) (Cohen et al. 2005); (2) IMC-A12 (ImClone), a fully human $IgG_1\kappa$ MAb ($K_d \sim 0.04\,nM$) (Burtrum et al. 2003); (3) h7C10 MAb (Merck), a humanized $IgG_1\kappa$ MAb ($K_d \sim 1.5\,nM$) (Goetsch et al. 2005); and (4) AVE1642 MAb (Sanofi-Aventis/ImmunoGen), a humanized $IgG_1\kappa$ MAb (Kd $\sim 1.5\,nM$) (Maloney et al. 2003).

Different findings suggest the involvement of IGF-IR and its ligands in development and maintenance of PCa. Elevated levels of plasma IGF-I and reduced levels of the main serum binding protein IGF-BP3, have been shown to be associated with an increased risk of PCa (Djavan et al. 2001). IGF IR expression is maintained throughout all stages of the disease and inhibition of its expression in prostate cancer cell lines by antisense oligonucleotides reduced cell growth and migration in vitro and in vivo (Grzmil et al. 2004). Blocking of ligand binding by an IGF-like peptide resulted in growth inhibition of different PCa cell lines (Pietrzkowski et al. 1993). A12 MAb significantly inhibited the growth of both androgen-dependent and androgen–independent PCa xenografts by induction of G1- or G2-M cell cycle arrest, respectively (Wu et al. 2005). Enhanced activity was demonstrated when the MAb treatment was combined with docetaxel (Wu et al. 2006).

At present, only CP-751,871 MAb is being evaluated in PCa patients. In a randomized two-arm phase II study, treatment of HPRC patients with CP-751,871 in combination with docetaxel and prednisone is being compared to chemotherapy alone. The primary endpoints of the study are antitumor efficacy measured as objective responses using PSA and RECIST criteria.

3.2 Antibodies to Emerging Targets

3.2.1 Discovery of Novel Targets in Prostate Cancer

During the last decade, utilization of various genomics and proteomics methodologies has yielded numerous novel sequences with upregulated expression in prostate cancer. Their validation as therapeutic targets required meeting the following desirable features: significant and homogeneous expression in a majority of patients with advanced, metastatic disease; minimal expression in normal vital tissues; and involvement in disease pathogenesis. This section will focus on the novel cell surface targets in PCa that have been validated as attractive targets for either naked or payload antibody-based therapy and are currently advancing to or are already in clinical trials.

3.2.2 Prostate-Specific Membrane Antigen (PSMA)

Prostate-Specific Membrane Antigen (PSMA) is a 100-kDa cell surface glycoprotein identified as the enzyme glutamate carboxypeptidase II, which is involved in cellular uptake of dietary folate and regulation of neurotransmitter release in the brain (Pinto et al. 1996). Among normal tissues, PSMA expression has been detected in prostate, small intestine, kidney, salivary glands, and in the central nervous system (Silver et al. 1997). Significant PSMA expression was detected across all stages of PCa with a strong correlation between target density and progression to advanced, higher grade, hormone-independent and metastatic disease and poor prognosis (Ross et al. 2005). Abundant PSMA expression was also detected on the neovasculature of various solid tumors but not on normal vasculature (Chang et al. 1999). Characterization of mice in which PSMA expression has been knocked out has suggested that it plays a role in endothelial cell invasion through extracellular matrix (Conway et al. 2006). The role of PSMA enzymatic activity in prostate cancer progression has not been established yet and inhibition of enzymatic activity in vitro or in vivo did not inhibit tumor cell growth (Ross et al. 2005). Various anti-PSMA antibodies were evaluated in different therapeutic and diagnostic settings. A mouse MAb, 7E11/CYT-356 (ProstaScint®, Cytogen), is marketed for imaging of PCa soft tissue metastases (Kahn et al. 1998). However, being directed to an intracellular epitope, this MAb has limited therapeutic applications. Antibodies directed to PSMA extracellular epitopes have shown good targeting to PCa tumors in xenograft models but no antitumor activity (Bander et al. 2003). The lack of efficacy by naked antibodies, combined with the rapid internalization of PSMA antibody complexes, led to the development of antibodies armed with either toxins or radioisotopes as the predominant therapeutic strategy for PSMA.

   The most extensive preclinical and clinical work has been performed with the mouse MAb J591 and its humanlike (de-immunized) derivative $IgG_1\kappa$ HuJ591, which binds to the extracellular domain of PSMA with 1 nM affinity (Ross et al. 2005). In studies with established PCa xenografts, the antibody conjugated to either radioisotopes or to the antimicrotubule toxin DM1, a derivative of maytansinoid, demonstrated significant antitumor activity (Smith-Jones et al. 2003, Henry et al. 2004).

A series of phase I clinical studies were performed in HPRC patients treated with HuJ591 conjugated to different payloads: (1) Indium-111 (^{111}In); (2) Yttrium-90 (^{90}Y); (3) Lutetium-177 (^{177}Lu); and (4) DM1 toxin. Studies with the radiolabeled antibodies indicated that the conjugates were well tolerated with MTD established as $17.5\,\mathrm{mCi\,m^{-2}}$ and $30\,\mathrm{mCi\,m^{-2}}$ for repeat dosing of ^{90}Y and ^{177}Lu, respectively (Nanus et al. 2003, Milowsky et al. 2004, Bander et al. 2005). In most patients, the antibody localized well to established tumor sites, including bone and soft tissue metastases. In both studies, antitumor activity, including PSA decline and/or measurable disease responses, were seen in about 10% of patients. Phase II studies with ^{177}Lu HuJ591 are underway.

A phase I/II clinical study, which explored escalating doses $(18–343\,\mathrm{mg\,m^{-2}})$ of huJ591-DM1 (MLN2704, Millennium) in HPRC patients, indicated that the ADC was tolerated in most patients, including those who received multiple doses. Durable antitumor activity, based on either PSA decline or partial tumor response, was detected in two patients treated at 264 and $343\,\mathrm{mg\,m^{-2}}$ dose, respectively (Galsky et al. 2005). In a follow-up phase I/II study in progressing HPRC patients, multiple ascending doses of MLN2704 at different dosing schedules were tested for tolerability and efficacy. Dose-dependent antitumor effects were seen, most notably PSA decline of 49–88% in 4 out of 6 patients at the $330\,\mathrm{mg\,m^{-2}}$ dose. However, the frequency of grade 2–3 peripheral neuropathy limited the continuous treatment at these dose levels (Milowsky et al. 2006). At present, further development of MLN2704 has been discontinued.

Another anti-PSMA ADC progressing to the clinic is an $IgG_1\,\kappa$ fully human MAb conjugated to auristatin E toxin (Progenics Pharmaceuticals). Treatment of mice bearing established human prostate tumors with this ADC prolonged their survival and led to tumor eradication in a subset of the mice (Ma et al. 2006).

3.2.3 Prostate Stem Cell Antigen (PSCA)

PSCA is a 123-amino acid cell surface glycoprotein, a member of the Thy-1/Ly-6 family of glycosylphosphatidylinositol (GPI)- anchored antigens. PSCA was cloned by gene expression profiling using PCa lymph node-derived xenografts (Reiter et al. 1998). In normal tissues, PSCA expression is restricted predominantly to the prostate, stomach, bladder, and ureter. IHC analysis has demonstrated PSCA expression in the majority of patients with prostate (Gu et al. 2000, Han et al. 2004, Lam et al. 2005), pancreatic (Argani et al. 2001), and bladder (Amara et al. 2001) cancers. In prostate cancer, PSCA protein expression has been detected in all stages of the disease, including high-grade prostatic intraepithelial neoplasia (PIN), primary androgen-dependent and hormone-refractory disease. PSCA expression has been detected in over 90% of primary prostate tumors analyzed, and increased expression levels (for both intensity and frequency) have been correlated with Gleason score, tumor stage, grade, and progression to androgen-independent disease (Gu et al. 2000). In addition, PSCA overexpression has been linked to an increased risk of biochemical recurrence (Han et al. 2004). Significant and uniform expression has also been detected in the majority of PCa metastatic lesions, including over 85% of bone metastases and over 65% of lymph node and liver metastases, with higher staining intensity observed in bone lesions (Lam et al. 2005). This expression profile makes PSCA a compelling therapeutic target in different PCa patient populations.

The function of PSCA is not fully understood and insights into the relevance of PSCA to PCa development and progression have been derived predominantly from in vivo studies with mouse and human anti-PSCA MAbs. 1G8 is a mouse $IgG_1\kappa$ MAb that binds to the PSCA extracellular domain with affinity of 1 nM (Saffran et al. 2001). Treatment with 1G8 of mice bearing PCa bone metastasis-derived LAPC9 xenografts, established subcutaneously or orthotopically, led to a significant inhibition of tumor growth. Tumor growth inhibition was detected with both androgen-dependent and androgen–independent tumors as well as those derived from PC3 cells engineered to express PSCA. Inhibition of orthotropic tumor growth resulted in significant prolongation of survival of 1G8-treated mice as compared to mice treated with a control antibody. Furthermore, the MAb demonstrated a dramatic inhibitory effect on the spread of local prostate tumors to distal sites, even in the presence of a large tumor burden (Saffran et al. 2001). 1G8 bears the mouse IgG_1 isotype that is incapable of mediating CDC or ADCC, thus suggesting that the MAb antitumor effect stems from an intrinsic antibody activity on modulating PSCA function in tumor growth and spread. The minimal contribution, if any, from the antibody effector function was corroborated by the demonstration that 1G8-derived $F(ab')_2$ fragments inhibited the growth of prostate tumor cells both in vivo and in vitro (Gu et al. 2005).

The compelling in vivo efficacy data obtained with mouse MAbs provided the rationale for the generation of AGS-PSCA, a fully human $IgG_1\kappa$ MAb that specifically binds to PSCA with high affinity ($K_d \sim 0.2\,nM$). AGS-PSCA significantly inhibited the growth of established LAPC9 androgen- independent and androgen-dependent tumors grown subcutaneously or orthotopically. Enhanced activity on established tumors was demonstrated when AGS-PSCA was administered in combination with docetaxol (Jakobovits et al. 2005). The significant antitumor activity of AGS-PSCA as a monotherapy and in combination with the approved chemotherapeutic agent supported the initiation of phase I clinical study in patients with advanced prostate cancer (Agensys/Merck).

The restricted expression of PSCA in normal tissues and its internalization upon binding to antibodies led to its evaluation as a target for ADC approach. Mouse MAbs conjugated to the maytansinoid derivative DM1 demonstrated in vitro cytotoxicity of PSCA-expressing cells and marked in vivo efficacy with complete regression of established tumors in a large subset of mice bearing PC3-PSCA tumors (Ross et al. 2002).

3.2.4 Cytotoxic T Lymphocyte-Associated Antigen 4 (CTAL-4)

Unlike the other described targets that are expressed by tumors or their associated endothelial cells, Cytotoxic T lymphocyte-associated antigen 4 (CTLA-4) is expressed on activated T cells as a second counter-receptor for the B7 family of costimulatory molecules. CTLA-4 functions as a negative regulator of T cell activation (Allison 1994) leading to attenuation of T cell response to tumor cells. Blocking CTLA-4 function by MAbs resulted in enhanced immune responses and tumor rejection in mice (Leach et al. 1996). Two anti-CTLA-4 fully human MAbs, IgG$_1$κ ipilimumab (Medarex/Bristol-Myers Squibb) and IgG$_2$κ CP-675,206 (Pfizer) are being evaluated for clinical efficacy in different cancer indications. In PCa patients, ipilimumab has been evaluated both as a monotherapy and in combination with chemotherapy or vaccine agents. In a randomized phase II study in HPRC patients, which compared the treatment of ipilimumab (3 mg kg^{-1}, every 4 weeks) as a single agent to its combination with a single dose of docetaxel, PSA responses, but no radiologic responses, were observed in three patients in each arm (13% and 15%, respectively), indicating no apparent enhancement of activity by docetaxel. Three patients experienced severe adverse effects related to immune breakthrough events (Small et al. 2006). Two major studies are underway: (1) a phase I/II dose escalating study in HPRC patients aimed at evaluating ipilimumab at 3, 5, 7.5, and 10 mg kg^{-1} every 3 weeks for 4 doses, for safety and antitumor assessment; (2) a phase I trial in HPRC patients to study the combination of GM-CSF-gene-transduced allogeneic PCa cellular immunotherapy (GVAX) and ipilimumab (0.3, 1, 3, or 5 mg kg^{-1}, every 4 weeks). Preliminary data have suggested a relationship between PSA response and the antibody dose level (Gerritsen et al. 2006).

3.2.5 Six-Transmembrane Epithelial Antigen of the Prostate-1 (STEAP-1)

STEAP-1 is a novel 339 amino acid cell surface antigen identified by differential gene expression profiling of PCa bone lesion-derived (Hubert et al. 1999). IHC analysis demonstrated significant and homogeneous STEAP-1 expression in all stages of PCa, including early, advanced, and hormone refractory diseases and in all lymph nodes and bone metastases (Hubert et al. 1999). In normal tissues, STEAP-1 is expressed predominantly in the prostate. The function of STEAP-1 in not fully understated, but studies in our laboratories have shown its involvement in intercellular communication in tumor cells in vitro (Challita-Eid et al. 2004). These findings concur with the hypothesis that STEAP-1 may function as a channel/transporter protein, based on its localization at cell–cell junctions and its six-transmembrane topology. Two MAbs, specific to STEAP-1 extracellular loops, were shown to inhibit STEAP-1-mediated intercellular transport in vitro and significantly inhibited in vivo growth of prostate tumor xenografts, as manifested by both tumor volume and PSA levels (Challita-Eid et al. 2004, 2007). These results support the involvement of STEAP-1 in the growth of PCa and indicate the ability of naked STEAP-1 antibodies to modulate this function.

3.2.6 Tomoregulin

Tomoregulin (TMEFF2) is a cell surface target for PCa that was identified by gene expression profiling and bioinformatics analysis (Afar et al. 2004, Zhao et al. 2005). In normal human tissues, tomoregulin is predominantly expressed in the prostate and central nervous system. In PCa, the protein was shown to be expressed in the majority of primary tumors and lymph node and bone metastatic lesions that represent both hormone-naïve and hormone-resistant diseases (Glynne-Jones et al. 2001, Afar et al. 2004, Zhao et al. 2005).

Although tomoregulin was shown to be associated with cell proliferation and emergence of hormone independence (Glynne-Jones et al. 2001, Gery et al. 2002), no antitumor activity by naked tomoregulin MAbs was demonstrated in PCa xenograft models and payload-conjugated antibody approach was pursued by different laboratories (Afar et al. 2004, Zhao et al. 2005). Tomoregulin was selected as a candidate for an ADC-based therapeutic approach due to its expression profiling and its rapid internalization when ligated with an antibody. When auristatin E was conjugated to antitomoregulin mouse MAb Pr-1, the ADC specifically killed target-expressing cells in vitro and significantly inhibited PCa xenograft growth in vivo (Afar et al. 2004). No signs of overt toxicity by the ADC, which cross-reacts with mouse tomoregulin, were observed. A humanized version of Pr-1 ADC (huPr-1-vcMMAE, Protein Design Labs) is being targeted to advance to clinical studies. Another tomoregulin mouse MAb, 2H8, armed with radioisotopes has been tested for antitumor activity. ^{111}In-labeled 2H8 MAb showed tumor-specific accumulation and the ^{90}Y-conjugated MAb inhibited tumor growth in PCa xenograft models (Zhao et al. 2005).

4 Conclusions

The numerous efforts to develop antibody-based therapies for PCa reflect the lack of effective treatments for advanced, metastatic PCa and the desire to identify safer and less toxic therapies for earlier stages of the disease. The 10 antibody products described in this review, progressing in PCa preclinical and clinical development, signify the emergence of MAbs as one of the leading targeted therapeutic modalities in PCa. These activities reflect both better characterization of established targets in PCa patients and the large number of novel validated targets in the disease. Proven clinical benefits of MAbs directed to growth factors (e.g., VEGF) and growth factor receptors (e.g., HER2, EGFR) in cancers of the colon, lung, breast, and head and neck have led to their regulatory approval and successful commercialization. Characterization of these targets for expression and function in PCa provided the rationale for evaluation of trastuzumab, cetuximab, panitumumab, and bevacizumab in HPRC patients. However, the limited clinical benefit observed with HER2- and EGFR-targeted MAbs in PCa suggests that these growth factor receptors do not play the critical role in PCa as they do in other cancer indications. On the other hand, this outcome points out at challenges in selection of HPRC patients with the desirable target expression, who are most likely to benefit from the treatment. Due to the difficulty in obtaining metastatic tissues, patient profiling relies predominantly on archived primary tumors, which may not be representative of target expression in advanced stages of PCa. Until new screening methodologies are available, development of MAb products in PCa can be facilitated by focusing on targets that exhibit significant and uniform expression in all stages of the disease, such as PSMA, PSCA, and STEAP-1, and do not dictate patient selection. Products to such targets would be applicable to advanced as well as early disease. Of special interest are MAbs directed to targets whose expression is not modulated by androgen, and which can be administered in combination with hormone therapy to further delay disease recurrence. The targets described in this review represent different biological pathways and mechanisms that impact PCa, including growth, survival, metastatic spread, angiogenesis, and immune response. Therefore, MAbs directed to these targets can provide treatments that affect different aspects of the disease. In addition, many of the described targets exhibit highly restricted expression in normal tissues, thus allowing the development of payload-conjugated MAbs. The current multitude of MAb products under development, together with encouraging results emerging for some of them, indicate that MAb-based therapy will play an important role in future treatments of PCa.

References

Adams GP, Weiner LM (2005) Monoclonal antibody therapy of cancer. Nat Biotechnol. 23(9):1147–1157

Adams TE, Epa VC, Garrett TP, Ward CW (2000) Structure and function of the type 1 insulin-like growth factor receptor. Cell Mol Life Sci. 57(7):1050–1093

Afar DE, Bhaskar V, Ibsen E et al. (2004) Preclinical validation of anti-TMEFF2-auristatin E-conjugated antibodies in the treatment of prostate cancer. Mol Cancer Ther. 3(8):921–932

Agus DB, Scher HI, Higgins B et al. (1999) Response of prostate cancer to anti Her-2/neu in androgen-dependent and independent human xenograft models. Cancer Res. 62:5485–5488

Agus DB, Akita RW, Fox WD et al. (2002) Targeting ligand-activated ErbB2 signaling inhibits breast and prostate tumor growth. Cancer Cell 2(2):127–137

Agus DB, Gordon M, Taylor RB et al. (2003) Clinical activity in a phase I trail of HER-2 targeted rhuMAb 2C4 (pertuzumab) in patients with advanced solid malignances (AST). Proc Am Soc Clin Oncol 22 (abstr 771)

Agus DB, Sweeney CJ, Morris M et al. (2005) Efficacy and safety of single agent pertuzumab (rhuMAb 2C4), a HER dimerization inhibitor, in hormone refractory prostate cancer after failure of taxane-based therapy. J Clin Oncol. 23(16S):4624

Allison JP (1994) CD28-B7 interactions in T-cell activation. Curr Opin Immunol. 6(3):414–419

Amara N, Palapattu GS, Schrage M et al. (2001) Prostate Stem Cell Antigen is overexpressed in human transitional cell carcinoma. Cancer Res 61:4660–4665

Argani P, Rosty C, Reiter RE et al. (2001) Discovery of new markers of cancer through serial analysis of gene expression: Prostate Stem Cell Antigen is overexpressed in pancreatic adenocarcinoma. Cancer Res 61:4320–4324

Bander NH, Nanus DM, Milowsky MI et al. (2003) Targeted systemic therapy of prostate cancer with a monoclonal antibody to prostate-specific membrane antigen. Semin Oncol. 30(5):667–676

Bander NH, Nanus DM, Milowsky MI et al. (2005) Phase I trail of[177] Lutetium-labeled J591, a monoclonal antibody to prostate-specific membrane antigen, independent prostate cancer. J Clon Oncol 23(21):4591–4601

Baselga J (2001) The EGFR as a target for anticancer therapy-focus on cetuximab. Eur J Cancer 37(Suppl 4):S16–S22

Bok RA, Halabi S, Fei DT et al. (2001) Vascular endothelial growth factor and basic fibroblast growth factor urine levels as predictors of outcome in hormone-refractory prostate cancer patients: a cancer and leukemia group B study. Cancer Res. 61(6):2533–2536

Bonner JA, Giralt J, Harari PM et al. (2004) Cetuximab prolongs survival in patients with locoregionally advanced squamous cell carcinoma of head and neck: A phase III study of high dose radiation therapy with or without cetuximab. J Clin Oncol 22:5507

Borgstrom P, Bourdon MA, Hillan KJ (1998) Neutralizing anti-vascular endothelial growth factor antibody completely inhibits angiogenesis and growth of human prostate carcinoma micro tumors in vivo. Prostate 35(1):1–10

Burtrum D, Zhu Z, Lu D et al. (2003) A fully human monoclonal antibody to the insulin-like growth factor I receptor blocks ligand-dependent signaling and inhibits human tumor growth in vivo. Cancer Res. 63(24):8912–8921

Burtscher I, Christofori G (1999) The IGF/IGF-1 receptor signaling pathway as a potential target for cancer therapy. Drug Resist Updat 2(1):3–8

Challita-Eid PM, Soudabeh E, Zili A et al. (2004) Targeting STEAP-1 with Monoclonal Antibodies Inhibits Growth of Human Cancer Xenografts in Mice. AACR annual meeting: late-breaking abstract

Challita-Eid PM, Morrison KR, Etessami S et al. (2007) Monoclonal Antibodies to STEAP-1 Inhibit Intercellular Communication in vitro and Growth of Human Tumor Xenografts in vivo. *Cancer Res.* 67:5798–5805

Chang SS, O'Keefe DS, Bacich DJ et al. (1999) Prostate-specific membrane antigen is produced in tumor-associated neovasculature. Clin Cancer Res 5(10):2674–2681

Citri A, Yarden Y (2006) EGF-ERBB signaling: towards the systems level. Nat Rev Mol Cell Biol 7(7):505–516

Cohen BD, Baker DA, Soderstrom C et al. (2005) Combination therapy enhances the inhibition of tumor growth with the fully human anti-type 1 insulin-like growth factor receptor monoclonal antibody CP-751,871. Clin Cancer Res 11(5):2063–2073

Conway RE, Petrovic N, Li Z et al. (2006) Prostate-specific membrane antigen regulates angiogenesis by modulating integrin signal transduction. Mol Cell Biol 26(14):5310–5324

Craft N, Shostak Y, Carey M, Sawyers CL (1999) A mechanism for hormone-independent prostate cancer through modulation of androgen receptor signaling by the HER-2/neu tyrosine kinase. Nat Med 5(3):264–265

Cunningham D, Humblet Y, Siena S et al. (2004) Cetuximab monotherapy and cetuximab plus irinotecan in irinotecan-refractory metastatic colorectal cancer. N Engl J Med 351(4):337–345

Di Lorenzo G, Tortora G, D'Armiento FP et al. (2002) Expression of epidermal growth factor receptor correlates with disease relapse and progression to androgen-independence in human prostate cancer. Clin Cancer Res 8(11):3438–3444

Di Marco E, Pierce JH, Fleming TP et al. (1989) Autocrine interaction between TGF alpha and the EGF-receptor: quantitative requirements for induction of the malignant phenotype. Oncogene 4(7):831–838

Djavan B, Waldert M, Seitz C, Marberger M (2001) Insulin-like growth factors and prostate cancer. World J Urol (4):225–233

Doronina SO, Toki BE, Torgov MY et al. (2003) Development of potent monoclonal antibody auristatin conjugates for cancer therapy. Nat Biotechnol 21:778–784

Duque JL, Loughlin KR, Adam RM et al. (1999) Plasma levels of vascular endothelial growth factor are increased in patients with metastatic prostate cancer. Urology 54(3):523–527

Ferrara N, Gerber HP, LeCouter J (2003) The biology of VEGF and its receptors. Nat Med 9(6):669

Ferrara N, Hillan KJ, Gerber HP et al. (2004) Discovery and development of bevacizumab, an anti-VEGF antibody for treating cancer. Nat Rev Drug Discov 3(5):391–400

Fishwild DM, O'Donnell SL, Bengoechea T et al. (1996) High-avidity human IgG kappa mono-clonal antibodies from a novel strain of minilocus transgenic mice. Nat Biotechnol 14(7):845–851

Galsky MD, Eisenberger M, Cooper-Moore et al. (2005) Phase 1/2 dose escalation trial of the prostate specific membrane antigen (PSMA)-targeted immunocojugate, MLN2704, in patients with progressive metastatic androgen-dependent prostate cancer. Proc Am Soc Clin Oncol 24:2005

Gerritsen W, Van Den Eertwegh AJ, Giaccone G (2006) A dose escalation trail GM-CSF gene transduced allogeneic prostate cancer cellular immunotherapy in combination with fully human anti-CTLA antibody (MDX-010, ipilimumab) in patients with metastatic hormone-refractory prostate cancer (mHRPC). J Clin Oncol 24(18S):2500

Gery S, Sawyers CL, Agus DB et al. (2002) TMEFF2 is an androgen-regulated gene exhibiting antiproliferative effects in prostate cancer cells. Oncogene 21:4739–4746

Glynne-Jones E, Harper ME, Seery LT et al. (2001) TENB2, a proteoglycan identified in prostate cancer that is associated with disease progression and androgen independence. Int J Cancer 94:178–184

Goetsch L, Gonzalez A, Leger O et al. (2005) A recombinant humanized anti-insulin-like growth factor receptor type I antibody (h7C10) enhances the antitumor activity of vinorelbine and anti-epidermal growth factor receptor therapy against human cancer xenografts. Int J Cancer 113(2):316–328

Griffiths AD, Hoogenboom HR (1993) Building an in vitro immune system in: protein engineer-ing of antibody molecules for prophylactic and therapeutic antibodies in man. Clark M (eds) Nottingham Academic Titles, pp 45–64

Grothey A, Voigt W, Schober C et al. (1999) The role of insulin-like growth factor I and its receptor in cell growth, transformation, apoptosis, and chemoresistance in solid tumors. J Cancer Res Clin Oncol 125(3–4):166–73

Grzmil M, Hemmerlein B, Thelen P et al. (2004) Blockade of the type I IGF receptor expression in human prostate cancer cells inhibits proliferation and invasion, up-regulates IGF binding protein-3, and suppresses MMP-2 expression. J Pathol 202(1):50–59

Gu Z, Thomas G, Yamashiro J et al. (2000) Prostate stem cell antigen (PSCA) expression increases with high gleason score, advanced stage and bone metastasis in prostate cancer. Oncogene 19(10):1288–1296

Gu Z, Yamashiro J, Kono E, Reiter RE (2005) Anti-prostate stem cell antigen monoclonal anti-body 1G8 induces cell death in vitro and inhibits tumor growth in vivo via a Fc-independent mechanism. Cancer Res 65(20):9495–9500

Han KR, Seligson DB, Liu X et al. (2004) Prostate stem cell antigen expression is associated with gleason score, seminal vesicle invasion and capsular invasion in prostate cancer. J Urol 171(3):1117–11121

Henry MD, Wen S, Silva MD (2004) A prostate-specific membrane antigen-targeted monoclonal antibody-chemotherapeutic conjugate designed for the treatment of prostate cancer. Cancer Res 64(21):7995–8001

Hubert RS, Vivanco I, Chen E et al. (1999) STEAP: a prostate-specific cell-surface antigen highly expressed in human prostate tumors. Proc Natl Acad Sci USA 96(25):14523–14528

Hurwitz H, Fehrenbacher L, Novotny W et al. (2004) Bevacizumab plus irinotecan, fluorouracil, and leucovorin for metastatic colorectal cancer. N Engl J Med 350(23):2335–2342

Jakobovits A (1998) The long-awaited magic bullets: therapeutic human monoclonal antibodies from transgenic mice. Expert Opin Investig Drugs 7(4):607–614

Jakobovits A, Gudas JM, Kanner SB et al. (2005) Therapeutic potential of AGS-PSCA: A fully human monoclonal antibody to prostate stem cell antigen (PSCA) for the treatment of prostate pancreatic cancers. J Clin Oncol 23(16S):4722

Jemel A, Murray T, Ward E et al. (2005) Cancer Statistics, 2005. CA Cancer J Clin 55:10–30

Kahn D, Williams RD, Manyak MJ et al. (1998) 111 Indium-capromab pendetide in the evaluation of patients with residual or recurrent prostate cancer after radical prostatectomy. The Prosta Scint Study Group J Urol 159(6):2041–2046

Kirschenbaum A, Wang JP, Ren M et al. (1997) Inhibition of vascular endothelial cell growth factor suppresses the in vivo growth of human prostate tumors. Urol Oncol 3:3–10

Koeppen HKW, Wright BD, Burt AD et al. (2001) Overexpression of HER-2 in solid tumors: an immunohistochemical survey. Histopathology 3:96–104

Kohler G, Milstein C (1975) Continuous cultures of fused cells secreting antibody of predefined specificity. Nature 256:495–497

Lam JS, Yamashiro J, Shintaku IP et al. (2005) Prostate stem cell antigen is over expressed in prostate cancer metastases. Clin Cancer Res 11(7):2591–2596

Lara PN Jr, Chee KG, Longmate J et al. (2004) Trastuzumab plus docetaxel in HER-2/neu-positive prostate carcinoma: final results from the California Cancer Consortium screening and Phase II trial. Cancer 100:2125–2131

Leach DR, Krummel MF, Allison JP (1996) Enhancement of antitumor immunity by CTLA-4 blockade. Science 271:1734–1736

Lonberg N (2005) Human antibodies from transgenic animals. Nat Biotechnol 9:1117–1125

Ma D, Hopf CE, Malewicz AD et al. (2006) Potent antitumor activity of an auristatin-conjugated, fully human monoclonal antibody to prostate-specific membrane antigen. Clin Cancer Res.12(8):2591–2596

Maloney EK, McLaughlin JL, Dagdigian NE (2003) An anti-insulin-like growth factor I receptor antibody that is a potent inhibitor of cancer cell proliferation. Cancer Res. 63(16):5073–83

Marengo SR, Sikes RA, Anezinis P et al. (1997) Metastasis induced by overexpression of p185neu-T after orthotropic injection into a prostatic epithelial cell line (NbE). Mol Carcinog. 19(3):165–175

Melnyk O, Zimmerman M, Kim KJ et al. (1999) Neutralizing anti-vascular endothelial growth factor antibody inhibits further growth of established prostate cancer and metastases in a pre-clinical model. J Urol 161(3):960–963

Mendelsohn J, Baselga J (2006) Epidermal growth factor receptor targeting in cancer. Semi Oncol 33:369–385

Mendez MJ, Green LL, Corvalan JR et al. (1997) Functional transplant of megabase human immunoglobulin loci recapitulates human antibody response in mice. Nat Genet 15(2):146–156

Milowsky MI, Nanus DM, Kostakoglu L et al. (2004) Phase I trial of yttrium-90-labeled anti-prostate-specific membrane antigen monoclonal antibody J591 for androgen-independent prostate cancer. J Clin Oncol 22(13):2522–2531

Milowsky MI, Galasky, George DJ et al. (2006) Phase I/II trail of the prostate-specific membrane antigen (PSMA)-targeted immunoconjugate MLN 2704 in patients (pts) with progressive metastatic castratin resistant prostate cancer (CRPC). J Clin Oncol:4500

Morris MJ, Reuter VE, Kelly WK (2002): HER-2 profiling and targeting in prostate carcinoma: a Phase II trial of trastuzumab alone and with paclitaxel. Cancer 94:980–986

Morrison SL, Oi VT (1975) Chimeric immunoglobulin genes. Academic, London, UK, pp 260–274

Nanus DM, Milowsky MI, Kostakoglu L et al. (2003) Clinical use of monoclonal antibody HuJ591 therapy: targeting prostate specific membrane antigen. J Urol 170(6 Pt 2):S84–S88

Nishio Y, Yamada Y, Kokubo H et al. (2006) Prognostic significance of immunohistochemical expression of the HER-2/neu oncoprotein in bone metastatic prostate cancer. Urology 68(1):110–115

Olayioye MA, Neve RM, Lane HA, Haynes NE (2000) The ErbB signaling network receptor heterodimerization in development and cancer. EMBO J 19:3159–3167

Pauletti G, Dandekar S, Rong H et al. (2000) Assessment of methods for tissue-based detection of the HER-2/neu alteration in human breast cancer: a direct comparison of fluorescence in situ hybridization and immunohistochemistry. J Clin Oncol 18(21):3651–3664

Peeters M, Van Cutsem E, Siena S et al. (2006) A phase 3 multicenter, randomized controlled trial (RCT) of panitumumab plus best supportive care (BSC) vs BSC alone in patients (pts) with metastatic colorectal cancer (mCRC). Proc Am Assoc Cancer Res 47:Abstract CP-1

Pegram M, Slamon D (2000) Biological rationale for HER2/neu (c-erbB2) as a target for mono-clonal antibody therapy. Semin Oncol 27(Suppl 9):13–9

Picus J, Halabi S, Rini B et al. (2003) The use of bevacizumab (B) with docetaxel (D) and estra-mustine (E) in hormone refractory prostate cancer (HRPC): initial results of CALGB 90006. Proc Am Soc Clin Oncol 22:393

Pietrzkowski Z, Mulholland G, Gomella L et al. (1993) Inhibition of growth of prostatic cancer cell lines by peptide analogues of insulin-like growth factor. Cancer Res 53(5):1102–1106

Pinto JT, Suffoletto BP, Berzin TM et al. (1996) Prostate-specific membrane antigen: a novel folate hydrolase in human prostatic carcinoma cells. Clin Cancer Res. 2(9):1445–1451

Pound CR, Partin AW, Eisenberger MA et al. (1999) Natural history of progression after PSA elevation following radical prostatectomy. JAMA 281:1591–1597

Prewett M, Rockwell P, Rockwell RF et al. (1996) The biologic effects of C225, a chimeric mon-oclonal antibody to the EGFR, on human prostate carcinoma. J Immunother Emphasis Tumor Immunol (6):419–427

Reese DM, Fratesi P, Corry M et al. (2001) A phase II trail of humanized anti-vascular endothe-lial growth factor antibody for the treatment of androgen-independent prostate cancer. Pros J 3(2):65–70

Reiter RE, Gu Z, Watabe T et al. (1998) Prostate stem cell antigen: a cell surface marker overex-pressed in prostate cancer. Proc. Natl. Acad. Sci. USA 95:1735–1740

Riechmann L, Clark M, Waldmann H et al. (1988) Reshaping human antibodies for therapy. Nature 332(24):323–327

Ross JS, Gray KE, Webb IJ et al. (2005) Antibody-based therapeutics: focus on prostate cancer. Cancer Metastasis Rev 24(4):521–537

Ross S, Spencer SD, Holcomb I (2002) Prostate Stem Cell Antigen as Therapy Target: Tissue Expression and in Vivo Efficacy of an immunoconjugate. Cancer Res 62:2546–2553

Saad F, Schulman CC (2004) Role of bisphosphonates in prostate cancer. Eur Urol 45:26–34

Saffran DC, Raitano AB, Hubert RS et al. (2001) Anti-PSCA monoclonal antibodies inhibit tumor growth and metastasis formation and prolong the survival of mice bearing human prostate can-cer xenografts Proc Natl Acad Sci USA 98(5):2658–2663

Scher HI, (2000) HER2 in prostate cancer–a viable target or innocent bystander? J Natl Cancer Inst 92(23):1866–1868

Sherwood ER, Lee C (1995) Epidermal growth factor-related peptides and the epidermal growth factor receptor in normal and malignant prostate. World J Urol 13(5):290–296

Sebastian S, Settleman J, Reshkin SJ et al. (2006) The complexity of targeting EGFR signaling in cancer: from expression to turnover. Biochim Biophys Acta 1766(1):120–139

Signoretti S, Rodolfo M, Manola J et al. (2000) Her-2-neu expression and progression toward androgen independence in human prostate cancer. J Natl Cancer Inst 92(23):1866–1888

Silberman MA, Partin AW, Veltri RW, Epstein JI (1997) Tumor angiogenesis correlates with pro-gression after radical prostatectomy but not with pathologic stage in gleason sum 5 to 7 adeno-carcinoma of the prostate. Cancer 79(4):772–779

Silver DA, Pellicer I, Fair WR et al. (1997) Prostate-specific membrane antigen expression in normal and malignant human tissues. Clin Cancer Res (1):81–85

Slamon DJ, Leyland-Jones B, Shak S et al. (2001) Use of chemotherapy plus a monoclonal anti-body against HER2 for metastatic breast cancer that overexpresses HER2. N Engl J Med 344(11):783–792

Slovin SF, Kelly WK, Cohen R et al. (1997) Epidermal growth factor receptor (EGFr) monoclonal antibody (MoAb) C225 and doxorubicin (DOC) in androgen-dependent (AI) prostate cancer (PC): results of phase Ib/IIa study. Proc Am Soc Clin Oncol 16(311a):Abstract 1108

Small E, Higano C, Tchekmedyian et al. (2006) Randomized phase II study comparing 4 monthly doses of ipilimumab (MDX-010) as a single agent or in combination with a single dose of docetaxel in patients with hormone-refractory prostate cancer. J Clin Oncol 24(18S):4609

Smith SV (2004) Technology evaluation: cetuximab mertansine. ImmunoGen. Curr Opin Mol Therap 6:666–674

Smith-Jones PM, Vallabhajosula S, Navarro V et al. (2003) Radiolabeled monoclonal antibodies specific to the extracellular domain of prostate-specific membrane antigen: preclinical studies in nude mice bearing LNCaP human prostate tumor. J Nucl Med 44(4):610–617

Solit DB, Angus DB (2001) HER-kinase-directed therapy of prostate cancer. Prostate J 3:53–58

Tannock IF, de Wit R, Berry WR et al. (2004) Docetaxel plus prednisone or mitoxantrone plus prednisone for advanced prostate cancer. N Engl J Med 351:1502–1512

Valentinis B, Baserga R (2001) IGF-I receptor signaling in transformation and differentiation. Mol Pathol 54(3):133–137

Van Cutsem E, Peeters M, Siena S et al. (2007) An open-label, randomized, phase 3 clinical trial of panitumumab plus best supportive care versus best supportive care in patients with chemotherapy-refractory metastatic colorectal cancer. J Clin Oncol 25:1658–1664

Weidner N, Carroll PR, Flax J et al. (1993) Tumor angiogenesis correlates with metastasis in invasive prostate carcinoma. Am J Pathol 143(2):401–409

Wu AM, Senter PD (2005) Arming antibodies: prospects and challenges for immunoconjugates. Nat Biotechnol 23(9):1137–1146

Wu JD, Odman A, Higgins LM et al. (2005) In vivo effects of the human type I insulin-like growth factor receptor antibody A12 on androgen-dependent and androgen-independent xenograft human prostate tumors. Clin Cancer Res 11(8):3065–3074

Wu JD, Haugk K, Coleman I et al. (2006) Combined in vivo effect of A12, a type 1 insulin-like growth factor receptor antibody, and docetaxel against prostate cancer tumors. Clin Cancer Res 12(20):6153–6160

Wujcik D (2006) EGFR as a target: rationale for therapy. Semin Oncol Nurs. 22(1):5–9

Yang XD, Jia XC, Corvalan JR et al. (1999) Eradication of established tumors by a fully human monoclonal antibody to the epidermal growth factor receptor without concomitant chemotherapy. Cancer Res 59(6):1236–1243

Yang XD, Jia XC, Corvalan JR, Wang P, Davis CG (2001) Development of ABX-EGF, a fully human anti-EGF receptor monoclonal antibody, for cancer therapy. Crit Rev Oncol Hematol 38(1):17–23

Yang XD, Roskos L, Davis G et al. (2005) From XenoMouse technology to panitumumab (ABX-EGF). The Oncogenomics Handbook, pp 647–657

Yeon CH, Pegram MD (2005) Anti-erbB-2 antibody trastuzumab in the treatment of HER2-amplified breast cancer. Invest New Drugs 23(5):391–409

Zhao XY, Schneider D, Biroc SL et al. (2005) Targeting Tomoregulin for Radioimmunotherapy of prostate cancer. Cancer Res 7:2846

Anti-IgE and Other Antibody Targets in Asthma

J. Singh and M. Kraft(⊠)

1 Asthma Background 258
   1.1 Asthma Epidemiology 258
   1.2 The Biology of Asthma 258
   1.3 Current Treatments for Asthma..................................... 260
2 Anti-IgE Antibodies for Asthma 262
   2.1 Role of Immunoglobulin E in Asthma Pathogenesis 262
   2.2 Anti-IgE as a Therapeutic Strategy 264
   2.3 The Development of Anti-IgE Antibodies and the Emergence of Omalizumab
        (Xolair^{TM}) 265
   2.4 Pharmacokinetics and Dosing of Omalizumab 266
   2.5 Clinical Efficacy of Omalizumab 269
   2.6 Adverse Events and Safety Issues of Omalizumab 273
   2.7 Practical Aspects of Omalizumab 275
3 Anti-TNF-α Therapy for Asthma 277
   3.1 Role of Tumor Necrosis Factor-Alpha (TNF-α) in Asthma Pathogenesis 277
   3.2 The Use of Anti-TNF Therapy in Asthma 278
   3.3 Additional Issues Regarding Anti-TNF Therapy in Asthma 279
4 Other Antibody-Mediated Therapies for Asthma........................... 280
   4.1 Antibodies to Interleukin-5 280
   4.2 Antibodies to Interleukin-4 and Interleukin 13 281
   4.3 Other Antibody-Based Therapies in Development 281
5 Summary 282
References 282

Abstract Asthma is a heterogeneous disorder of unknown etiology that manifests as recurrent episodes of coughing, wheezing, and breathlessness. These symptoms are often debilitating and exacerbations usually are unexpected, resulting in work

M. Kraft

Duke Asthma, Allergy and Airway Center, Duke University Medical Center, Durham, NC 27710, USA

e-mail: Jaspal.Singh@duke.edu

Y. Chernajovsky, A. Nissim (eds.) *Therapeutic Antibodies. Handbook of Experimental Pharmacology 181.*

or school absences, limitations in activity, reduced quality of life, and personal and economic hardships.

Over the past several decades, a great deal has been learned about asthma pathophysiology, and currently available therapies have revolutionized asthma treatment. However, asthma remains a global public health problem, and the hope is that newer therapies targeting specific biological mediators of asthma, particularly antibody-mediated therapies, offer exciting new modes to the control of this disease. We will review some of these therapies, with the majority of attention devoted to anti-IgE therapy which has been approved for treatment of adult and childhood asthma by the US Food and Drug Administration (FDA) since 2003.

1 Asthma Background

1.1 Asthma Epidemiology

Roughly 17 million Americans are affected by asthma, one-third of whom are children (Gold and Wright 2005). Worldwide estimates of asthma prevalence range from 2 to 36% of various international populations (Braman 2006). Currently, the incidence and prevalence of asthma in the US population overall appears to have reached a plateau, but there may well be increases within certain racial and ethnic groups (Cohen et al. 2006; Lugogo and Kraft 2006). Many patients with asthma also make frequent visits to their ambulatory care provider or the emergency department. There has been a recent increase in the rates of outpatient and emergency room visits from 1980 to 1999 as reported in the Morbidity and Mortality Weekly Report (Mannino et al. 2000), indicating that asthma control is suboptimal in the US population. Hospitalizations for asthma are a significant factor in asthma-related cost. Patient absenteeism from work likely also has an important impact on productivity. Thus, asthma remains an important public health problem both nationally and globally (Eder et al. 2006).

1.2 The Biology of Asthma

Over the last several decades, much has been learned about asthma physiology and pathogenesis. For decades, the paradigm was relatively simple: exposure from an environmental allergen in a susceptible host resulted in inflammation in the airways; the inflammation was then felt to result in the symptoms of the disease. However, what became increasingly clear is that the symptoms of the disease and the asthma clinical severity were only loosely connected in many individuals with asthma. Today, a number of cells and molecular determinants were felt to play important roles in asthma pathogenesis. Our current understanding is that the immunopathology of asthma is complex and involves a dynamic interplay among various components of the adaptive and innate immune systems, the environment, and host

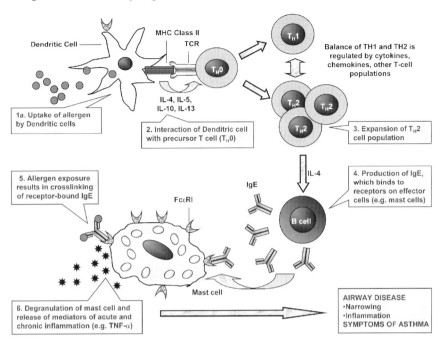

Fig. 1 Classical mechanisms of allergic asthma. Allergens are taken up by dendritic cells and presented to T cells. The T-cell response is balanced between the T_H1 and T_H2 response, and this interaction is balanced by numerous other factors. The T_H2 response classically results in clonal expansion of the T_H2 cell population, which manifests by activation of B lymphocytes. These activated B cells transform and produce allergen-specific IgE, which then binds to the FcεRI receptor on effector cells (e.g., mast cells, basophils). Crosslinking of allergen to receptor-bound IgE results in degranulation and subsequent release of numerous inflammatory mediators. The resulting acute and chronic inflammation results in airway disease and the symptoms of asthma

susceptibility. Certain factors may modify these effects to result in overt clinical disease, and subclinical disease may progress despite excellent therapy targeted against asthma.

The classical paradigm of asthma is depicted in Fig. 1. After a dendritic cell or other antigen-presenting cell encounters an allergen, the cell triggers the naive T cell population to undergo a specific clonal expansion. Through numerous complex mechanisms which involve isotype class switching, this T_H2-mediated reaction results in the production of B cells which secrete allergen-specific immunoglobulin E (IgE). These IgE molecules have the ability to bind to receptors on effector cells such as mast cells. On subsequent allergen re-exposure, the allergen, IgE molecules, and FcεRI receptor interact to result in mast cell degranulation, the release of numerous inflammatory mediators, and the subsequent symptoms of asthma. Within this paradigm, antibody targets that inhibit important mediators and effectors appear particularly promising for the treatment of asthma and other allergic diseases. To date, these therapies generally center on the adaptive immune system and its production of immunoglubilins (e.g., IgE) and cytokines (e.g., TNF-α) that are felt to drive many of the mechanisms of asthma. We will review a few of these potentially therapeutic antibodies in detail below.

1.3 Current Treatments for Asthma

Numerous guidelines for the diagnosis and treatment of asthma have been published since the 1980s. In the United States, in 1991, the National Heart, Lung, and Blood Institute (NHLBI) published its first set of guidelines (NHLBI 1991), which were subsequently updated by the National Asthma Education and Prevention Program in 1997 (NAEEP 1997) and again in 2002 (NAEEP 2002). The most famous of the global guidelines were originally published by the Global Initiative for Asthma (GINA) (NHLBI/WHO 2002), a joint consortium of the NHLBI and the World Health Organization that updates its guidelines at least annually. A recent update of the GINA guidelines was just released in 2006, with new NHLBI guidelines expected in 2007. Updated guidelines can be found on the GINA website (http://www.ginasthma.com/).

Essentially, the treatment of asthma centers around the control of or response to patient symptomatology with particular attention to symptoms of dyspnea, cough, and wheezing. Therefore, patient well-being, number and severity of exacerbations, and improvement in quality of life (e.g., fewer missed days of work/school) are the most common assessments of response to treatment. Treatment effectiveness may also be objectively quantified by physiological measurements such as measures of pulmonary function. Common physiological parameters include peak expiratory flow rate (PEF) with forced exhalation as well as the forced expiratory lung volume in 1 s (FEV1); both may be reduced from baseline during disease flares, but the results are not consistent among or within cohorts of asthmatics. Notably, the actual airway inflammation and remodeling that ensue are not well-measured by current methodologies. There has been some excitement recently about using quantitative measurements of exhaled nitric oxide as a surrogate marker for airway inflammation, but this has not been universally accepted nor available. Therefore, symptoms and patient tolerance dictate current guidelines to asthma treatment, also reflecting a shift toward improving or maintaining symptom control rather than trying to alter disease severity. Importantly, the newer asthma treatment guidelines represent a shift in thought from categories of asthma severity to categories of control, regardless of severity. Therapy is stepped up or down depending on overall control.

Available therapies are generally divided into nonpharmacologic and pharmacologic categories. Nonpharmacologic therapies in asthma center around avoidance of asthma triggers. Triggers may be discrete allergens for which the patient has a known allergic predisposition (e.g., a positive skin-prick test on skin testing). For example, certain species of house dust mite are known environmental allergens, and many experts recommend that patients cover their mattresses with plastic covers so as to avoid direct exposure to as much house dust mite antigen as possible. Avoidance of the offending allergen makes intuitive sense, but many of the allergens are ubiquitous in the environment, difficult to avoid, or difficult to determine. Other nonallergen triggers include exposure to environmental tobacco smoke, cold air, and exercise, none of which may be easy to avoid. Clearly, trigger avoidance, though of great importance, is markedly insufficient as sole therapy for the majority of asthmatics.

The mainstays of pharmacological therapies for asthma have been bronchodilators and corticosteroids. Bronchodilators, particularly β-agonists, dilate the small airways and can have short or long-lasting effects, depending on the formulation. These are not generally thought to treat the underlying inflammation, but rather provide symptomatic relief. Given that the hallmark of allergic asthma is inflammation, the underlying inflammation of acute and chronic asthma is treated with corticosteroids. Corticosteroids decrease inflammation through numerous proposed mechanisms, and to date oral or parentally administered corticosteroids are the mainstay of treatment for patients with severe asthma, especially during a flare requiring hospitalization. The major advance in asthma pharmacotherapy in the last two decades has been the introduction and widespread use of inhaled corticosteroids in patients with mild to moderate asthma. Though they are generally well-tolerated, inhaled corticosteroids have potential adverse effects. These have usually been thought to be mild and easily treatable (e.g., throat pain, oral thrush), but recent evidence suggests that inhaled corticosteroids reach the systemic circulation and may have untoward effects on bone growth and suppression of the hypothalamic–pituitary axis leading to possible adrenal gland dysfunction and osteoporosis (Gulliver and Eid 2005). Moreover, the combination of inhaled corticosteroids and long-acting β-agonists may be insufficient to treat patients with severe asthma. It is being increasingly recognized that a small number of patients, generally those with severe persistent asthma, are the most difficult to treat and are responsible for a large segment of the costs of asthma (Dolan et al. 2004). These patients demonstrate a need for additional therapeutic options to achieve enhanced asthma control.

Second-line agents for the control of asthma, such as mast-cell stabilizing agents, leukotriene inhibitors and methylxanthines, have variable roles in the daily management of asthma. Desensitization immunization with antigens (allergens), which is used mainly in the United States for allergic rhinitis, is not effective for the majority of asthma patients. Overall, these therapies have benefited subsets of patients; therefore, new therapeutic targets are needed. Many of these therapies are targeted toward specific aspects of the innate and adaptive immune response. More recently, the approval and use of anti-IgE antibodies has generated much excitement, as has the potential uses of other antibodies targeting asthma mediators. We will review the pathophysiology, mechanisms, and pharmacologic considerations of the latter agents in detail in this chapter.

2 Anti-IgE Antibodies for Asthma

2.1 Role of Immunoglobulin E in Asthma Pathogenesis

Immunoglobulin E (IgE) has been known to be a key mediator of asthma and other allergic disorders for over 30 years and plays a central role in allergic responses to allergens in patients with asthma and rhinitis. IgE was officially recognized by the WHO as a new immunoglobulin in 1968. Its receptor was first identified in 1974 (Kulczycki et al. 1974) while more detail on the receptor's molecular weight and valence was published in 1977. After further characterization over the ensuing decades, Kinet identified the IgE-mast cell interaction as a paradigm for the antigen–antibody relationship. Current evidence suggests that the majority of asthma has an allergic basis (Holt et al. 1999), and that IgE is central to the initiation of both allergic and nonallergic asthma. Elevated serum levels of specific IgE toward common environmental allergens characterize allergic diseases such as asthma and rhinitis as illustrated by several lines of evidence. Elevated serum IgE in the first year of life, IgE sensitization, and exposure to airborne allergens are all risk factors for the development of childhood and lifelong asthma (Sporik et al. 1990; Martinez et al. 1995). Concordantly, increased IgE levels are associated with increasing asthma disease severity in patients with moderate to severe persistent asthma (Borish et al. 2005). This is conceptually supported by the correlation of elevated serum IgE with sputum eosinophilia (Covar et al. 2004) and elevated levels of nitric oxide in airways of asthmatics (Strunk et al. 2003).

IgE is produced by B cells after sensitization and has a short half-life. Despite low serum concentrations, IgE is immunologically highly active due to the large number of high-affinity IgE receptors on mast cells and basophils. In addition, IgE upregulates receptors on several cell type, including basophils and mast cells. The binding of IgE to the receptors on these cells results in the formation of cross-links between the allergen and the IgE molecule, thereby initiating an inflammatory cascade through release of a variety of mediators, including histamine, prostaglandins, leukotrienes, chemokines, and platelet-activating factor. In some individuals with allergic asthma, higher than normal IgE levels may increase persistent airway inflammation and bronchial hyperresponsiveness, presumably through ongoing chronic allergic activation of this complex system.

As in other antibodies, the antigen-binding site of IgE is contained in the Fab fragment. The $C\varepsilon3$ domains of the Fc fragment bind either of the two known IgE receptors, the high-affinity receptor ($FC\varepsilon RI$) or the low-affinity receptor ($FC\varepsilon RII$) (Buhl 2004). Importantly, the IgE-mediated allergic cascade involves a biphasic response with an immediate or early allergic response and a late allergic response (Dolovich et al. 1973). The early response occurs acutely, usually within 1 h of exposure to allergen, whereas the late response occurs 4–24 h later. IgE plays a critical role in both the early and late phase responses via interaction with the $Fc\varepsilon RI$ and $Fc\varepsilon RII$ receptors.

The early allergic response results from IgE-mediated mast cell degranulation. Interaction of receptor-bound IgE antibodies with soluble multivalent allergen leads to receptor aggregation (Bradding et al. 2006). By signal transduction, a complex series of events ensues culminating in rapid degranulation and release of the stored contents of cytoplasmic granules and newly formed mediators. Acute allergic symptoms are generated by interaction of these receptor mediators with specific receptors on target tissues; clinically, this cascade results in bronchospasm or acute asthma. Moreover, the severity of this response likely has a great deal to do with the mast cell density in the airways (Bradding et al. 2006). Disruption of the initial binding of IgE antibodies, thereby preventing activation of mast cells and other airway effector cells, is an important potential mechanism by which anti-IgE antibodies may attenuate the early allergic response.

Continued expression of mediators elicits an inflammatory response designated as the late-phase reaction, though the precise cause and significance of this late phase are less well understood. Eosinophils likely play a role, and in response to IgE binding to the FcεRI receptor, eosinophilic cytoplasmic granules and a number of cytokines and lipid mediators are synthesized and released by degranulation. However, the low level of FcεRI expression on eosinophils means this may not be the major pathway in the late phase response (Prussin and Metcalfe 2006). Given that IgE also enhances antigen presentation to T cells via FcεRI receptors on antigen-presenting cells (Maurer et al. 1995), this may explain the pathogenesis for the role of IgE in the late-phase response. Regardless of mechanism, this late phase response results in persistent symptoms, airway hyperresponsiveness, and bronchospasm (Strunk and Bloomberg 2006).

Additional effects of IgE and its binding to the FcεRII receptor are not fully understood but are being investigated heavily. Importantly, the expression of FcεRI in basophils correlates with serum IgE levels (Malveaux et al. 1978), suggesting that lowering IgE levels may attenuate the early asthmatic reaction. In turn, IgE can also directly or indirectly maintain the mast cell pool by protecting the cell from apoptosis (Kitaura et al. 2003), thereby proposing a mechanism whereby continued suppression of IgE may lead to persistent attenuation of allergic asthma symptoms. It is also likely that IgE may facilitate sensitization to allergens via effects on different cell types. For example, asthmatic airway smooth muscle expresses surface FcεRII and expression is upregulated by IgE-FcεRII binding (Hakonarson et al. 1999), so FcεRII may be involved in transepithelial migration (Buhl 2004). FcεRII is also implicated in the IgE-mediated presentation of allergen to antigen-presenting cells, and allergen presentation to T cells is enhanced by IgE-FcεRI complexes on antigen-presenting cells (Maurer et al. 1995). This allergen presentation leads to classic Th2 cell-mediated allergic reactions with resulting inflammation. Also after allergen inhalation, the number of dendritic cells recruited to the airway epithelia is increased in asthma, and the expression of FcεRI by these cells is also significantly increased compared to controls (Geiger et al. 2000). Allergens can thus be internalized and presented to dendritic cells via cross-linking of allergen-IgE antibodies bound to the alpha chain of FcεRI (Upham 2003). In regard to B cells, IgeE binds to FcεRII receptors on B cells, where it alters differentiation and regulation of further IgE synthesis (Broide 2001; Oettgen and Geha 2001). In summary, the IgE molecule probably plays a number of unique roles in the allergic response, many of which require further elucidation.

2.2 Anti-IgE as a Therapeutic Strategy

Given the above clinical, epidemiologic, and biological evidence indicating the role of IgE in asthma pathogenesis, it is not surprising that anti-IgE therapies have been developed to treat allergic asthma and related disorders. The rationale for this was first published by Chang in 1987, who proposed that chimeric or humanized anti-IgE antibodies with a set of unique binding properties could be used for the isotype-specific control of IgE, and thus would be a logical therapeutic approach to IgE-mediated diseases (Chang 2000). IgE binding to its Fc receptors mediates both FecRI-mediated mast cell degranulation and FcεRII-mediated enhancement of

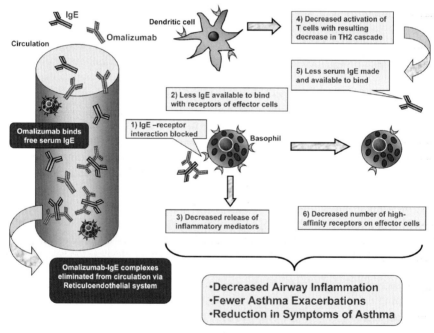

Fig. 2 Mechanisms of action of omalizumab. Omalizumab binds free IgE to form omalizumab-IgE complexes. The binding of omalizumab to the Fc portion of the IgE molecule: (1) prevents the binding of IgE with the high-affinity receptors of effector cells, including basophils, dendritic cells, and mast cells; (2) since these complexes are eliminated, there is then less free IgE available for the remaining receptors; (3) there is a resulting decreased release in inflammatory mediators; (4) a decrease in the allergic cascade results in fewer T_H cell reactions resulting in (5) less serum IgE being produced. (6) downregulation of high-affinity receptors on effector cells. The net effect then of omalizumab is decreased airway inflammation, fewer exacerbations, and a reduction in asthmatic symptoms

antigen presentation in the allergic reaction; both roles thus make anti-IgE therapy a potentially ideal target. A monoclonal anti-IgE antibody that binds free but not receptor-bound IgE would therefore be postulated to inhibit the initiation of the allergic cascade by preventing IgE binding to receptors.

The potential downstream effects of blocking IgE receptor binding are numerous. Blocking IgE binding to FcεRI receptors on dendritic cells could reduce the efficiency of antigen presentation to T cells, whereas blocking binding to those on mast cells and basophils could prevent allergen-induced degranulation and the release of inflammatory mediators (Fig. 2). It then becomes logical that if the inflammatory mediators are not released, the progression of an asthmatic reaction would be attenuated and a patient's symptoms improved. Moreover, if new immune cells such as basophils are created to replenish the patient's systemic supply during routine cell turnover, these new cells would not have gone through upregulation of their FcεRI receptors because of the low plasma free IgE concentration (Chang 2000). As discussed later, this latter effect may explain why anti-IgE therapy takes several weeks to achieve maximal benefit.

2.3 The Development of Anti-IgE Antibodies and the Emergence of Omalizumab (Xolair^{TM})

As intriguing as the prospect is for an anti-IgE monoclonal antibody, there are a number of considerations involved in the development of therapeutic monoclonal antibodies. First of all, the antibody must be nonimmunogenic and nonaphylactogenic, issues which hindered the development of murine monoclonal antibodies for decades (Dillman 1989). Secondly, the binding of the therapeutic antibody to the IgE molecule should occur with a high degree of specificity and affinity. Moreover, the binding affinity between IgE and the antibody should favor the formation of immune complexes small enough to result in a reasonable degree of clearance without adverse reactions. Lastly, for therapeutic efficacy, a dose of anti-IgE capable of almost completely removing free IgE might be necessary, because only 2000 IgE molecules are required for half-maximal histamine release from basophils exposed to allergen (MacGlashan 1993).

Based on the above, two recombinant humanized monoclonal antibodies have been developed against the IgE molecule. The antibodies are made with a human IgG1 framework and a complementarity-determining region from a murine anti-IgE antibody (Presta et al. 1993). Overall, less than 5% of the amino acid residues are murine, which is why the molecules are considered to have low potential for immunogenicity. The antibodies recognize the Cε3 domain of free human IgE, the same Fc site as the high-affinity receptor binding site. Specifically, the FcεRI binding site within the Cε3 domain depends on six exposed amino acids localized in three loops: Arg408, Ser411, Lys414, Glu452, Arg465, and Met469 (Presta et al. 1994). When the IgE antibody binds to this region, the interaction between IgE and effector cells is blocked (Fig. 2). Moreover, the antibody-IgE complexes formed as a result of treatment are small and not thought to be able to trigger complement activation nor give rise to immune complex-mediated pathology (Liu et al. 1995). Importantly, the antibodies only bind free IgE, not cell-surface-bound IgE. This ensures that there is no crosslinking of effector cells, and hence the effector cells are not activated. This may seem to be intuitively obvious, but has been an important challenge in the development of antibody-mediated therapies (Roskos et al. 2004). To test this concept, in vitro experiments have shown that anti-IgE did not induce histamine release from IgE-loaded human basophils (Shields et al. 1995).

Omalizumab (also referred to as rhu-Mab-E25, rhu-mab in the literature), is a recombinant humanized monoclonal antibody that was first cloned in 1992 by Genentech (Presta et al. 1993; Adis 2002). It was commercialized with Novartis and Tanox under the trade name Xolair. The second anti-IgE molecule developed is the CGP51901 or TNX-901 monoclonal antibody independently developed by Tanox (Chang 2000). The latter has been successfully used to treat subjects with peanut allergy in a phase II trial but is not yet commercially available (Leung et al. 2003). The two antibody development programs were combined in 1996, which targeted omalizumab for further development. Therefore, the vast majority of medical literature on clinical and biological data regarding anti-IgE therapies is based on omalizumab. As detailed later, omalizumab has been shown to reduce serum concentrations of free IgE, resulting in significant reductions in early and late asthmatic responses following allergen inhalation and improved asthma symptom control. In 2003, the FDA granted approval for the use of omalizumab in moderate to severe atopic asthmatic patients.

2.4 Pharmacokinetics and Dosing of Omalizumab

Developing a dosing regimen for omalizumab takes into account the pharmacokinetic properties and the goals of serum IgE reduction. Given subcutaneously, the drug is absorbed slowly, with an absolute bioavailability of 62%, and peak serum concentrations are reached 7–8 days following the injection (Genentech 2003). Interval of dosing is predicated on the long average terminal half-life of omalizumab of 19–22 days (Hochhaus et al. 2003). The serum concentration of total IgE in the nonatopic, nonasthmatic population is $<100\,IU\,ml^{-1}$ ($<240\,ng\,ml^{-1}$); however, in allergic individuals, this concentration varies from normal range to several hundred $IU\,ml^{-1}$. Clinical benefit with omalizumab is observed when free IgE levels in serum are reduced to $50\,ng\,ml^{-1}$ or less, but little additional benefit is gained with levels $<12\,ng\,ml^{-1}$ (Hochhaus et al. 2003). It was then determined that omalizumab must be given at molar excess of 15–20:1 relative to baseline total IgE to achieve such a reduction in free IgE (Casale et al. 1997). Therefore, the ability of omalizumab to reduce free IgE levels to less than 10% of pretreatment level depends on the dose and the patient's weight and baseline IgE level (Boulet et al. 1997; Hochhaus et al. 2003). A pooled analysis of two previous studies with 859 patients with asthma found that administration of the minimum dose calculated to achieve a mean free IgE level of $25\,ng\,ml^{-1}$ resulted in free IgE levels of $<50\,ng\,ml^{-1}$ in more

Table 1 Dosing of Omalizumab

Pre-treatment serum IgE (IU ml^{-1})	Body Weight (kg)			
	30–60	> 60–70	> 70–90	> 90–150
30–100	150 mg every 4 weeks	150 mg every 4 weeks	150 mg every 4 weeks	300 mg every 4 weeks
>100–200	300 mg every 4 weeks	300 mg every 4 weeks	300 mg every 4 weeks	225 mg every 2 weeks
>200–300	300 mg every 4 weeks	225 mg every 2 weeks	225 mg every 2 weeks	300 mg every 2 weeks
>300–400	225 mg every 2 weeks	225 mg every 2 weeks	300 mg every 2 weeks	Do not dose
>400–500	300 mg every 2 weeks	300 mg every 2 weeks	375 mg every 2 weeks	Do not dose
>500–600	300 mg every 2 weeks	375 mg every 2 weeks	Do not dose	Do not dose
>600–700	375 mg every 2 weeks	Do not dose	Do not dose	Do not dose

than 95% of patients (Hochhaus et al. 2003). As a footnote, there was no change in the serum IgE levels after inhalation of aerosolized omalizumab (Fahy et al. 1999), which leads one to suspect that the lack of efficacy of this route of administration may have somehow been due to its ineffectiveness at obtaining systemic levels.

Taking the above factors into account, an individualized tiered dosing table was developed to ensure that free IgE reduction is achieved (Hochhaus et al. 2003). The recommended dose is 0.016 mg per kilogram of body weight per international unit of IgE every four weeks, administered subcutaneously at either two-week or four-week intervals. The actual dose depends mainly on current body weight and pretreatment total IgE level; the corresponding dosing table (Table 1) takes into account the broad range of pretreatment total IgE levels and the patient body weights likely to be encountered in clinical practice. Patients requiring a monthly dose of ≤300 mg are treated once every 4 weeks while those requiring a higher dose receive two equal doses administered every 2 weeks. There is presently no recommended dose for patients with body weight greater than 150 kg and/or total IgE 700 IU ml^{-1} or greater.

The tiered dosing strategy has proven overall to be successful in meeting the targeted objectives. Results from large, placebo-controlled phase III clinical studies in patients with moderate-to-severe allergic asthma show overall consistent suppression of free IgE, with median serum free IgE levels well below the target of 25 ng ml^{-1} (10.4 IU ml^{-1}) across the omalizumab dose range (Busse et al. 2001; Milgrom et al. 2001; Soler et al. 2001). The clinical effectiveness of this strategy is detailed later in this chapter, but overall, the results indicate improved asthma symptom control in subjects with allergic asthma. Moreover, a retrospective pooled analysis of two of these studies was conducted to study the range of individualized doses and free IgE suppression in relation to clinical effectiveness. This analysis showed no additional clinical benefit at higher omalizumab doses or at serum free IgE levels lower than the average target of 25 ng ml^{-1} (10.4 IU ml^{-1}) (Hochhaus et al. 2003). However, this latter aspect is controversial as others argue that higher dosing, particularly to achieve near-saturation of high-affinity receptors, has been poorly studied and may be of direct clinical benefit.

Biologically, following either intravenous or subcutaneous injection of omalizumab, a substantial reduction in the free serum IgE concentrations was demonstrated after a single injection (Casale et al. 1997). Notably, the magnitude of reduction was typically 89–99% from the pretreatment levels (Schulman 2001), and that this effect occurred regardless of different dosing regimens. Low levels of free serum IgE appeared to be sustained throughout the trials. Proof-of-concept studies have shown decreased numbers of eosinophils in sputum samples and bronchial biopsies (Djukanovic et al. 2004). Important studies have also shown a reduction in FcεRI receptor density on basophils, and a decrease in basophil responsiveness to stimulation by allergen of approximately 90% (MacGlashan et al. 1997). This indicates that FcεRI-receptor density is regulated by circulating levels of free IgE, and that reducing free IgE with omalizumab is very effective in decreasing FcεRI expression. Similar downregulation of FcεRI receptors has been noted with mast cells (Beck et al. 2004) and dendritic cells (Prussin et al. 2003), implying that the effector cell response to IgE is not only mediated by the IgE-FcεRI binding, but that the effects of IgE antagonism extend into later phases of the asthmatic response (Fig. 2). Concordantly, studies have shown decreased numbers of eosinophils in sputum samples and bronchial biopsies (Djukanovic et al. 2004), further supporting evidence that the underlying inflammatory response is being appropriately suppressed in asthmatic airways.

Additional considerations for dosing, beyond weight and pretreatment total IgE, do not appear to require dose adjustments. Specifically there is no need to adjust based on additional demographic factors such as age, gender, and ethnicity. There is also no need for adjustment based on renal impairment, as drug metabolism and elimination is via the reticulendothelial system of the liver and spleen. Though cases of hepatic and/or renal toxicity have not been reported, drug dosing in liver impairment has not been studied. Treatment duration itself is controversial. Bousquet and colleagues noted that, among patients who responded to 16 weeks' treatment with omalizumab, only 61% responded at 4 weeks whereas 87% had responded at 12 weeks (Bousquet et al. 2005). Although the mechanism of this delayed onset of action is unknown, it is likely that the downstream anti-inflammatory effects of anti-IgE activity require several weeks to achieve maximum efficacy. Therefore, a minimum duration of 12 weeks is currently recommended before determining the level of omalizumab response. Interestingly, after discontinuation of omalizumab therapy, changes in free IgE concentrations, basophil FcεRI expression, and allergen-induced histamine release from basophils slowly returned to pretreatment levels within 2–10 months (Saini et al. 1999). Based on this premise, some authors advocate treatment for years or possibly even lifelong (Chang 2000), but this concept is very controversial particularly in light of the high cost of omalizumab and unknown long-term risks associated with this medication.

2.5 Clinical Efficacy of Omalizumab

2.5.1 Overview

A number of phase II and III studies have been published to date on the effectiveness of omalizumab. Published studies to date have come from the United States, Europe, and Japan, with the majority of human subjects being adults with allergic asthma. Primary outcomes in the majority of studies included (1) a reduction or termination in steroid usage and (2) decreased frequency of exacerbations (as defined by either hospital admissions, emergency room visits, days lost from work/school, unscheduled doctor visits, and/or increase in medicine). Secondary outcomes varied in the studies, but generally included assessments of asthma symptoms, health-related quality of life indices, rescue medication usage, physiological measures of pulmonary function testing, and adverse events. The results of the above analyses have been pooled and recently published by the Cochrane Collaboration (Walker et al. 2006), which evaluated 3,143 subjects with mild to severe allergic asthma enrolled in 14 published and unpublished studies. Essentially, there have been key phase III clinical trials in 1651 patients (age, 6–76 years) (Busse et al. 2001; Milgrom et al. 2001; Soler et al. 2001; Holgate et al. 2004). Moreover, a number of other exploratory and secondary analyses have been performed to date and are summarized below.

2.5.2 Patient Selection and Study Design

In four randomized, double-blind, placebo-controlled trials (Busse et al. 2001; Milgrom et al. 2001; Soler et al. 2001; Holgate et al. 2004), patients had asthma for at least one year and required treatment with inhaled corticosteroids. All patients were nonsmokers and had at least one positive skin test to a perennial aeroallergen (specifically, dust mites, cockroaches, or dog and cat dander), as well as a serum IgE between 50–$700\,\text{IU ml}^{-1}$. Each trial followed a similar overall structure: (1) after patient enrollment, a 4–10 week *run-in period* was used to optimize and stabilize current therapies including adjustments of inhaled corticosteroids; (2) a *stable-steroid phase* for 12–16 weeks during which inhaled corticosteroids were maintained at a stable dose, followed by (3) a *steroid-reduction phase* during which inhaled corticosteroids were lowered to the lowest range required for asthma control.

The majority of patients were adults with moderate to severe persistent asthma (requiring doses of inhaled beclomethasone, or its equivalent, ranging from 168 to 1200 mcg per day) (Strunk and Bloomberg 2006). Two of these trials included adolescents and adults (Busse et al. 2001; Soler et al. 2001), and one was a study of children 6–12 years of age (Milgrom et al. 1999b). The fourth trial evaluated patients with more severe asthma who required high-dose inhaled corticosteroids for symptom control (fluticasone, $\geq$ mcg per day) (Holgate et al. 2004). A more recent trial involved patients who required at least 1000 mcg per day of inhaled beclomethasone plus a long-acting bronchodilator for symptom control (Humbert et al. 2005). These issues are important, given that the use of first-line therapies (i.e., inhaled corticosteroids) in these patients with asthma were surprisingly low, especially in the earlier trials. Since omalizumab is only FDA-approved as a second-line agent in the current treatment of asthma, it is very possible that studies may have had a biased effect toward efficacy if steroid doses were indeed not optimized prior to administration of omalizumab.

Omalizumab has been given via intravenous, subcutaneous, and inhalational routes. In asthmatic adults, both intravenous and subcutaneous routes were efficacious (Boulet et al. 1997; Fahy et al. 1997; Milgrom et al. 1999a; Busse et al. 2001; Soler et al. 2001; Holgate et al. 2004; Vignola et al. 2004), whereas the inhalation route showed no efficacy and did not reduce serum-free IgE (Fahy et al. 1999). Therefore, the subcutaneous route was selected as the most practical for clinical use, being used in the largest trials and subsequently receiving FDA approval.

2.5.3 Results

The results of the major clinical trials, as compiled by the Cochrane Collaboration and summarized in Table 2, are detailed below. When Omalizumab was used as an add-on therapy to inhaled or oral corticosteroids in patients with stable asthma, there seemed to be a significant reduction in the risk of asthma exacerbations, particularly in the severe asthma group (Busse et al. 2001). Moreover, the exacerbations appeared to be of lesser duration and severity. Also, patients treated with omalizumab were significantly more likely to be able to decrease the dose of inhaled corticosteroids, often decreasing dosage by greater than 50% or even being able to discontinue inhaled corticosteroids completely (Milgrom et al. 1999a; Busse et al. 2001; Soler et al. 2001). Interestingly, treatment with omalizumab was also associated with shorter duration of exacerbations in adults with moderate to severe asthma (Busse et al. 2001), but not in a pediatric subgroup (Lemanske et al. 2002). Concordantly, there was a reduction in β-2 agonist usage in adolescents and adults with moderate to severe asthma, both in the subcutaneous and high-dose IV formulations. In patients taking oral corticosteroids, there was not a significant difference in the number of patients being able to withdraw from oral steroid therapy between omalizumab and placebo treatment (Holgate et al. 2004).

Omalizumab reduced free IgE by 89–99% in asthmatic subjects (Walker et al. 2006), which indicates that the antibody is indeed binding to free IgE. Though this may intuitively seem adequate in its ability to suppress asthma symptoms, some authors suggest that this inability to reach 99% suppression of free IgE may reflect undertreatment in the clinical trials (Avila 2007). Therefore, it is conceivable that omalizumab may have greater efficacy than was demonstrated in the clinical trials.

The effects of omalizumab on lung function and airway hyperresponsiveness were small and did not reach statistical or clinical significance (Djukanovic et al. 2004). Only one published study showed statistically significant improvement in lung function as measured by the forced expiratory volume over 1 s (FEV1) (Vignola et al. 2004), with the magnitude of improvement being of dubious clinical significance. This lack of significant improvement is not surprising, given that other studies

Table 2 Clinical efficacy of omalizumab based on Cochrane Analysis (Avila 2007)

Clinical outcome	Superiority of Omalizumab vs. placebo
Reduction in free serum IgE (range)	89–99%
Odds ratio of having exacerbation	0.60 (95% CI 0.42–0.86)
Rate of exacerbations per subject	−0.18 (95% CI −0.10 to −0.25)
Duration of exacerbation	7.8 vs. 12.7 days ($p < 0.001$)
Rescue short-acting bronchodilator use	−0.63 puffs/day (95% CI −0.90 to −0.36)
Peak expiratory flow (ml min^{-1})	3.6 ml min^{-1} (95% CI −23.5 to 160.1)
End of treatment FEV1 (ml)	68.3 ml (95% CI −23.5 to 160.1)
Change in FEV1 (ml)	73 ml ($p = 0.03$) or 2.8% ($p = 0.04$) better
End of treatment asthma symptom score change	−0.046 (95% CI −0.75 to −0.29)
Reduction in symptom score ≥ 50%	2.99 (95% CI 1.64–5.44)
Improvement in asthma quality-of-life scores	0.32 (95% CI 0.22–0.43)
Rate of subjects achieving asthma control	59% vs. 41% ($p < 0.001$)
Odds ratio of achieving good or excellent asthma control	2.6 (95% CI 1.9–3.4)
Odds ratio of complete inhaled corticosteroid withdrawal	2.5 (95% CI 2.0–3.1)
Rate of complete steroid withdrawal	34% vs. 14% ($p < 0.001$)
Inhaled corticosteroid reduction	−118 mcg BDP (95% CI −154 to −84)
Likelihood of reducing ICS ≥ 50%	2.5 (95% CI 2.0–3.1)
Odds ratio of withdrawing oral corticosteroid	1.18 (95% CI 0.53–2.63)
Median relative reduction in oral corticosteroid use	69% vs. 75% ($p = 0.68$)
Odds ratio of being hospitalized for asthma	0.11 (95% CI 0.93–0.48)
Number need to treat to:	**Number (95% CI)**
Prevent one exacerbation	11 (9–16)
Enable one patient to stop steroid therapy	6 (5–8)
Enable one patient to reduce steroid therapy by >50%	5 (5–7)
Prevent one hospitalization for exacerbation	57 (52–98)
Enable one patient to rate his/ her asthma in good or excellent control	5 (4–6)

have previously shown no relationship between lung function and hospital admissions (Qureshi et al. 1998) as well as poor relationships between lung function and health-related quality of life (Wijnhoven et al. 2001). The most impressive benefit of omalizumab observed in the trials has been reduction in frequency of hospitalizations, where it reduced hospitalizations by 93.6% compared with placebo during the 12–16 weeks of the extension phase in three trials (1/767 omalizumab vs. 13/638 placebo; $p = 0.003$) (Busse et al. 2001; Milgrom et al. 2001; Soler et al. 2001; Avila 2007).

2.5.4 Impact of Omalizumab on Health-Related Quality of Life

An important secondary outcome in the studies, and one that is obviously of primary importance to the clinician, is improvement in heath-related quality of life. Traditionally, most studies in asthma have not focused on this aspect of outcome, rather focusing on conventional measurements of airway function such as spirometry, symptoms, medication usage, and degrees of airway hyperresponsiveness. Yet it is widely known that asthma exerts profound and variable effects on quality of life, and that such effects may be missed by measuring only conventional outcomes (Juniper 1999). Over the last two decades, the development and validation of several disease-specific instruments designed to assess quality of life have been developed. Moreover, these questionnaires are now widely available, easy to complete in 5–10 min, and found in multiple languages (Buhl 2003). Among the most widely used is the Asthma Quality of Life Questionnaire (AQLQ) (Juniper et al. 1992), a 32-item questionnaire that seeks to identify four basic domains in which asthma impacts one's quality of life: activity limitations, emotions, symptoms, and exposure to environmental stimuli. Each question is answered by the patient on a 7-point scale, from 1 (extremely impaired) to 7 (no impairment). Results are generally expressed in terms of a mean score for each domain, along with an overall score. An increase in domain or overall score of 0.5 or greater is generally accepted as clinically significant, and differences of 1.5 or greater reflecting a large improvement (Hajiro and Nishimura 2002; Jones 2002).

Initially, it appeared that use of omalizumab resulted in substantial improvement in health-related quality of life. This was evident by two of the four main clinical trials (Busse et al. 2001; Soler et al. 2001); these two studies not only utilized the AQLQ, but their similarities in study design allowed pooling of the data. Overall, patients treated with omalizumab experienced clinically relevant improvements in their asthma-related quality of life, as shown by improvements in mean scores of ≥ 0.5 in all four domains of the AQLQ, as well as the overall score (Buhl 2003). However, when more recent data were included in the analysis and the results pooled by the Cochrane Collaboration, the administration of subcutaneous omalizumab did not reach 0.5 (Walker et al. 2006), raising doubts about the significance of improvements in quality of life measures described above. Currently, it is still unclear as to what degree omalizumab improves quality of life measures in patients with asthma.

2.5.5 Summary of Efficacy in Asthma

Overall, the reduction in daily inhaled steroid use following treatment with omalizumab was modest but significant. However, the baseline steroid doses, the impressive effects of placebo treatment, and the mean difference in steroid consumption between treatment and placebo, bring in to question the true size of the steroid-sparing effects of omalizumab (Walker et al. 2006). An important caveat to the clinical trial data published so far is that, generally speaking, the majority of the data pertained to mild and moderate asthmatic subjects. Given that omalizumab is generally used to treat patients with severe or difficult-to-treat asthma, it has not been studied as extensively in this population. Therefore, several investigators have formed a consortium known as The Epidemiology and Natural History of Asthma: Outcomes and Treatment Regimens (TENOR) to study the natural history of such patients and the effects of advanced therapies such as omalizumab (Dolan et al. 2004).

2.5.6 Non-Asthma Atopic Diseases

In atopic diseases related to asthma, and specifically related to IgE, omalizumab has proven safe and effective. It attenuates early and late responses to allergen challenge to the skin (Beck et al. 2004; Ong et al. 2005) and early response to nasal allergen challenges (Kuehr et al. 2002) (late responses were not assessed). The magnitude of these reductions ranged from 20% to 70%. In addition, these reductions were associated with concomitant attenuation in local inflammatory diseases. It has been successfully used to treat allergic rhinitis alone and in combination with immunotherapy (Parks and Casale 2006). Recently, pretreatment of rush immunotherapy with omalizumab was found to decrease severity of anaphylaxis during therapy as well as decrease symptoms of ragweed-induced allergic rhinitis (Casale et al. 2006). Further clinical studies are needed in the use of omalizumab in the treatment of other atopic diseases such as atopic dermatitis, urticaria, and food allergies. Indeed, if omalizumab can control comorbid atopic conditions, this may be of particular benefit to asthmatic subjects who suffer from these related conditions; such benefit may, in some instances, justify the current high costs associated with the medication's administration.

2.6 Adverse Events and Safety Issues of Omalizumab

Omalizumab has so far been deemed to be a relatively safe medication, though information from phase IV trials are lacking in published form. The overall rate of any side effects in the phase III clinical trials was 80% for omalizumab-treated subjects and 77% for placebo-treated subjects, with injection-site reactions (45% treated, 43% placebo), viral infections (23% treated, 26% placebo), and upper-respiratory infections (20% treated, 20% placebo) accounting for the vast majority of these effects (Walker et al. 2006). Injection-site reactions were generally mild and included pain, induration, erythema, warmth, burning sensation, and localized hive formation.

Serious side effects occurred at similar rates between groups treated with omalizumab vs. placebo, yet particular concern is given to the development of anaphylaxis and malignancy. Anaphylaxis occurred in three subjects within 2 h of omalizumab injections, but none in the placebo arms (Genentech-Inc 2003; Rieves 2003). One patient developed large injection-site edema and mild pharyngeal edema. Another developed urticaria, skin pruritus and dyspnea hours after the initial treatment

(Avila 2007). Events resolved with epinephrine injections, oral antihistamines, and systemic corticosteroid administration. These reactions obviate the need for the ability to treat anaphylaxis in facilities that administer omalizumab. Moreover, the delayed anaphylaxis requires that patient and/or parent education be provided to recognize signs and symptoms of anaphylaxis.

There was a slightly increased risk of malignancy in patients treated with omalizumab, though this did not reach statistical significance. Malignancies occurred in 20 out of 4,127 (0.5%) of omalizumab-treated subjects and in 5 out of 2,236 (0.2%) of placebo-treated subjects (Genentech-Inc 2003; Rieves 2003; Avila 2007). In the omalizumab group, subjects were diagnosed with nonmelanoma skin cancer (5 subjects; one of these also had melanoma), breast cancer (5 subjects), prostate cancer (2), melanoma (2), parotid cancer (2), bladder cancer (2), non-Hodgkins lymphoma (1), pancreatic cancer (1), rectal cancer (1), and thyroid cancer (1). In the placebo group, subjects were diagnosed with nonmelanoma skin cancer (3 subjects), glioma (1), and testicular cancer (1). When expressed as events per exposure, there were 6.3 malignancies per patient-year in the omalizumab group and 3.3. in the placebo group for a rate difference of 3.0 and a rate ratio of 1.9 cancers per patient-year, both of which are not statistically significant. Moreover, the rate of cancer in the omalizumab group was similar to the expected rate for subjects of similar age and gender according to the National Cancer Institute's Surveillance, Epidemiology, and End Results database, which collects cancer statistics from 14% of the US population (Genentech-Inc 2003). Nevertheless, due to this heightened concern, Genentech has initiated the Epidemiologic Study of Xolair in Patients with Moderate to Severe Asthma (EXCELS) study and other surveillance evaluations to assess the natural medical history of patients with severe asthma, including rates of malignancies (Dolan et al. 2004; Borish et al. 2005; Slavin et al. 2006).

The development of immune complex disease and deposition seems to be a theoretical concern for many antibody-based therapies (Dillman 1989). If immune complexes are large, deposition can occur in multiple body tissues especially synovial joint spaces, the renal parenchyma, skin, and gastrointestinal tract. However, the humanization of the monoclonal antibody has resulted in less than 5% of amino acids being of murine origin, making the molecule less immunogenic. Moreover, if antibodies do develop, the resulting complexes are generally small and of low serum concentration (Liu et al. 1995). Among 1,723 subjects exposed to omalizumab, only one subject, who received the drug by inhalation, developed antibodies to omalizumab; none developed immune complex disease (Fahy et al. 1999). Overall, this appears to be less of a concern than was previously thought, but long-term data are not available as yet to clearly delineate this issue.

Though omalizumab has been studied and approved by the FDA for use in adolescents and adults, there are limited data in children under the age of 12, elderly subjects, and pregnant and nursing women. The latter issue deserves particular attention. In monkeys, omalizumab given at 12 times the dose used in clinical trials did not cause maternal toxicity, embryotoxicity, or teratogenicity. In human studies, 17 subjects became pregnant while receiving omalizumab, of whom 11 had normal deliveries and the others had spontaneous (3) or elective (3) abortions. In the placebo group, 10 subjects became pregnant, of whom 6 had normal deliveries, 2 had spontaneous abortions, and 2 had unknown outcomes (Avila 2007). Omalizumab was stopped as soon as pregnancy was noticed. Though the FDA classified omalizumab as a category B drug for use in pregnancy, as an IgG1 molecule, omalizumab can cross the placenta and its effects are unknown. Therefore, at the time of this writing, we advise that omalizumab be stopped in the event of pregnancy.

Another safety concern for anti-IgE therapy is a theoretical risk of increased parasitic infections in patients treated with omalizumab. Parasitic infections result in increased IgE, though it is unclear if this effect is protective or simply a secondary marker of active parasite infection (Mingomataj et al. 2006). To test this hypothesis, anti-IgE-treated mice were infected with *Nippostrogylus brasiliensis* (Amiri et al. 1994). In this model, omalizumab treatment resulted in decreased worm load and enhanced parasite clearance. A related concern is that anti-IgE therapy, by affecting the body's response to parasitic infections, especially early in life, may modulate the development of asthma and atopy (Yazdanbakhsh et al. 2001). These concerns are not well-answered at this timepoint, especially given that published clinical trials to date have occurred in well-developed countries, where the incidence of parasitic infections remains low in comparison to lesser-developed regions.

Overall, it appears that administration of omalizumab appears relatively safe, especially when administered by a skilled staff that is able to recognize and treat anaphylaxis immediately. However, phase IV clinical trial data are needed, especially if anti-IgE therapy is to be continued lifelong.

2.7 Practical Aspects of Omalizumab

Despite the improvements seen in asthma exacerbations and quality of life with omalizumab, the exact role of omalizumab in clinical practice has yet to be defined (Avila 2007). As discussed earlier in the chapter, a number of pharmacologic, environmental, and possibly immunologic treatment options exist. Moreover, recently a number of studies have advocated the use of adjunctive therapies or focus on coexisting conditions (Roberts et al. 2006), such as allergic rhinitis and sinusitis (Dixon et al. 2006), gastroesophageal reflux disease (Harding 2005), vocal cord dysfunction (Jain et al. 2006), obesity (Chinn 2006), and obstructive sleep apnea (Yigla et al. 2003). Although national guidelines for asthma management have been in place and advocated for several years, it is clear that adherence to these guidelines is suboptimal (Reeves et al. 2006). Therefore, many critics of omalizumab feel that if commonly used treatment options are implemented that conform to national guidelines and coexisting conditions are managed effectively, many patients with moderate to severe asthma would be symptomatically well-controlled. This is particularly evident in the impressive placebo responses noted in the above-described trials. Although placebo effects have been observed with virtually any medication, it is likely that with asthma particular attention to peak flow measurements, education about inhaler usage and techniques, and prompt treatment of disease exacerbations likely led to a strong placebo response. Given the suboptimal compliance observed in asthma medications, this could be seen as an advantage for omalizumab – a treatment that is administered periodically under clinical supervision has obvious benefits in this regard.

Despite the above criticisms, it is clear that better care is needed for the large number of patients with allergic asthma who are refractory to current therapies. What is not clear is which patients would specifically benefit from omalizumab. Patients who are particularly likely to benefit include those with evidence of sensitization to perennial aeroallergens who require high doses of inhaled corticosteroids and those with frequent exacerbations. Analyses of pooled data from published clinical trials have indicated that patients who had a response to omalizumab had a ratio of observed to expected FEV1 of less than 65% (normal ≥70%), were taking doses of inhaled corticosteroids equivalent to more than 800 mcg of beclomethasone diproprionate per day, and had had at least one visit to the emergency department in the past year (Bousquet et al. 2004; Bousquet et al. 2005). In general, current asthma symptoms are not a contraindication to the administration of omalizumab.

Dosing of omalizumab was discussed earlier and follows the normogram depicted in Table 1. A pretreatment total IgE is required, and dose adjustment made on the recommendation of 0.016 mg kg^{-1} of body weight per international unit of IgE. The drug is supplied as a lyophilized, sterile powder in single-use, 5-ml vials designed to deliver either 150 or 75 mg on reconstitution with sterile water for injection. The powder requires 15–20 min or more to dissolve, and the resulting viscous solution takes several seconds to both draw into the syringe and subsequently inject. Once prepared, the drug must be used within 4 h at room temperature or 8 h if refrigerated. Since doses can require several vials to be drawn and injected, the staff and facility demands for routine omalizumab injections can be beyond the capabilities of many clinicians' offices (Marcus 2006). From a subspecialty perspective, administration of omalizumab has been easier for allergists than pulmonologists for several reasons: (1) allergen skin testing (a requirement for administration of omalizumab) is routinely done in an allergist's office; (2) allergist offices routinely have patients do walk-in subcutaneous injections as done for immunotherapy; (3) allergists' staff are trained to quickly treat anaphylaxis (Marcus 2006; Avila 2007).

Omalizumab is considerably more expensive than conventional asthma therapy. At present, the cost of a single 150 mg vial is approximately $470, and accordingly yearly costs range from $6,100 to $36,600 per year (Marcus 2006). This compares with approximate annual costs of $1,280 for montelukast (Singulair, Merck), $2,160 for the combination of fluticasone diproprionate and salmeterol (Advair, GlaxoSmithKline), and $680 for extended-release theophylline (e.g., Uniphyl^{TM}) (Strunk and Bloomberg 2006). Given the expense, it is not surprising that many third-party payers are carefully surveying usage of omalizumab and that occasionally the approval process from Medicare and other payers may involve substantial administrative responsibilities (Marcus 2006). The only currently available cost-effectiveness analysis of omalizumab was limited to direct payer's costs and did not take into account indirect costs (Oba and Salzman 2004). The authors concluded that omalizumab is cost-effective in asthmatic subjects who experience ≥5 hospitalizations or ≥ 20 inpatient days for exacerbations per year. Clearly, a real-world cost-effectiveness analysis needs to be performed which accounts for not only direct and indirect costs of omalizumab administration, but also the health and societal effects of asthma control in patients optimized on various forms of asthma therapy.

Monitoring of total serum IgE levels during the course of therapy with omalizumab in not indicated, because these levels will be elevated as a result of the presence of circulating IgE-anti-IgE complexes. To date, free serum IgE levels are not routine and are prohibitively expensive for most laboratories. It is unclear if monitoring the free, circulating levels will have an effect on patient treatment and response, though assays are being investigated and developed for commercial availability and more widespread use.

3 Anti-TNF-α Therapy for Asthma

3.1 Role of Tumor Necrosis Factor-Alpha (TNF-α) in Asthma Pathogenesis

Tumor necrosis factor alpha (TNF-α) is an important cytokine in asthma pathogenesis. Extensive genetic, biologic, and physiologic evidence indicates that TNF-α may play a critical role in the initiation and amplification of airway inflammation in patients with asthma (Erzurum 2006). Preformed TNF-α is stored by mast cells and rapidly released during IgE-mediated reactions that typify the asthmatic response to allergens (Howarth et al. 2005; Mukhopadhyay et al. 2006) (Fig. 1). Elevated levels of TNF-α have been observed in induced sputum from patients with asthma (Keatings et al. 1997); moreover, the expression of TNF-α in asthmatic airways correlates with asthma disease severity (Howarth et al. 2005). Interestingly, inhalation of TNF-α by normal individuals increased airway responsiveness and neutrophil counts in induced sputum (Thomas et al. 1995) and TNF-α inhalation in patients with mild asthma causes airway hyperresponsiveness and sputum neutrophilia and eosinophilia (Thomas and Heywood 2002). TNF-α is a known candidate gene for asthma (Ober and Hoffjan 2006), and polymorphisms of the gene may be associated with the development of childhood asthma (Li et al. 2006).

Although it is clear that TNF-α is involved in asthma pathogenesis, the exact manner in which TNF-α effects its responses is complex and multifaceted. Macrophage activation in the late asthmatic response has been known to be a key pathway (Gosset et al. 1991), but TNF-α also upregulates adhesion molecule expression and activity, which leads to increased migration of eosinophils and neutrophils into the airways (Ohkawara et al. 1997). Airway epithelial cells are also activated by TNF-α to release cytotoxic mediators and reactive nitrogen and oxygen species that result in airway injury (Bayram et al. 2001; Bosson et al. 2003). The end result of chronic, unresolved inflammation is a structural change in the airway, termed airway remodeling. TNF-α may contribute to all aspects of remodeling, including the proliferation and activation of fibroblasts, the increased production of extracellular matrix glycoproteins, subepithelial fibrosis, and mucous-cell hyperplasia (Erzurum 2006). Independent of its effect on inflammation, TNF-α also has direct effects on bronchial hyperreactivity to methacholine and allergen (Pennings et al. 1998).

3.2 The Use of Anti-TNF Therapy in Asthma

Humanized anti-TNF-α monoclonal antibodies (infliximab, adalimumab) and soluble TNF receptor blockers (etanercept) have been developed and shown to be effective in other inflammatory diseases such as Crohn's disease (Hyams et al. 2000) and rheumatoid arthritis (Scott and Kingsley 2006). In a murine model of asthma, treatment with anti-TNF-α monoclonal antibodies reduces pulmonary inflammation and airway hyperresponsiveness, perhaps via a decrease in eotaxin levels (Kim et al. 2006). Over the past several years, a number of studies have been undertaken to evaluate the potential benefits of anti-TNF therapy in diseases such as asthma (Howarth et al. 2005; Berry et al. 2006; Erin et al. 2006), chronic obstructive pulmonary disease (van der Vaart et al. 2005), and other diseases of lung and airway injury (Mukhopadhyay et al. 2006).

In a UK study, 17 subjects with severe corticosteroid-dependent asthma were administered subcutaneous etanercept (Enbrel^{TM}, Wyeth Laboratories, Berkshire, UK) in an open-label fashion and assessed for clinical and biological response. Administration of etanercept was associated with improvement in asthma symptoms, lung function, and bronchial hyperresponsiveness (Howarth et al. 2005). These effects were maintained 2–4 weeks after cessation of therapy, after which the benefits were lost. This trial prompted a follow-up study in which 10 patients with refractory asthma were randomized to etanercept in a crossover pilot study (Berry et al. 2006). In this study, 10 weeks of treatment with etanercept was associated with a significant improvement in methacholine responsiveness, asthma-related quality of life score, and post-bronchodilator FEV1.

Recently, another study was published investigating the usage of a different anti-TNF agent, infliximab (Remicade^{TM}, Centocorp Inc., Malvern, PA, USA). In this study, 38 patients with moderate-to-severe persistent asthma currently being treated with inhaled corticosteroids, were randomized to treatment with intravenous infliximab or placebo (Erin et al. 2006). Infliximab was well-tolerated and associated with a decrease in mean diurnal variation of peak expiratory flow (a marker of airway obstruction) and fewer numbers of patients with asthma exacerbations among the treated group. Concordantly, there were lower levels of TNF-α and other inflammatory markers in the sputum of treated subjects. Importantly, there were no treatment-related statistically significant effects of morning peak expiratory flow, exhaled nitric oxide levels, or blood or sputum eosinophilia. This was merely a pilot study, and larger studies are needed to understand the effects of TNF-α inhibition in asthmatics.

3.3 Additional Issues Regarding Anti-TNF Therapy in Asthma

The above data regarding the usage of anti-TNF therapies for asthma are quite preliminary as the number of study subjects are small and larger controlled trials are needed. Injection site reactions were common with administration of infliximab and etanercept, but were mild and easily treated.

The greatest concern in the use of these antibody-mediated therapies is the potential risks for acquiring serious infections. Animal studies have long shown an essential role of TNF-α in fighting infection; therefore, suppression of this arm of host defense may significantly hamper one's ability to fight pathogens. Serious infections with anti-TNF therapies have been associated with all the anti-TNF therapies to date (Giles and Bathon 2004). These can be either usual bacterial infections (Kroesen et al. 2003), but may also include tuberculosis (Keane et al. 2001; Bresnihan and Cunnane 2003), serious fungal infections (Wood et al. 2003), and other less-commonly seen pathogens. It is perhaps the alarming incidence of tuberculosis that has most healthcare workers concerned about the use of anti-TNF therapies, as disease has great public health and treatment-related consequences (Rychly and DiPiro 2005). Recently, a systematic review was published addressing this concern – 9 clinical trials of over 3,900 patients with rheumatoid arthritis treated for 12 weeks or longer with anti-TNF therapies were compared to 1,512 patients who received placebo (Bongartz et al. 2006). In patients treated for 3–12 months, the odds ratio for serious infections in the treated group was 2.0 (95% CI 1.3 to 3.1), meaning essentially double the incidence of serious infections in the treated group vs. control group. The incidence of serious infection was almost 1 in 60 treated subjects based upon this analysis. This is not as high as others would have predicted, but is still clinically relevant.

Another important concern in the use of anti-TNF therapies is the theoretical increased incidence in the development of malignancy. TNF was originally named for the recognition of its ability to kill tumor cells in vitro and is important in natural killer cell and CD8 lymphocyte-mediated killing of tumor cells. In the above-mentioned meta-analysis by Bongartz et al., the pooled odds ratio for the development of malignancy in these patients with rheumatoid arthritis was 3.3 (95% CI 1.2–9.1), and the authors estimated that roughly one malignancy would develop for every 154 patients treated with anti-TNF therapies (treatment period of 3–12 months). Moreover, this is dose-dependent as studies utilizing higher doses were associated with greater incidences of malignancy formation.

Other potential adverse effects associated with anti-TNF therapies include the development of congestive heart failure, demyelinating diseases, and systemic lupus erythematosus, but in most cases these can be identified and managed (Hochberg et al. 2005). As an aside, adalimumab was associated, paradoxically, with the development of asthma in a single case report (Bennett et al. 2005), though the mechanism for this remains speculative.

Overall, anti-TNF therapies are important in the treatment of many immunologically mediated diseases, though their roles in asthma remain uncertain as yet given the paucity of clinical data. Needless to say, more data are needed to gain better understanding of potential benefits in patients with asthma. Moreover, concerns for infection, malignancy, and other serious adverse effects remain particularly important in the evaluation of these therapies. Like anti-IgE therapy, anti-TNF therapies share many concerns for parenteral administration, costs, and identifying patients who would most benefit from these therapies.

4 Other Antibody-Mediated Therapies for Asthma

There are numerous other potential antibody targets in asthma (Walsh 2005; Walsh 2006). Since much asthmatic inflammation is thought to be a consequence of uncontrolled inflammation, it follows that a number of targets are being developed that modulate inflammatory pathways.

4.1 Antibodies to Interleukin-5

Interleukin-5 (IL-5) is a cytokine that is crucial to the development and release of eosinophils and the subsequent release of eosinophils from the bone marrow, their enhanced adhesion to endothelials cells lining the postcapillary tissues. Several animal models of asthma, including primates, have provided good evidence that inhibiting the effects of IL-5 using specific monoclonal antibodies inhibited eosinophilic inflammation and airway hyperresponsiveness. Given its central role in regulating eosinophil development and function, IL-5 was therefore chosen as a potentially attractive target to prevent or blunt eosinophil-mediated inflammation in patients with asthma.

To date, clinical trials with anti-IL5 monoclonal antibodies have not reported substantial efficacy. The first study of mepolizumab (Leckie et al. 2000) was criticized for lack of power and validity of patient selection. A later placebo-controlled study found that treatment of mild asthmatic patients with mepolizumab abolished circulating eosinophils and reduced airway and bone marrow eosinophils (Flood-Page et al. 2003b); however, there were no significant improvements in clinical measures of asthma. Interestingly, lung biopsy samples from the treatment group contained intact tissue eosinophils and large quantities of eosinophil granule proteins, likely explaining the lack of clinical benefit. Similar findings were reported with the anti-IL5 monoclonal antibody SCH55700 in patients with severe asthma that had not been controlled by inhaled corticosteroid use (Kips et al. 2003). These authors reported profound reductions in circulating eosinophils, but no significant improvement was observed in either asthma symptoms or lung function. Interestingly, anti-IL-5 therapy reduced deposition of extracellular membrane proteins in the bronchial subepithelial basement membrane of mild allergic asthmatics, hence implying that this therapy may improve airway remodeling in asthma (Flood-Page et al. 2003a).

4.2 Antibodies to Interleukin-4 and Interleukin 13

Another cytokine important in eosinophil accumulation is Interleukin-4 (IL-4), and together with its close relative, Interleukin-13 (IL-13), it is important in IgE synthesis by B cells. Both cytokines signal through a shared surface receptor, IL-4α, which then activates the transcription factor, STAT-6 (Jiang et al. 2000). Studies with soluble IL-4 given in a nebulized form demonstrated that the fall in lung function induced by withdrawal of inhaled corticosteroids was prevented in patients with moderately severe asthma (Borish et al. 2001). However, despite these promising findings, subsequent trials have not been as successful and consequently this treatment is no longer being developed (Walsh 2005). Other approaches for blocking the IL-4 receptor include administration of antibodies against the receptor and mutant IL-4 proteins. Interrupting IL-4 receptor signaling by targeting transcription factors such as STAT-6, GATA-3, or FOG-1 might also be possible (Barnes 2003).

IL-13 has been found in bronchoalveolar lavage fluid following allergen provocation of asthmatic subjects, which strongly correlated with the increase in eosinophil numbers (Kroegel et al. 1996) and mRNA expression was detected in bronchial biopsies from allergic and nonallergic asthmatic subjects (Humbert et al. 1997). In animal models, IL-13 mimics many of the pro-inflammatory changes associated with asthma (Grunig et al. 1998). Two receptors for IL-13 have been described – IL-13Rα1 and IL-13Rα2. The latter exists in soluble form and has a high affinity for IL-13, which by competitive inhibition of IL-13 results in decreases in IgE production, pulmonary eosinophilia, and airway hyperresponsiveness (Wills-Karp et al. 1998). A humanized IL-13Rα2 is in clinical development as a novel therapy for asthma, but results so far have been inconclusive about its benefits (Walsh 2006).

4.3 Other Antibody-Based Therapies in Development

A number of potential antibody-mediated therapies are probably worth mentioning but beyond the scope of this chapter, as data are too preliminary on their potential for clinical effectiveness. The majority of these therapies invariably involve control of the inflammatory cascade. The spectrum of potential sites of action is diverse, and may involve targeting of intracellular adhesion molecules located on inflammatory cells and airway epithelia (e.g., VCAM), specific therapies against mast cells and their mediators (e.g., tryptase, prostaglandins), regulation of apoptosis of inflammatory cells (e.g., via inhibition of NF-κB), regulation of cell cycling and signaling cascades, and even gene-based therapies that target transcriptional activation of the inflammatory cascade (Walsh 2005).

5 Summary

Asthma remains a disease of great public health importance, and though current therapies have dramatically improved asthma control in the vast percentage of patients with asthma, current treatments remain inadequate in certain segments of the asthma population. Antibody-mediated therapies, specifically anti-IgE therapy, are proving to be viable tools in the management of asthma and related inflammatory disorders. Though their current roles are still being determined, and long-term efficacy and safety data still being accumulated, we believe that such targeted therapies will ultimately change the daily management of asthma.

References

Adis (2002) Omalizumab. Biodrugs 16:380–386

Amiri P, Haak-Frendscho M, Robbins K, McKerrow JH, Stewart T, Jardieu P (1994) Anti-immunoglobulin E treatment decreases worm burden and egg production in Schistosoma mansoni-infected normal and interferon gamma knockout mice. J Exp Med 180:43–51

Avila PC (2007) Does Anti-IgE Therapy Help in Asthma? Efficacy and Controversies. Annu Rev Med 58

Barnes PJ (2003) Cytokine-directed therapies for the treatment of chronic airway diseases. Cytokine Growth Factor Rev 14:511–522

Bayram H, Sapsford RJ, Abdelaziz MM, Khair OA (2001) Effect of ozone and nitrogen dioxide on the release of proinflammatory mediators from bronchial epithelial cells of nonatopic nonasthmatic subjects and atopic asthmatic patients in vitro. J Allergy Clin Immunol 107:287–294

Beck LA, Marcotte GV, MacGlashan JD, Togias A, Saini S (2004) Omalizumab-induced reductions in mast cell FcεRI expression and function. J Allergy Clin Immunol 114:527–530

Bennett AN, Wong M, Zain A, Panayi G, Kirkham B (2005) Adalimumab-induced asthma. Rheumatology 44:1199–1200

Berry MA, Hargadon B, Shelley M, Parker D, Shaw DE, Green RH, Bradding P, Brightling CE, Wardlaw AJ, Pavord ID (2006) Evidence of a role of tumor necrosis factor {alpha} in refractory asthma. N Engl J Med 354:697–708

Bongartz T, Sutton AJ, Sweeting MJ, Buchan I, Matteson EL, Montori V (2006) Anti-TNF antibody therapy in rheumatoid arthritis and the risk of serious infections and malignancies: systematic review and meta-analysis of rare harmful effects in randomized controlled trials. JAMA 295:2275–2285

Borish L, Chipps B, Deniz Y, Gujrathi S, Zheng B, Dolan C (2005) Total serum IgE levels in a large cohort of patients with severe or difficult-to-treat asthma. Ann Allergy Asthma Immunol 95:247–253

Borish LC, Nelson HS, Corren J, Bensch G, Busse WW (2001) Efficacy of soluble IL-4 receptor for the treatment of adults with asthma. J Allergy Clin Immunol 107:963–970

Bosson J, Stenfors N, Bucht A, Helleday R, Pourazar J, Holgate ST, Kelly FJ, Sandstrom T, Wilson S, Frew AJ, Blomberg A (2003) Ozone-induced bronchial epithelial cytokine expression differs between healthy and asthmatic subjects. Clin Exp Allergy 33:777–782

Boulet L-P, Chapman KR, Cote J, Kalra S, Bhagat R, Swystun VA, Laviolette M, Cleland LD, Deschesnes F, Su JQ, Devault A, Fick RB, Cockcroft DW (1997) Inhibitory effects of an Anti-IgE antibody E25 on allergen-induced early asthmatic response. Am J Respir Crit Care Med 155:1835–1840

Bousquet J, Cabrera P, Berkman N, Buhl R, Holgate S, Wenzel S, Fox H, Hedgecock S, Blogg M, Cioppa GD (2005) The effect of treatment with omalizumab, an anti-IgE antibody, on asthma exacerbations and emergency medical visits in patients with severe persistent asthma. Allergy 60:302–308

Bousquet J, Wenzel S, Holgate S, Lumry W, Freeman P, Fox H (2004) Predicting Response to Omalizumab, an Anti-IgE Antibody, in Patients With Allergic Asthma. Chest 125:1378–1386

Bradding P, Walls AF, Holgate ST (2006) The role of the mast cell in the pathophysiology of asthma. J Allergy Clin Immunol 117:1277–1284

Braman SS (2006) The Global Burden of Asthma. Chest 130:4S-12

Bresnihan B, Cunnane G (2003) Infection complications associated with the use of biologic agents. Rheum Dis Clin North Am 29:185–202

Broide DH (2001) Molecular and cellular mechanisms of allergic disease. J Allergy Clin Immunol 108:S65–S71

Buhl R (2003) Omalizumab (Xolair) improves quality of life in adult patients with allergic asthma: a review. Respir Med 97:123–129

Buhl R (2004) Anti-IgE antibodies for the treatment of asthma. Curr Opin Pulm Med 11:27–34

Busse W, Corren J, Lanier BQ, McAlary M, Fowler-Taylor A, Cioppa GD, van As A, Gupta N (2001) Omalizumab, anti-IgE recombinant humanized monoclonal antibody, for the treatment of severe allergic asthma. J Allergy Clin Immunol 108:184–190

Casale TB, Bernstein IL, Busse WW, LaForce CF, Tinkelman DG, Stoltz RR, Dockhorn RJ, Reimann J, Su JQ (1997) Use of an anti-IgE humanized monoclonal antibody in ragweed-induced allergic rhinitis. J Allergy Clin Immunol 100:110–121

Casale TB, Busse WW, Kline JN, Ballas ZK, Moss MH, Townley RG, Mokhtarani M, Seyfert-Margolis V, Asare A, Bateman K (2006) Omalizumab pretreatment decreases acute reactions after rush immunotherapy for ragweed-induced seasonal allergic rhinitis. J Allergy Clin Immunol 117:134–140

Chang TW (2000) The pharmacological basis of anti-IgE therapy. Nat Biotech 18:157–162

Chinn S (2006) Obesity and asthma. Paediatr Respir Rev 7:223–228

Cohen RT, Celedon JC, Hinckson VJ, Ramsey CD, Wakefield DB, Weiss ST, Cloutier MM (2006) Health-Care Use Among Puerto Rican and African-American Children With Asthma. Chest 130:463–471

Covar RA, Spahn JD, Martin RJ, Silkoff PE, Sundstrom DA, Murphy J, Szefler SJ (2004) Safety and application of induced sputum analysis in childhood asthma. J Allergy Clin Immunol 114:575–582

Dillman R (1989) Monoclonal antibodies for treating cancer. Ann Intern Med 111:592–603

Dixon AE, Kaminsky DA, Holbrook JT, Wise RA, Shade DM, Irvin CG (2006) Allergic rhinitis and sinusitis in asthma: Differential effects on symptoms and pulmonary function. Chest 130:429–435

Djukanovic R, Wilson SJ, Kraft M, Jarjour NN, Steel M, Chung KF, Bao W, Fowler-Taylor A, Matthews J, Busse WW, Holgate ST, Fahy JV (2004) Effects of treatment with anti-immunoglobulin E antibody omalizumab on airway inflammation in allergic asthma. Am J Respir Crit Care Med 170:583–593

Dolan C, Fraher K, Bleecker E, Borish LC, B, Hayden M, Weiss S, Zheng B, Johnson C, Wenzel S (2004) Design and baseline characteristics of the epidemiology and natural history of asthma: Outcomes and Treatment Regimens (TENOR) study: a large cohort of patients with severe or difficult-to-treat asthma. Ann Allergy Asthma Immunol 92:32–39

Dolovich J, Hargreave FE, Chalmers R, Shier KJ, Gauldie J, Bienenstock J (1973) Late cutaneous allergic responses in isolated IgE-dependent reactions. J Allergy Clin Immunol 52:38–46

Eder W, Ege MJ, von Mutius E (2006) The asthma epidemic. N Engl J Med 355:2226–2235

Erin EM, Leaker BR, Nicholson GC, Tan AJ, Green LM, Neighbour H, Zacharasiewicz AS, Turner J, Barnathan ES, Kon OM, Barnes PJ, Hansel TT (2006) The effects of a monoclonal antibody directed against tumor necrosis factor-alpha in asthma. Am J Respir Crit. Care Med 174:753–762

Erzurum SC (2006) Inhibition of tumor necrosis factor α for refractory asthma. N Engl J Med 354:754–758

Fahy J, Cockcroft D, Boulet L, Wong H, Deschesnes F, Dvid E, Ruppel J, Su J, Adelman D (1999) Effect of aerosolized anti-IgE (E25) on airway responses to inhaled allergen in asthmatic subjects. Am J Respir Crit Care Med 160

Fahy JV, Fleming HE, Wong HH, Liu JT, Su JQ, Reimann J, Fick RB, Boushey HA (1997) The effect of an anti-IgE monoclonal antibody on the early- and late-phase responses to allergen inhalation in asthmatic subjects. Am J Respir Crit Care Med 155:1828–1834

Flood-Page P, Menzies-Gow A, Phipps S, Ying S, Wangoo A, Ludwig MS, Barnes N, Robinson D, Kay AB (2003a) Anti-IL-5 treatment reduces deposition of ECM proteins in the bronchial subepithelial basement membrane of mild atopic asthmatics. J Clin Invest 112:1029–1036

Flood-Page PT, Menzies-Gow AN, Kay AB, Robinson DS (2003b) Eosinophil's role remains uncertain as anti-interleukin-5 only partially depletes numbers in asthmatic airway. Am J Respir Crit Care Med 167:199–204

Geiger E, Magerstaedt R, Weendorf JHM, Kraft S, Hanau D, Bieber T (2000) IL-4 induces the intracellular expression of the α chain of the high-affinity receptor for IgE in in vitro-generated dendritic cells. J Allergy Clin Immunol 105:150–156

Genentech-Inc (2003) Briefing document on safety of omalizumab (Xolair) for treatment of allergic asthma (BLA STN 103976/0). Food and Drug Administration, Washington, DC

Genentech (2003) Omalizumab prescribing information. South San Francisco, CA

Giles JT, Bathon JM (2004) Serious Infections Associated with Anticytokine Therapies in the Rheumatic Diseases. J Intensive Care Med 19:320–334

Gold DR, Wright R (2005) Population disparities in asthma. Ann Rev Public Health 26:89–113

Gosset P, Tsicopoulos A, Wallaert B, Vannimenus C, Joseph M, Tonnel A-B, Capron A (1991) Increased secretion of tumor necrosis factor α and interleukin-6 by alveolar macrophages consecutive to the development of the late asthmatic reaction. J Allergy Clin Immunol 88:561–571

Grunig G, Warnock M, Wakil AE, Venkayya R, Brombacher F, Rennick DM, Sheppard D, Mohrs M, Donaldson DD, Locksley RM, Corry DB (1998) Requirement for IL-13 independently of IL-4 in experimental asthma. Science 282:2261–2263

Gulliver T, Eid N (2005) Effects of glucocorticoids on the hypothalamic-pituitary-adrenal axis in children and adults. Immunol Allergy Clin North Am 25:541–555

Hajiro T, Nishimura K (2002) Minimal clinically significant difference in health status: the thorny path of health status measures? Eur Respir J 19:390–391

Hakonarson H, Carter C, Kim C, Grunstein M (1999) Altered expression and action of the low-affinity IgE receptor FcεRII (CD23) in asthmatic airway smooth muscle. J Allergy Clin Immunol 104:575–584

Harding (2005) Gastroesophageal reflux: a potential asthma trigger. Immunol Allergy Clin N Am 25:131–148

Hochberg MC, Lebwohl MG, Plevy SE, Hobbs KF, Yocum DE (2005) The benefit/risk profile of TNF-blocking agents: findings of a consensus panel. Semin Arthritis Rheum 34:819–836

Hochhaus G, Brookman L, Fox H, Johnson C, Matthews J, Ren S, Deniz Y (2003) Pharmacodynamics of omalizumab: implications for optimised dosing strategies and clinical efficacy in the treatment of allergic asthma. Curr Med Res Opin 19:491–498

Holgate ST, Chuchalin AG, Hebert J, Lotvall J, Persson GB, Chung KF, Bousquet J, Kerstjens HA, Fox H, Thirlwell J, Cioppa GD (2004) Efficacy and safety of a recombinant anti-immunoglobulin E antibody (omalizumab) in severe allergic asthma. Clin Exp Allergy 34:632–638

Holt P, Macaubas C, Stumbles P, Sly P (1999) The role of allergy in the development of asthma. Nature 402:B12–B17

Howarth PH, Babu KS, Arshad HS, Lau L, Buckley M, McConnell W, Beckett P, Al Ali M, Chauhan A, Wilson SJ, Reynolds A, Davies DE, Holgate ST (2005) Tumour necrosis factor (TNFα) as a novel therapeutic target in symptomatic corticosteroid dependent asthma. Thorax 60:1012–1018

Humbert M, Beasley R, Ayres J, Slavin R, Hebert J, Bousquet J, Beeh KM, Ramos S, Canonica GW, Hedgecock S, Fox H, Blogg M, Surrey K (2005) Benefits of omalizumab as add-on therapy in patients with severe persistent asthma who are inadequately controlled despite best available therapy (GINA 2002 step 4 treatment): INNOVATE. Allergy 60:309–316

Humbert M, Durham SR, Kimmitt P, Powell N, Assoufi B, Pfister R, Menz G, Kay AB, Corrigan CJ (1997) Elevated expression of messenger ribonucleic acid encoding IL-13 in the bronchial mucosa of atopic and nonatopic subjects with asthma. J Allergy Clin Immunol 99:657–665

Hyams JS, Markowitz J, Wyllie R (2000) Use of infliximab in the treatment of Crohn's disease in children and adolescents. J Pediatr 137:192–196

Jain S, Bandi V, Officer T, Wolley M, Guntupalli K (2006) Role of vocal cord function and dysfunction in patients presenting with symptoms of acute asthma exacerbation. J Asthma 43:207–212

Jiang H, Harris MB, Rothman P (2000) IL-4/IL-13 signaling beyond JAK/STAT. J Allergy Clin Immunol 105:1063–1070

Jones PW (2002) Interpreting thresholds for a clinically significant change in health status in asthma and COPD. Eur Respir J 19:398–404

Juniper E (1999) Health-related quality of life in asthma. Curr Opin Pulm Med 5:105–110

Juniper E, Guyatt G, Epstein R, Ferrie P, Jaeschke R, Hiller T (1992) Evaluation of impairment of health-related quality of life in asthma: development of a questionnaire for use in clinical trials. Thorax 47:76–83

Keane J, Gershon S, Wise RP, Mirabile-Levens E, Kasznica J, Schwieterman WD, Siegel JN, Braun MM (2001) Tuberculosis associated with infliximab, a tumor necrosis factor α-neutralizing agent. N Engl J Med 345:1098–1104

Keatings VM, Jatakanon A, Worsdell YM, Barnes PJ (1997) Effects of inhaled and oral glucocorticoids on inflammatory indices in asthma and COPD. Am J Respir Crit Care Med 155:542–548

Kim J, McKinley L, Natarajan S, Bolgos GL, Siddiqui J, Copeland S, Remick DG (2006) Anti-tumor necrosis factor-alpha antibody treatment reduces pulmonary inflammation and methacholine hyper-responsiveness in a murine asthma model induced by house dust. Clin Exp Allergy 36:122–132

Kips JC, O'Connor BJ, Langley SJ, Woodcock A, Kerstjens HAM, Postma DS, Danzig M, Cuss F, Pauwels RA (2003) Effect of SCH55700, a humanized anti-human interleukin-5 antibody, in severe persistent asthma: a pilot study. Am J Respir Crit Care Med 167:1655–1659

Kitaura J, Song J, Tsai M, Asai K, Maeda-Yamamoto M, Mocsai A, Kawakami Y, Liu F-T, Lowell CA, Barisas BG, Galli SJ, Kawakami T (2003) Evidence that IgE molecules mediate a spectrum of effects on mast cell survival and activation via aggregation of the FcεRI. PNAS 100:12911–12916

Kroegel C, Julius P, Matthys H, Virchow Jc, Jr., Luttmann W (1996) Endobronchial secretion of interleukin-13 following local allergen challenge in atopic asthma: relationship to interleukin-4 and eosinophil counts. Eur Respir J 9:899–904

Kroesen S, Widmer AF, Tyndall A, Hasler P (2003) Serious bacterial infections in patients with rheumatoid arthritis under anti-TNF-α therapy. Rheumatology 42:617–621

Kuehr J, Brauburger J, Zielen S, Schauer U, Kamin W, Von Berg A, Leupold W, Bergmann K-C, Rolinck-Werninghaus C, Grave M (2002) Efficacy of combination treatment with anti-IgE plus specific immunotherapy in polysensitized children and adolescents with seasonal allergic rhinitis. J Allergy Clin Immunol 109:274–280

Kulczycki A, Isersky C, Metzger H (1974) The interaction of IgE with rat basophilic leukemia cells. I. Evidence for specific binding of IgE. J Exp Med 139:600–616

Leckie MJ, Brinke At, Khan J, Diamant Z, O'Connor BJ, Walls CM, Mathur AK, Cowley HC, Chung KF, Djukanovic R (2000) Effects of an interleukin-5 blocking monoclonal antibody on eosinophils, airway hyper-responsiveness, and the late asthmatic response. Lancet 356:2144–2148

Lemanske RF, Jr., Nayak A, McAlary M, Everhard F, Fowler-Taylor A, Gupta N (2002) Omalizumab improves asthma-related quality of life in children with allergic asthma. Pediatrics
110:e55

Leung DYM, Sampson HA, Yunginger JW, Burks AW, Jr., Schneider LC, Wortel CH, Davis FM,
Hyun JD, Shanahan WR, Jr., the TNXPASG (2003) Effect of anti-IgE therapy in patients with
peanut allergy. N Engl J Med 348:986–993

Li Y-F, Gauderman WJ, Avol E, Dubeau L, Gilliland FD (2006) Associations of tumor necrosis
factor G-308A with childhood asthma and wheezing. Am J Respir Crit Care Med 173:970–976

Liu J, Lester P, Builder S, Shire SJ (1995) Characterization of Complex formation by humanized
anti-IgE monoclonal antibody and monoclonal human IgE. Biochemistry 34:10474–10482

Lugogo NL, Kraft M (2006) Epidemiology of asthma. Clin Chest Med 27:1–15

MacGlashan D (1993) Releasability of human basophils: cellular sensitivity and maximal histamine release are independent variables. J Allergy Clin Immunol 91:605–615

MacGlashan DW, Jr., Bochner BS, Adelman DC, Jardieu PM, Togias A, McKenzie-White J,
Sterbinsky SA, Hamilton RG, Lichtenstein LM (1997) Down-regulation of FcεRI expres-
sion on human basophils during in vivo treatment of atopic patients with anti-IgE antibody.
J Immunol 158:1438–1445

Malveaux F, Conroy M, Adkinson NJ, LM L (1978) IgE receptors on human basophils. Relationship to serum IgE concentration. J Clin Invest 62:176–181

Mannino DM, Homa DM, Akinbami LJ, Moorman JE, Gwynn C, Redd SC (2000) Surveillance
for Asthma – United States, 1980–1999.

Marcus P (2006) Incorporating anti-IgE (omalizumab) therapy into pulmonary medicine practice:
practice management implications. Chest 129:466–474

Martinez FD, Wright AL, Taussig LM, Holberg CJ, Halonen M, Morgan WJ (1995) Asthma and
wheezing in the first six years of life. N Engl J Med 332:133–138

Maurer D, Ebner C, Reininger B, Fiebiger E, Kraft D, Kinet JP, Stingl G (1995) The high affinity
IgE receptor (FcεRI) mediates IgE-dependent allergen presentation. J Immunol 154:6285–6290

Milgrom H, Berger W, Nayak A, Gupta N, Pollard S, McAlary M, Taylor AF, Rohane P (2001)
Treatment of childhood asthma with anti-immunoglobulin E antibody (omalizumab). Pediatrics
108:e36

Milgrom H, Fick R, Su J, Reimann J, Bush R, Watrous M, Metzger W (1999a) Treatment of allergic
asthma with monoclonal anti-IgE antibody. N Engl J Med 341:1966–1973

Milgrom H, Fick RB, Su JQ, Reimann JD, Bush RK, Watrous ML, Metzger WJ, The rhu M-
ESG (1999b) Treatment of allergic asthma with monoclonal anti-IgE antibody. N Engl J Med
341:1966–1973

Mingomataj EC, Xhixha F, Gjata E (2006) Helminths can protect themselves against rejection
inhibiting hostile respiratory allergy symptoms. Allergy 61:400–406

Mukhopadhyay S, Hoidal J, Mukherjee T (2006) Role of TNFα in pulmonary pathophysiology.
Respir Res 7:125

NAEEP (1997) National Asthma Education and Prevention Program Expert Panel Report 2: Guidelines for the Diagnosis and Management of Asthma. NIH

NAEEP (2002) Expert Panel Report 2: Guidelines for the Diagnosis and Management of
Asthma – Update on Selected Topics (2002). NIH

NHLBI (1991) Guidelines for the Diagnosis and Management of Asthma: I. Definition and diagnosis. J Allergy Clin Immunol 88:427–438

NHLBI/WHO (2002) Global Initiative for asthma: global strategy for asthma management and
prevention. NIH

Oba Y, Salzman GA (2004) Cost-effectiveness analysis of omalizumab in adults and adolescents
with moderate-to-severe allergic asthma. J Allergy Clin Immunol 114:265–269

Ober C, Hoffjan S (2006) Asthma genetics 2006: the long and winding road to gene discovery.
Genes Immunol 7:95–100

Oettgen HC, Geha RS (2001) IgE regulation and roles in asthma pathogenesis. J Allergy Clin
Immunol 107:429–440

Ohkawara Y, Lei XF, Stampfli MR, Marshall JS, Xing Z, Jordana M (1997) Cytokine and eosinophil responses in the lung, peripheral blood, and bone marrow compartments in a murine model of allergen-induced airways inflammation. Am J Respir Cell Mol Biol 16:510–520

Ong YE, Menzies-Gow A, Barkans J, Benyahia F, Ou T-T, Ying S, Kay AB (2005) Anti-IgE (omalizumab) inhibits late-phase reactions and inflammatory cells after repeat skin allergen challenge. J Allergy Clin Immunol 116:558–564

Parks KW, Casale TB (2006) Anti–immunoglobulin E monoclonal antibody administered with immunotherapy. Allergy Asthma Proc 27:33–36

Pennings HJ, Kramer K, Bast A, Buurman WA, Wouters EF (1998) Tumour necrosis factor-alpha induces hyperreactivity in tracheal smooth muscle of the guinea-pig in vitro. Eur Respir J 12:45–49

Presta L, Shields R, O'Connell L, Lahr S, Porter J, Gorman C, Jardieu P (1994) The binding site on human immunoglobulin E for its high affinity receptor. J Biol Chem 269:26368–26373

Presta LG, Lahr SJ, Shields RL, Porter JP, Gorman CM, Fendly BM, Jardieu PM (1993) Humanization of an antibody directed against IgE. J Immunol 151:2623–2632

Prussin C, Griffith DT, Boesel KM, Lin H, Foster B, Casale TB (2003) Omalizumab treatment downregulates dendritic cell FcεRI expression. J Allergy Clin Immunol 112:1147–1154

Prussin C, Metcalfe DD (2006) IgE, mast cells, basophils, and eosinophils. J Allergy Clin Immunol 117:S450–S456

Qureshi F, Pestian J, Davis P, Zaritsky A (1998) Effect of nebulized ipratropium on the hospitalization rates of children with asthma. N Engl J Med 339:1030–1035

Reeves MJ, Bohm SR, Korzeniewski SJ, Brown MD (2006) Asthma care and management before an emergency department visit in children in Western Michigan: how well does care adhere to guidelines? Pediatrics 117:S118–126

Rieves D (2003) FDA medical officer's review of safety information on omalizumab in briefing BLA STN 103976/0. Food and Drug Administration, Washington, DC

Roberts NJ, Robinson DS, Partridge MR (2006) How is difficult asthma managed? Eur Respir J 28:968–973

Roskos LK, Davis CG, Schwab GM (2004) The clinical pharmacology of therapeutic monoclonal antibodies. Drug Development Res 61:108–120

Rychly D, DiPiro J (2005) Infections associated with tumor necrosis factor-alpha antagonists. Pharmacotherapy 25:1181–1192

Saini SS, MacGlashan DW, Jr., Sterbinsky SA, Togias A, Adelman DC, Lichtenstein LM, Bochner BS (1999) Down-regulation of human basophil IgE and FCεRIα surface densities and mediator release by anti-IgE-infusions is reversible in vitro and in vivo. J Immunol 162:5624–5630

Schulman ES (2001) Development of a monoclonal anti-immunoglobulin E antibody (Omalizumab) for the treatment of allergic respiratory disorders. Am J Respir Crit Care Med 164:6S–11

Scott DL, Kingsley GH (2006) Tumor necrosis factor inhibitors for rheumatoid arthritis. N Engl J Med 355:704–712

Shields R, Whether W, Zioncheck K, O'Connell L, Fendly B, Presta L, Thomas D, Saban R, Jardieu P (1995) Inhibition of allergic reactions with antibodies to IgE. Int Arch Allergy Immunol 107:308–312

Slavin RG, Haselkorn T, Lee JH, Zheng B, Deniz Y, Wenzel SE (2006) Asthma in older adults: observations from the epidemiology and natural history of asthma: outcomes and treatment regimens (TENOR) study. Ann Allergy, Asthma Immunol 96:406–414

Soler M, Matz J, Townley R, Buhl R, O'Brien J, Fox H, Thirlwell J, Gupta N, Della Cioppa G (2001) The anti-IgE antibody omalizumab reduces exacerbations and steroid requirement in allergic asthmatics. Eur Respir J 18:254–261

Sporik R, Holgate ST, Platts-Mills TA, Cogswell JJ (1990) Exposure to house-dust mite allergen (Der p I) and the development of asthma in childhood. A prospective study. N Engl J Med 323:502–507

Strunk RC, Bloomberg GR (2006) Omalizumab for Asthma. N Engl J Med 354:2689–2695

Strunk RC, Szefler SJ, Phillips BR, Zeiger RS, Chinchilli VM, Larsen G, Hodgdon K, Morgan W, Sorkness CA, Lemanske JRF (2003) Relationship of exhaled nitric oxide to clinical and inflammatory markers of persistent asthma in children. J Allergy Clin Immunol 112:883–892

Thomas P, Heywood G (2002) Effects of inhaled tumour necrosis factor alpha in subjects with mild asthma. Thorax 57:774–778

Thomas PS, Yates DH, Barnes PJ (1995) Tumor necrosis factor-alpha increases airway responsiveness and sputum neutrophilia in normal human subjects. Am J Respir Crit Care Med 152:76–80

Upham JW (2003) The role of dendritic cells in immune regulation and allergic airway inflammation. Respirology 8:140–148

van der Vaart H, Koeter GH, Postma DS, Kauffman HF, ten Hacken NHT (2005) First study of infliximab treatment in patients with chronic obstructive pulmonary disease. Am J Respir Crit Care Med 172:465–469

Vignola AM, Humbert M, Bousquet J, Boulet LP, Hedgecock S, Blogg M, Fox H, Surrey K (2004) Efficacy and tolerability of anti-immunoglobulin E therapy with omalizumab in patients with concomitant allergic asthma and persistent allergic rhinitis: SOLAR. Allergy 59:709–717

Walker S, Monteil M, Phelan K, Lasserson T, EHW (2006) Anti-IgE for chronic asthma in adults and children. Cochrane Database Syst Rev

Walsh GM (2005) Novel therapies for asthma – advances and problems. Curr Pharm Design 11:3027–3038

Walsh GM (2006) Targeting airway inflammation: novel therapies for the treatment of asthma. Curr Med Chem 13:3105–3111

Wijnhoven HAH, Kriegsman DMW, Hesselink AE, Penninx BWJH, de Haan M (2001) Determinants of different dimensions of disease severity in asthma and COPD: pulmonary function and health-related quality of life. Chest 119:1034–1042

Wills-Karp M, Luyimbazi J, Xu X, Schofield B, Neben TY, Karp CL, Donaldson DD (1998) Interleukin-13: central mediator of allergic asthma. Science 282:2258–2261

Wood KL, Hage CA, Knox KS, Kleiman MB, Sannuti A, Day RB, Wheat LJ, Twigg HL, III (2003) Histoplasmosis after Treatment with Anti-Tumor Necrosis Factor-α Therapy. Am J Respir Crit Care Med 167:1279–1282

Yazdanbakhsh M, van den Biggelaar A, Maizels RM (2001) Th2 responses without atopy: immunoregulation in chronic helminth infections and reduced allergic disease. Trends Immunol 22:372–377

Yigla M, Tov N, Solomonov A, Rubin A, Harlev D (2003) Difficult-to-control asthma and obstructive sleep apnea. J Asthma 40:865–871

Part V
Development of Antibody-Based Cellular and Molecular Therapies

Cytokine, Chemokine, and Co-Stimulatory Fusion Proteins for the Immunotherapy of Solid Tumors

L.A. Khawli, P. Hu, and A.L. Epstein(✉)

1 Introduction 292
2 Overview of Cancer Immunotherapy. 293
   2.1 Antibody-Targeted Immunotherapy 294
   2.2 Untargeted Soluble Fc Fusion Protein Immunotherapy 295
3 Immunoregulatory Molecules 296
   3.1 Cytokines. 296
   3.2 Chemokines. 299
   3.3 B7 Costimulation 305
   3.4 TNFSF Ligands 309
   3.5 Immunoregulatory T Cells (Treg) 314
4 Conclusions 320
References 324

Abstract This chapter describes the generation of novel reagents for the treatment of cancer using fusion proteins constructed with natural ligands of the immune system. Immunotherapy is a powerful therapeutic modality that has not been fully harnessed for the treatment of cancer. We and others have hypothesized that if the proper immunoregulatory ligands can be targeted to the tumor, an effective immune response can be mounted to treat both established primary tumors and distant metastatic lesions. Though it is generally believed that immunotherapy has the potential to treat only residual disease, we offer evidence that this approach can, by itself, destroy large tumor masses and produce lasting remissions of experimental solid tumors. From these studies, three major classes of immune activators, namely, cytokines, chemokines, and costimulatory molecules, have been shown to generate antitumor responses in animal models. In addition, the reversal of immune tolerance

A.L. Epstein
Department of Pathology, USC Keck School of Medicine, 2011 Zonal Avenue, HMR 205, Los Angeles, CA 90033, USA
e-mail: aepstein@usc.edu

Y. Chernajovsky, A. Nissim (eds.) *Therapeutic Antibodies. Handbook of Experimental Pharmacology 181.*
© Springer-Verlag Berlin Heidelberg 2008

by the deletion of T regulatory (Treg) cells has been shown to be equally important for effective immunotherapy. In an attempt to identify reagents that can provide an enhanced immune stimulation and treatment of cancer, our laboratory has developed a novel monoclonal antibody targeting approach, designated Tumor Necrosis Therapy (TNT), which utilizes stable intracellular antigens present in all cell types but which are only accessible in dead and/or dying cells. Since tumors contain necrotic and degenerating regions that account for 30–80% of the tumor mass, this targeting approach can be used to deliver therapeutic reagents to the core of tumors, a site abundant in tumor antigens. In our first set of reagents, a panel of cytokine fusion proteins was genetically engineered using monoclonal antibody chimeric TNT-3 (chTNT-3) directed against necrotic regions of tumors (single-stranded DNA) fused with IL-2, or GM-CSF, or TNFα, or IFNγ. Tested against different solid tumors, these reagents were found to mount an effective although transient immune response to tumor especially when used in combination. To improve upon these results, additional chTNT-3 fusion proteins using the liver-expression chemokine (LEC) and the costimulatory molecule B7.1 were constructed. Both of these reagents were found to work significantly better than the above cytokine fusion proteins due to their ability to stimulate multiple arms of the immune system deemed useful for cancer immunotherapy. Finally, the Tumor Necrosis Factor Superfamily (TNFSF) gene *CD137L* was used to generate chTNT-3 antibody (targeted) and soluble Fc (untargeted) fusion proteins. When used alone, both forms of costimulatory fusion proteins were found to produce in a dose-dependent manner, complete regression of murine solid tumors. Evidence is presented to show that Treg cells play an important role in suppressing antitumor immunity since the deletion of these cells, when used in combination with LEC or costimulatory fusion proteins, produced profound and effective treatment with sustained memory. It is hoped that these data will further the preclinical development of soluble Fc and antibody based fusion proteins for the immunotherapy of cancer.

1 Introduction

Immunotherapy is a powerful therapeutic modality that utilizes the patient's own immune system to attack and eliminate tumor cells. To ensure the clinical potential of this approach, our laboratory is investigating ways to enhance the antitumor response of the host at the tumor site, thereby minimizing systemic toxicity. To do so, we have genetically engineered fusion proteins composed of the Tumor Necrosis Therapy (TNT) monoclonal antibody, which targets single stranded DNA exposed in degenerating cells (Epstein et al. 1988, 1991; Chen et al. 1991; Miller et al. 1993; Hornick et al. 1998) linked to immune effector or ligands molecules. These fusion proteins are able to target solid tumors in immunocompetent mice, overcome peripheral tolerance, and incite an effective antitumor immune response that brings about tumor regression in solid tumor models. Our laboratory has successfully generated a number of new TNT fusion protein, including one with the CC liver-expression chemokine (LEC, CCL16), demonstrated to be a very potent chemoattractant to PMNs, T cells, macrophages, B-cells, and dendritic cells (Giovarelli et al. 2000; Hisayuki et al. 2001). These studies confirmed the ability of LEC/chTNT-3 to induce a multiarmed immune response against solid tumors by attracting APC and effector cells into the tumor to induce significant tumor regression (Li et al. 2003a). More recently, we have found that tumor regression can also be achieved through the use of the costimulatory molecule B7.1 (Liu et al. 2005), the APC molecule that activates T cells by delivering a second signal via binding to CD28. While investigating which T-cell subpopulations are required for LEC and B7.1 activity, we discovered that depletion of $CD4^+$ or $CD4^+CD25^+$ immunoregulatory T cells (Tregs) greatly enhanced LEC and B7.1 activity, resulting in complete and lasting remissions of established solid tumors in BALB/c mice (Li et al. 2003b, 2005). Finally, the laboratory has discovered that fusion proteins consisting of costimulatory proteins such as CD137L which enhance immunity are very effective in suppressing tumor growth in syngeneic tumor models of the mouse.

The overall goal of our laboratory is to develop reagents that can be successfully translated to the clinic for the treatment of solid tumors. In general, current treatment modalities of surgery, radiation, and chemotherapy are nonspecific, in that they remove or destroy normal cells along with the cancer cells. Other factors that limit the effectiveness of current therapeutic modalities include the presence of distant metastases, tumor cell heterogeneity, and the resistance of tumors to drugs and radiation (Mocellin et al. 2002) especially after repeated treatment. Systemic treatments for solid tumors with standard chemotherapy agents are largely ineffective, leaving the clinician few options to treat this lethal group of tumors. Therefore, new approaches to therapy are needed to provide the oncologist with viable treatment alternatives (Dy and Adjei 2002). Immunotherapy is a promising approach that utilizes the patient's own immune system to destroy evolving tumor. Once thought to be a method of treatment for minimal residual disease only, our laboratory and others now believe that this form of therapy has the potential to destroy larger primary tumors and distant metastatic lesions. The key immune molecules for accomplishing this have been identified and fall into three classes of potent modulators called cytokines, chemokines, and costimulatory molecules. In general, we have focused our studies on the identification of relevant cellular processes associated with effective solid tumor immunotherapy. Those cellular and molecular components of the immune system that have the capacity to treat tumor need to be harnessed and properly presented in order to generate effective cancer therapy.

2 Overview of Cancer Immunotherapy

The goal of cancer immunotherapy is to establish an effective immune response to tumors in patients. As part of the malignant phenotype, tumors have evolved to overcome innate and adaptive immune responses of the host in order to grow and metastasize (Smyth et al. 2001). Historically, investigators have been of the opinion that the immune response against tumors is inherently weak and has insufficient T effector cells to destroy large, established lesions. As evidenced by recent research, however, cancer immunotherapy may have sufficient therapeutic potential to treat and cure deep-seated and established malignancies if properly invoked (Waldmann et al. 2003; Parish 2003; Blattman and Greenberg 2004). For this to happen, however, two key events must occur, namely, the reversal of immune tolerance and the activation of effective immunity with memory. One of the most powerful methods nature has evolved to control the immune system is the generation of Treg cells, the same cells now believed to be one of the major mechanisms responsible for the protection of the fetus in the mother's womb (Aluvaihare et al. 2004). Recent histopathologic and flow cytometric studies, respectively, have shown an increase in Treg cells in the parenchyma of solid tumors or circulating in the blood or cavity fluids of cancer patients (Liyanage et al. 2002; Ichihara et al. 2003; Marshall et al. 2004). Experimentally, methods to suppress Treg cells in tumor-bearing mice using anti-CTLA-4 (Leach et al. 1996), anti-CD4 (North and Awwad 1990), or anti-CD25 (Tanaka et al. 2002; Pardoll 2003) antibodies have provided improved immunotherapy when used alone or with tumor vaccines. The second event that is required for active immunotherapy is the use of potent immunostimulatory agents to evoke an effective immune response against tumor antigens. More recently, our laboratory has shown that combination therapy with an anti-Treg cell antibody and several different fusion proteins is an effective method of reactivating the immune system to tumor (Li et al. 2003; Liu et al. 2005, 2006). By comparison, when these reagents are used alone, they produce only partial responses compared to untreated controls (Strumhoeful et al. 1999; Runyon et al. 2001). As reviewed by Chen (2004) and Yamaguchi et al. (2004), B7-CD28 costimulation (second signal) is an important and vital step in the activation of T cells. Recently, it has been demonstrated that B7-CD28 costimulation can activate both the Th1 and Th2 differentiation pathways and that the latter is dependent on the induction of IL-4. Used systemically, however, this approach can induce unwanted autoimmune side effects such as those seen with anti-CTLA-4 antibody treatment (Sutmuller et al. 2001). These toxic side effects may be substantially decreased if costimulation is targeted to the tumor site and not distributed systemically. In this chapter, we intend to show the effects of different fusion proteins consisting of active immunostimulatory molecules and compare their activity as targeted and untargeted reagents. It is hypothesized that proper immune activation, when used in combination with methods to reverse immune tolerance, can successfully treat established solid tumors.

2.1 Antibody-Targeted Immunotherapy

Immunotherapy has been used to treat tumor-bearing hosts for over a century (Ben-Efraim 1999). Unfortunately, the promise of effective cytokine-based immunotherapy for cancer remains largely unfulfilled. Despite numerous in vitro and in vivo studies demonstrating the stimulatory effects of various cytokines to induce active leukocyte responses against tumor cells, favorable and consistent responses have remained elusive in the actual treatment of human disease. The limitation in clinical efficacy is partly due to the toxic effects observed with traditional administration methods as well as the inability to recreate the microenvironmental conditions required for the generation of specific antitumor immune responses using these reagents (Parmiani et al. 2000; Di Cailo et al. 2001). Systemic infusion produces elevated cytokine levels that lead to a nonspecific activation of immune cells. Rather than a coordinated response limited to tumor, as is seen during naturally occurring immune responses, these bioactive compounds often lead to dysfunctional systemic activation with significant dose-limiting and potentially fatal toxicities (Ben-Efraim 1999). Additionally, treatment protocols that fail to localize these bioactive molecules may not only be unsuccessful in the generation of specific immune activity, but may actually predispose the patient to immunodeficiency states or tolerance (Bubenik et al. 2000). Most recently, it has become recognized that in addition to the induction of an effective immunologic response to tumor, it is also important to produce a lasting response by the development of immunologic memory (Di Cailo et al. 2001). Placed in the correct context, the immune system is capable of massive cell destruction as witnessed by graft vs. host responses and certain autoimmune states. Based upon these observations, it is highly feasible that once harnessed the immune system will be capable of destroying deep-seated primary tumors and metastatic lesions in cancer patients.

In an attempt to identify reagents that can elicit an effective antitumor immune response, we generated a panel of fusion proteins consisting of the tumor targeting monoclonal antibody chTNT-3 that binds to necrotic regions of tumors (Epstein et al. 1988; 1991) and cytokines, chemokines, and costimulatory molecules previously shown to be important components of an antitumor response. At the center of this approach is the TNT antibody, which has a number of important characteristics that make it an ideal delivery agent for immune modulators. These include its applicability to a wide range of human and animal cancers, its inability to bind normal tissues, its long retention time in tumors after targeting, and its ability to target necrotic regions centrally in both primary and metastatic lesions. Because of these attributes, TNT has been used to deliver radionuclides (Hornick et al. 1998), immunostimulatory molecules (Li et al. 2003; Liu et al. 2005; 2006), and vasopermeability agents (Hornick et al. 1999) to treat experimental and human tumors. To date over 250 patients have been treated with ^{131}I-chTNT-3 and the results show that all types of tumors tested can be targeted specifically (Chen et al. 2005; Yu et al. 2006). No uptake has been seen in normal tissues regardless of the age or condition of the patients tested. In June of 2003, ^{131}I-chTNT-3 became the second radiolabeled monoclonal antibody worldwide to obtain FDA approval. The antibody was approved for the treatment of lung cancer and is currently in clinical trials for the treatment of brain and other solid tumors.

2.2 Untargeted Soluble Fc Fusion Protein Immunotherapy

Optimal activation of naïve T cells requires both antigen-specific signaling and the induction of costimulatory pathways (Zou 2005). The absence of costimulatory signaling leads naïve T cells to fail to recognize antigens and become tolerant to cancer cells, a possible strategy by which tumors escape from host immunity (Mapara and Sykes 2004). To break immune tolerance and elicit effective antitumor responses, many strategies have been devised, including the expression of costimulatory molecules (Townsend and Allison 1993; Hodge et al. 1994), blockade of inhibitory signaling using anti-CTLA-4 antibody (Leach et al. 1996), and grafting T cells with the stimulatory receptor CD28 in adoptive immunotherapy (Maher and Davies 2004). In the above studies, suppression of tumor growth was achieved by presenting costimulatory signals directly on the tumor cell surface in transfected cells, by gene therapy and by similar approaches (Singh et al. 2003). All these strategies are promising but have only been met with limited success in experimental therapeutic models. In the past few years, soluble costimulatory proteins fused to the N-terminus of the Fc portion of antibodies have been developed and tested in mouse tumor models (Moro et al. 1999; Zheng et al. 2001). For example, Sturmhoefel et al. (1999) have reported that B7.2-Fc therapy as an adjuvant in cancer vaccines could produce complete tumor rejection in some tumor models, including the poorly-immunogenic B16/F10 tumor. It was concluded that tumor rejection induced by B7.2-Fc was mediated by type 2 CD8$^+$ T cells and was dependent on IL-4 induction (Yamaguchi et al. 2004). Soluble Fc fusion proteins represent a nontargeting approach to provide costimulation or immune activation systemically. Because they do not target tumor in vivo, however, they could produce autoimmune side effects, which may limit their clinical utility. To determine which reagent(s) are most promising for translation to man, we have chosen to generate and compare both tumor-targeted and nontargeted derivatives when possible.

3 Immunoregulatory Molecules

3.1 Cytokines

Cytokines are extracellular protein messenger molecules produced by cells involved in inflammation, immunity, differentiation, cell division, fibrosis, and repair (Smith 1993). Molecular characterization studies have revealed, however, that several cytokines also function as cell surface signaling molecules such as TNFα, IL-1α, TGFβ, and IL-2. A distinctive feature of cytokines is that they are not constitutively produced, but are generated in response to stimulation. Cytokine genes are highly inducible and a number of transcriptional factors such as NFκB, NF-AT, and AP-1 are involved in the regulation and production of their mRNA's (Oppenheim and Feldmann 2001). Typically, their production lasts a few hours to a few days and they usually have a short action radius associated with a very high affinity for receptors. Their high potency is also due to the fact that receptors only require a low occupancy (around 10%) to stimulate immune cells. The usual mechanism of action of cytokines is on neighboring cells and because of their short half-life, which is in the order of minutes, only small amounts ever enter the systemic circulation during inflammation. When administered systemically, cytokines are in general very toxic causing multiple symptoms, including fever, hypotension, headache, malaise, weakness, and capillary leak syndrome, thereby making it difficult to achieve clinically relevant dosages. Importantly, cytokines can act in networks and cascades influencing a number of different immune cells once secreted into an inflamed tissue. Because of their potency, a number of mechanisms exist to regulate their effects in tissues.

The first cytokine to obtain approval for cancer therapy was Interleukin-2 (IL-2) (Rao et al. 1997). IL-2 is a potent cytokine involved in both the cellular and humoral arms of the immune system. Its primary role is to stimulate the growth and proliferation of T lymphocytes. It has also been shown, however, to have stimulatory effects on a variety of immune cells, including natural killer (NK) cells, lymphokine-activated killer (LAK) cells, and tumor infiltrating lymphocytes (TIL) (Rao et al. 1997). While it has shown some promise in the treatment of renal cancer and melanoma (Silagi and Shaefer 1986), its potential is offset by the occurrence of serious adverse reactions with its use, including damage to the blood vessels of the body (capillary leak syndrome). Direct applications in which IL-2 is infused intratumorally has been somewhat more effective and has resulted in a higher level of therapeutic response, including the control of clinical complications, prevention of the growth of established tumors, and reduction in the size of the tumor mass (Sone and Ogura 1994). Unfortunately, this technique is not feasible for disseminated disease.

As mentioned previously, one approach to using these potent cytokines is to link them to tumor targeting MAbs to generate fusion proteins. Toward this end, our laboratory has generated a series of fusion proteins consisting of chTNT-3 and IL-2, murine GM-CSF, TNFα, and murine IFNγ. Gene transfection of transplantable tumors with the above cytokine DNAs has clearly demonstrated that the production of high local concentrations of these cytokines in tumors can stimulate effective antitumor immune responses (Ajani et al. 1989; Morikawa et al. 1989). Based upon this information, targeting these cytokines to the tumor parenchyma is a viable alternative that can be applied to patients once fully human derivatives are constructed. Our laboratory has completed the production of several fusion proteins consisting of chTNT-3 and human IL-2 (LeBerton et al. 1991; Khawli et al. 1994; 1997; Hornick et al. 1999), murine IFNγ (Mizokami et al. 2003), human IFNγ and TNFα (Sharifi et al. 2002), and muGM-CSF (unpublished) genetically linked to the C-terminal portion of chTNT-3. Their construction, testing, and use in immunotherapy experiments are briefly described further.

3.1.1 Cytokine Fusion Proteins

The chTNT-3 (IgG$_1$κ) was constructed and expressed as described previously (Hornick et al. 1999). PCR fragments containing either the human IL-2, IFNγ, or TNFα cDNA preceded by a noncleavable seven amino acid linker peptide was inserted into the NotI site previously appended immediately downstream of the human γ1 terminal codon, producing a TNT-3 VH/human γ1/human cytokine fusion gene. This resulted in the expression vectors pEE12/chTNT-3 HC/hIL-2, pEE12/chTNT-3 HC/muIFNγ, and pEE12/chTNT-3 HC/TNFα, encoding a fusion protein consisting of the chimeric TNT-3 heavy chain with human IL-2, murine IFNγ, or TNFα at its C-terminus. These expression vectors were cotransfected with the expression vector for the chimeric TNT-3 light chain, pEE6/chTNT-3 light chain. The fusion protein was expressed in NS0 murine myeloma cells using the Glutamine Synthetase Gene Amplification System (Lonza) and purified by tandom protein-A affinity and ion-exchange chromatography.

The biological activity of each of the cytokine moieties of the four fusion proteins was determined by in vitro assays. IL-2 bioactivity was demonstrated by testing its ability to support the proliferation of IL-2-dependent CTLL-2 cells (Gillis et al. 1978). For the muTNT-3/muGM-CSF fusion protein, the biological activity of the muGM-CSF moiety was determined by measuring its ability to support the proliferation of the cytokine dependent cell line FDC-P (Delta-Cruz et al. 2000). From this assay, the ED_{50} for muTNT-3/muGM-CSF was shown to be 0.4–1.0 ng ml^{-1}. For the muIFNγ moiety of the chTNT-3/muIFNγ fusion protein, an assay was performed to determine the induction of nitric oxide (NO) in RAW 264.7 murine macrophage cells (Kim and Son 1996). By this method, the specific activity of the chTNT-3/muIFN-γ fusion protein was calculated to be approximately 450 U μg^{-1}. ChTNT-3 was negative in all of the above assays. The biological activity of chTNT-3/muIFN-γ was also measured by up-regulation of MHC class II molecule expression in the WEHI-3 murine myelomonocytic cell line using flow cytometry. Cells were grown in complete media supplemented with recombinant muIFNγ, chTNT-3, or chTNT-3/muIFN-γ for 48 h and then assayed for MHC class II molecule expression by FACS. By this method, the specific activity of the fusion protein was 430 U/μg. In contrast, chTNT-3 was unable to induce MHC class II up-regulation. For the chTNT-3/huTNFα fusion protein, the biological activity of TNFα moiety was determined by the percent inhibition of Hep-2 cell growth as described previously (Hogan 1993). From this assay, the chTNT-3/TNFα fusion protein was found to have a specific activity of 10.8 U μg^{-1}.

Clearance and biodistribution studies were performed to determine pharmacokinetic clearance half-life and tumor uptake of all the fusion proteins. The results of these studies are shown in Table 1. Marked differences in clearance times are noted

Table 1 Summary of pharmacokinetic clearance and biodistribution studies with cytokine fusion proteins

Antibody or antibody/cytokine	Half-life (h)	Tumor model	% Injected dose/gm of tumor at 3 days
chTNT-3	134	MAD 109	13.5
chTNT-3/muIFN-γ	46	MAD 109	2.4
chTNT-3	134	LS174T	7.1
chTNT-3/huIFN-γ	9.1	LS174T	1.2
chTNT-3/huIL-2	12	LS 174 T	1.7
chTNT-3/huTNF-α	8	LS 174 T	1.3
muTNT-3	150	Colon 26	5.3
muTNT-3/muGM-CSF	15	Colon 26	1.27

between the muIFNγ fusion protein and the IL-2, TNFα, and muGM-CSF fusion proteins. The chTNT-3 was found to have an unusually long half-life in these studies. For all the fusion proteins, tumor uptake is significantly lower than that seen for chTNT-3. The tumor-to-organ ratios, however, which reflect normal organ uptake and provide an indication of possible toxicity, are either comparable or even slightly higher for all the fusion proteins.

In summary, the above characterization studies demonstrate that all the fusion proteins are able to maintain their binding affinity to antigen as well as their direct cytotoxic effect and immunomodulatory functions. In vivo, the fusion proteins were found to have a substantially shorter whole body half-life than parental chTNT-3, yet were able to target tumor as shown by biodistribution analyses. Because of their retention in tumor and rapid clearance from normal tissues, the fusion proteins were found to have equivalent or higher normal tissue/tumor ratios than chTNT-3.

3.1.2 Combination Therapy with Cytokine Fusion Proteins

The chTNT-3/cytokine fusion proteins were tested in three different solid tumor models of the BALB/c mouse, including the COLON 26 colon adenocarcinoma, the MAD109 lung carcinoma, and the RENCA renal cell carcinoma. Analysis of the cytokine activity of these fusion proteins using standard in vitro tests shows that they have between 50 and 85% of the activity of the comparable free cytokine tested in parallel. Despite these somewhat lower activity levels, these reagents produced good tumor suppression in the three tumor models during and directly after treatment but 5–7 days after therapy, the tumors continued to progress in size (Fig. 1). In two of these models, those mice receiving the combination of chTNT-3/IL-2, chTNT-3/TNFα, and chTNT-3/IFNγ had the best tumor regression estimated to be about 80% of control groups at day 17. Although individual fusion proteins had varying degrees of effectiveness in these tumor models, this combination or the one in which muTNT-3/muGM-CSF was substituted for the chTNT-3/IL-2 was most effective. Because of species differences associated with the use of a chimeric antibody and human cytokines in the construction of most of these fusion proteins, treatments were limited to daily doses for 4–5 days. Since the tumors were found to continue growing at about the same pace as control treated mice, the therapeutic effect of these treatments was found to be transient in nature. This incomplete immune response may have been due to the nongeneration of immune memory cells.

3.2 Chemokines

Chemokines are small (7–15 kDa), secreted, and structurally related soluble proteins that are involved in leukocyte and dendritic cell chemotaxis, PMN degranulation, and angiogenesis (Mackay 2001). Based on the position and number of cysteine residues, they are divided into four families: CXC (α), CC (β), C (γ), and CX_3C. Because of their important role in the immune system, chemokines have

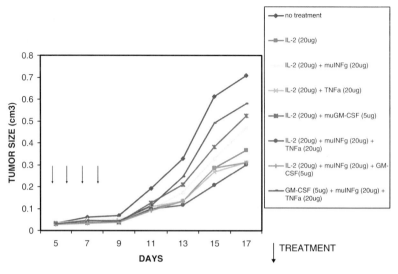

Fig. 1 Combination immunotherapy using TNT-3/cytokine fusion proteins in RENCA renal carcinoma tumor model. Each fusion protein is abbreviated in the chart by listing the cytokine moiety (IL-2, GM-CSF, IFNγ, and TNFα). For these studies, 6-week-old female BALB/C mice were injected subcutaneously with 5×10^6 tumor cells in the left flank. Five-seven days later when the tumors reached 0.5 cm in diameter ($0.2 \, \text{cm}^3$), groups of mice ($n = 5$) were injected daily for four consecutive days with intravenous injection of 0.1 ml inoculum of each fusion protein. The dose of the fusion proteins was 20 μg except for chTNT-3/muGM-CSF, which was more toxic necessitating the use of 5 μg/dose. Control groups received saline only or 20 μg of chTNT-3, which did not affect the growth curves of the three tumor models. A study of control groups from four individual experiments showed that the growth curves were very reproducible

been utilized to treat inflammatory and autoimmune diseases (Gerard and Rollins 2001), HIV, and cancer (Miyagishi et al. 1995). Because of their ability to recruit leukocytes into tumors, alter tumor vasculature structure, and stimulate host anti-cancer immune responses, chemokines are promising reagents in cancer therapy. The human chemokine LEC (liver-expression chemokine, CCL16, also known as NCC-4, LMC, and HCC-4) was originally found in an expression sequence tag library and later mapped to chromosome 17q in the CC chemokine cluster (Naruse et al. 1996). The *LEC* gene in the mouse is a pseudogene that has lost its function due to the insertion of an intron (Naruse et al. 1996). LEC (also known as NCC-4, LMC, and HCC-4) was also found to chemoattract monocytes, lymphocytes, and polymorphonuclear lymphocytes (PMNS) upon binding to CCR1 and CCR8 chemokine receptors (Howard et al. 2000). LEC is unique because unlike any other chemokine, it is the first chemokine whose mRNA expression is strongly increased and stabilized by the presence of IL-10. In vitro studies indicate that LEC requires a much higher concentration to induce maximum chemotaxis than it does for adhesion (Moser and Loetscher 2001). The potential therapeutic applications of LEC were first studied by Giovarelli et al. (2000), who showed that mammary carcinoma TSA cells engineered to express LEC inhibit the metastatic spread of tumor and induce tumor rejection due to an impressive infiltration of macrophages, dendritic cells, T cells, and PMNs, and the production of IFN-γ and IL-12. Furthermore, LEC is a potent chemotactic factor for both human monocytes and dendritic cells (APC cells) (Thelen 2001). Rejection of tumor by the secretion of LEC involves both CD8+ lymphocytes and PMNS (Giovarelli et al. 2000). In these mice, an anti-tumor immune memory was quickly established after rejection as shown by rechallenging experiments. The ability of LEC to improve markedly the recognition of poorly immunogenic tumor cells by promoting APC-T cell interaction establishes it as a prime candidate for targeted immunotherapy. As shown below, we describe the generation and testing of an antibody/chemokine fusion protein consisting of chTNT-3 and LEC, which targets central necrotic areas of tumor to chemoattract and amplify responding lymphoid and dendritic cells capable of inducing an effective antitumor immune response in three different experimental solid tumors of the mouse (Li et al. 2003a).

3.2.1 Chemokine Fusion Proteins

Since the N-terminus of chemokines is essential for bioactivity, we fused the C-terminus of the *LEC* gene to the N-terminus of the chTNT-3 heavy chain gene with a five amino acid universal linker (Gly4Ser). The fused LEC/chTNT-3 heavy chain gene (Fig. 2a) was translated under an antibody leader and the expressed fusion protein was found to retain its biological activities. The bioactivity of the

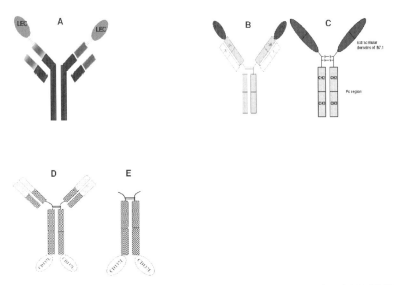

Fig. 2 Schematic diagram depicting the construction of different fusion proteins: (**a**) LEC/chTNT-3, (**b**) human B7.1/NHS76, (**c**) B7.1-Fc (N-terminal), (**d**) murine TNT-3/CD137L, and (**e**) murine Fc-CD137L (C-terminal)

302

L.A. Khawli et al.

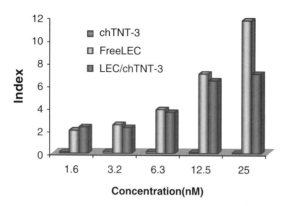

Fig. 3 Chemotaxic activity of LEC/chTNT-3. THP-1 human monocytic leukemia cells were used in a chemotaxis chamber (Neuroprobe, Gaithersburg, MD) to determine the biologic activity of the LEC/chTNT-3, free LEC, and chTNT-3 (negative control)

LEC fusion protein was demonstrated by measuring the migration of target cells in a 96-well microchemotaxis chamber. As shown in Fig. 3, free human recombinant LEC and the fusion protein induced human leukemia THP-1 cell migration. The migration of THP-1 cells exposed to the fusion protein was dose-dependent starting at a concentration as low as 1.6 nM and peaking at concentration of 12.5 nM. Free human recombinant LEC peaked at a higher concentration of about 25 nM in this assay. THP-1 cells exposed to the parental antibody (chTNT-3) did not show any migration verifying the biological activity of the LEC moiety of the fusion protein.

Biodistribution studies were performed to determine tumor uptake of the fusion protein. ^{125}I-LEC/chTNT-3 demonstrated a tumor uptake of 2.4% injected dose per gram (ID/g) at both 12 and 24 h post-injection (Fig. 4). The rapid clearance of ^{125}I-LEC/chTNT-3 also showed a decrease in radioactivity levels in blood and most of the other normal tissues at all time points, resulting in high tumor-to-organ ratios. These data demonstrate that the radiolabeled LEC/chTNT-3 specifically bound to tumor with excellent retention at the tumor site.

3.2.2 LEC Fusion Protein Treatment, Alone

The immunotherapeutic potential of LEC/chTNT-3 was demonstrated by treating groups of BALB/c mice that had been injected subcutaneously in the left flank with MAD109 murine lung carcinoma cells, COLON 26 cells, or RENCA cells. As shown in Fig. 5, LEC/chTNT-3 treatment produced a 55% tumor growth reduction in the COLON 26 tumor model, a 42% reduction in the RENCA tumor model, and a 37% reduction in the MAD109 lung tumor model, as compared to untreated controls. Importantly, LEC/chTNT-3 immunotherapy was found to be entirely nontoxic (even at 100 μg), in marked contrast to the use of chTNT-3/IL-2, chTNT-3/TNFα, and TNT-3/mGM-CSF fusion proteins, which demonstrated varying degrees of

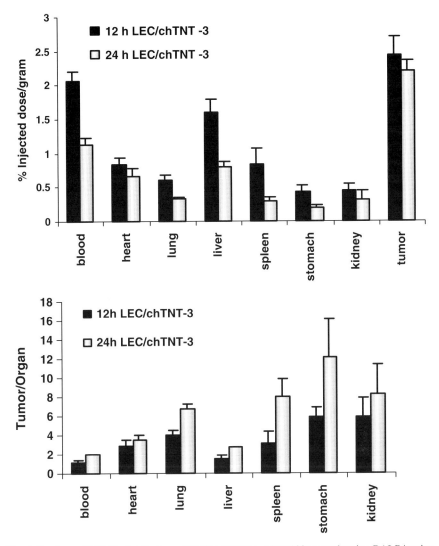

Fig. 4 Twelve and 24 h biodistribution of LEC/chTNT-3 in MAD109 tumor-bearing BALB/c mice. Tumor uptake was measured by (**a**) percent injected dose/gram of ^{125}I-labeled LEC/chTNT-3 and (**b**) tumor/normal organ ratio

toxicity when increased above 20 μg per dose. Treatment with these three fusion proteins at doses exceeding 20 μg made the mice lethargic, induced a ruffled fur appearance, produced a loss of appetite, and lowered activity levels of treated mice. Toxicity at the organ and cellular levels has not been investigated to date. Recently, a nontargeted LEC fusion protein consisting of human LEC and soluble Fc (LEC-Fc) was constructed and is currently being tested for potency and therapeutic potential.

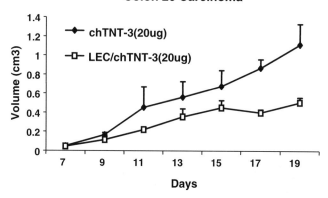

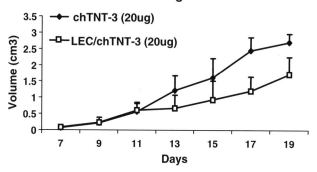

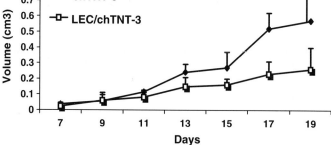

Fig. 5 LEC/chTNT-3 immunotherapy in three murine solid tumor models (Y axis is defined as Tumor Volume). This was demonstrated by treating groups ($n = 7$) of six-week old female BALB/c mice that had been injected subcutaneously in the left flank with 10^7 MAD109 murine lung carcinoma cells, COLON 26 cells, or RENCA cells. Tumors were grown until they reached 0.5 cm in diameter (5–7 days), and groups of mice were then treated daily for 5 days with intravenous injection of 0.1 ml LEC/chTNT-3 (20 µg), PBS, or control chTNT-3 (20 µg). Control studies showed that treatment with chTNT-3 antibody alone does yields no effect

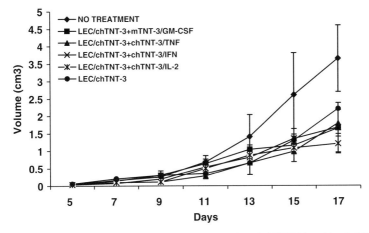

Fig. 6 Combination immunotherapy studies of LEC/chTNT-3 and chTNT-3/cytokine in MAD109-bearing BALB/c mice (*Y* axis is defined as Tumor Volume)

3.2.3 Combination Therapy with LEC and Cytokine Fusion Proteins

To enhance the therapeutic effectiveness of the LEC/chTNT-3, we focused our attention on combining this reagent with other fusion proteins that we and others have found to be critical components of cancer immunotherapy. For these studies, six-week-old female BALB/c mice were inoculated subcutaneously with approximately 5×10^6 MAD109 murine lung adenocarcinoma cells. Five days later when tumors reached 0.5 cm in diameter, the mice were injected with 0.1 ml of inoculum containing 20 µg of LEC/chTNT-3 alone or with 20 µg of chTNT-3/IFNγ, chTNT-3/TNFα, chTNT 3/GM CSF, or chTNT-3/IL-2. All groups were treated daily for 5 days and tumor growth was monitored every other day by caliper measurement in three dimensions. As shown in Fig. 6, combination therapy with LEC/chTNT-3 and each of the four chTNT-3/cytokine fusion proteins produced only minimal improvement but the combination containing the chTNT-3/IL-2 did show flattening of the growth curve by day 17.

3.3 B7 Costimulation

The growth and metastasis of tumors depends to a large extent on their capacity to evade host immune surveillance and overcome host defenses. Most tumors express antigens that can be recognized to a variable extent by the host immune system, but in many cases, an inadequate immune response is elicited because of the ineffective activation of effector T cells. Studies showed that the weak immunogenicity of tumor antigens might be due to inappropriate or absent expression of costimulatory molecules on tumor cells (Abken et al. 2002). For most T cells, proliferation and IL-2 production will not occur unless a costimulatory signal is also provided. In the absence of costimulatory signals during TCR engagement, T cells enter a functionally unresponsive state, referred to as clonal anergy. One of the major signaling pathways involved in delivering the costimulatory signal is mediated by interaction between CD28 on T cells and the B7 family members, including B7.1 (CD80) and B7.2 (CD86) on APC (Hatcock et al. 1994).

B7.1 was first discovered as a B-cell antigen in 1989 and it has been the most intensively investigated costimulatory molecule to date. T cell-mediated rejection of tumors is achieved by presenting costimulatory signals directly on the tumor cells surface. Transfection of several murine tumor cells with B7.1 or B7.2 genes induced T cell-dependent rejection of B7-expressing tumors in mice and protected against tumor challenge with parental tumor cells. These data suggest that the presentation of B7 molecules on the tumor cell surface in vivo might be a promising novel approach for cancer immunotherapy. Other strategies to decorate tumor cells with the costimulatory B7.1 molecule include those by McHuge et al. (1999) who constructed a recombinant glycol-lipid-anchored protein attached to the extracellular domain of human B7.1. This fusion protein was inserted in the tumor cell membrane and provided the necessary signal for the proliferation of cytotoxic T cells in a mixed lymphocyte reaction. In the late 1990s, a new form of B7.1 and B7.2, namely the generation of soluble B7-Ig, was studied and found to be very effective for the immunotherapy of solid tumors (Sturmhoefel et al. 1999), but little work with these reagents were done past these initial studies.

3.3.1 B7.1 Fusion Proteins

B7.1 is the prototypic costimulatory molecule and has the ability to provide T cells with the "second signal" that ensures T cell activation supersedes T cell anergy. We thus chose B7.1 as our first costimulatory fusion protein. To target B7.1, we linked the molecule to NHS76, a human TNT monoclonal antibody generated by phage display that is capable of binding intracellular antigens accessible and abundant in necrotic regions of tumors (Sharifi et al. 2001). These intracellular antigens show preferential localization in malignant tumors due to the presence of abnormally permeable, degenerating cells not found in normal tissues. Because the N-terminus of B7.1 is critical for interaction with its counter-receptors, the C-terminus of B7.1 was linked to the N-terminus of NHS76 (Fig. 2b). Studies confirmed that the B7.1/NHS76 fusion protein retained both the costimulatory activity of B7.1 and the tumor-targeting ability of NHS76 antibody (Liu et al. 2006). For comparison, we also constructed a B7.1 fusion protein consisting of human B7.1 and the Fc portion of human IgG$_1$, referred to as B7.1-Fc (Fig. 2c) (Liu et al. 2005).

Relative tumor uptake of the fusion protein was determined by tissue biodistribution studies in COLON 26 tumor-bearing BALB/c mice. Tumor and normal tissue uptake was measured 24 and 48 h after the i.v. administration of radiolabeled B7.1/NHS76. As shown in Fig. 7a, the uptake of the fusion protein per gram of

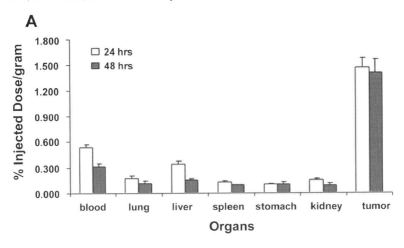

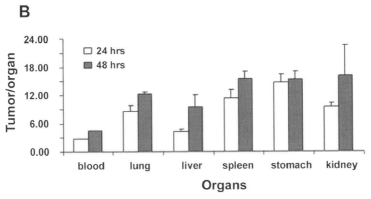

Fig. 7 In vivo biodistribution of ^{125}I-labeled B7.1/NHS76 in COLON 26-bearing BALB/c mice at 24 and 48 h post injection. Data were expressed for each mouse as (**a**) %ID/g (percentage injected dose per gram of organ) and (**b**) tumor/organ ratios

tumor (%ID/g) was significantly higher than the normal organs at both 24 and 48 h post-injection. The rapid clearance of ^{125}I-B7.1/NHS76 also demonstrated a marked decrease in radioactivity levels in blood, liver, and kidney with time, resulting in increasing tumor/organ ratios in Fig. 7b. These data demonstrate that B7.1/NHS76 targets the tumor with good retention as compared to normal organs and blood.

3.3.2 B7.1 Fusion Protein Treatment, Alone

Since human B7.1 can interact functionally with murine B7.1 counter-receptors, the immunotherapeutic potential of this fusion protein was tested in three mouse tumor models; COLON 26, RENCA, and MAD109. In testing the targeted molecule, mice treated with B7.1/NHS76 alone showed a 35–55% reduction in tumor volume

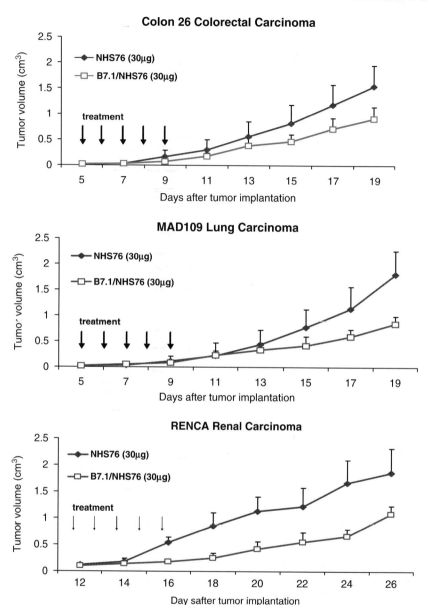

Fig. 8 Human B7.1/NHS76 immunotherapy in three different murine solid models. Control studies showed that pretreatment with NHS76 antibody alone does not show any effect

(Fig. 8). Identical treatment studies performed with the soluble B7.1-Fc fusion protein showed complete regression of COLON 26 tumors after a 5-day treatment regimen (Fig. 9). This was true even in mice with established MAD109 tumors, which are known to be poorly immunogenic.

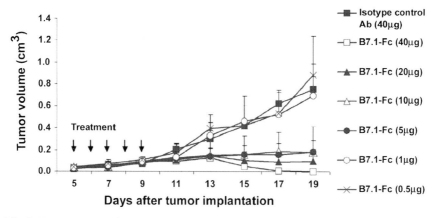

Fig. 9 Dose response of B7.1-Fc immunotherapy in COLON 26 tumor-bearing BALB/c mice. Antitumor effects of B7.1-Fc fusion protein show a dosing threshold, with doses greater than 5 μg per day inducing dramatic regression of mouse tumors, whereas doses less than 5 μg per day produced no antitumor effects

3.4 TNFSF Ligands

The members of Tumor Necrosis Factor Superfamily (TNFSF) are type II cell surface glycoproteins that are normally expressed on APCs. Their receptors are type I transmembrane proteins, characterized by cysteine-rich motifs in their extracellular domains, and are transiently expressed on T cells after initial activation. Several members of the TNFSF family, including OX40L, CD137L, and GITRL, upon binding to their receptors, provide critical signals for T cells to sustain their response after initial activation (immunological memory).

3.4.1 CD137L Costimulation

As described earlier, the B7-CD28 interaction has been widely studied as the primary pathway for delivering costimulatory signals to resting T cells (Yamaguchi et al. 2004). In addition, 4-1BB (CD137) is another important costimulatory pathway that has been recently described (Alderson et al. 1994; Futugawa et al. 2002; Wen et al. 2002). CD137 and its natural ligand CD137L are both members of the TNF superfamilies (Gruss et al. 1996). Generally, CD137 is found on activated T cells, and CD137L on activated B cells, activated macrophages, and differentiated dendritic cells (Futugawa et al. 2002). In mice, the expression of CD137 takes several hours following TCR stimulation, peaking at 60 h and declining again by 110 h. CD137L has been shown to costimulate T cell responses independently of signals through the CD28 molecule (Vinay and Kwon 1998) and can stimulate both

primary (Gramaglia et al. 2000) and secondary (DeBenedette et al. 1995) responses
of both CD4$^+$ and CD8$^+$ T cells (Cannons et al. 2001). Furthermore, enhanced
CD137/CD137L interactions amplify T cell-mediated antitumor immunity in several mouse models (Mogi et al. 2000). Similar experiments have shown that systemic administration of the agonistic anti-CD137 2A antibody eradicates established
subcutaneous tumors in mice (Melero et al. 1997) and a human 2A antibody is currently under development for the treatment of cancer.

Besides its relationship with conventional T cells, CD137 signaling on CD4$^+$
CD25$^+$ Treg cells, although presumed, has been controversial. For example, Zheng
et al. (2004) have verified the expression of CD137 on Treg cells isolated from mice,
and demonstrated that CD137L ligation augmented the proliferation of functional
Treg cells. Choi et al. (2004), however, using the agonist 2A antibody, showed that
CD137 signaling resulted in negligible enhancement of proliferation of Treg cells
and actually inhibited Treg cell function in vitro and in vivo.

3.4.2 CD137L Fusion Proteins

Taking into account the importance of the extracellular C-terminus of CD137L for
its bioactivity, the N-terminus of the extracellular CD137L gene was fused to the
C-terminus of the mTNT-3 heavy chain gene to construct both TNT-3/CD137L and
Fc-CD137L fusion genes (Figs. 2d and 2e) (Zhang 2007). Whole-body clearance
studies were performed in healthy BALB/c mice to establish the in vivo half-life
of TNT-3/CD137L and Fc-CD137L, which was found to be 18 and 24 h, respectively. Tissue biodistribution studies in COLON 26 tumor-bearing BALB/c mice
were performed to determine the relative tumor uptake of each fusion protein.
Tumor and normal tissue uptake was measured 24 and 48 h after i.v. administration
of radiolabeled TNT-3/CD137L and Fc-CD137L. As shown in Fig. 10, the uptake
of TNT-3/CD137L per gram of tumor was significantly higher than the uptake in
normal organs at 24 h and showed even higher retention at 48 h post-injection. As
expected, Fc-CD137L demonstrated low tumor retention over time. Examination
of the tumor draining lymph nodes, an important site for tumor immunotherapy,
revealed that TNT-3/CD137L had slightly better uptake than Fc-CD137L at 24
and 48 h post-injection (Fig. 10). However, the average tumor draining lymph node
retention of TNT-3/CD137L was still much lower than that measured in tumor.

A dosing study was performed in COLON 26-bearing BALB/c mice with
different doses ranging from 10 pmol/dose to 1 nmol/dose of TNT-3/CD137L,
Fc-CD137L, and anti-CD137 agonist antibody 2A (Fig. 11) (1 pmole is equivalent to 0.2, 0.1, and 0.15 µg of TNT-3/CD137L, Fc-CD137L, and 2A, respectively). At 10 pmol/dose (2, 1, and 1.5 µg of TNT-3/CD137L, Fc-CD137L, and
2A, respectively), no significant tumor reduction was observed in any of the treatment groups. At 100 pmol/dose (20, 10, and 15 µg of TNT-3/CD137L, Fc-CD137L,
and 2A, respectively) and 250 pmol/dose (50, 25, and 37.5 µg of TNT-3/CD137L,
Fc-CD137L, and 2A, respectively), 2A treated mice demonstrated 95% tumor

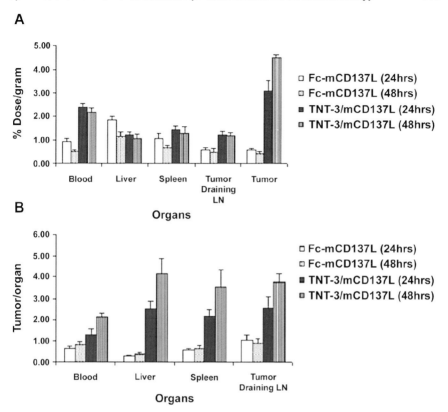

Fig. 10 Tissue biodistribution and tumor uptake of TNT-3/CD137L and Fc-CD137L at 24 and 48 h post-injection in COLON 26-bearing BALB/c mice. Tumor uptake was measured by percent injected dose per gram of ^{125}I-labeled TNT-3/CD137L or Fc-CD137L (*upper*) and tumor/normal organ ratios (*lower*); *columns* show the mean and *bars* indicate SD

volume reduction, while TNT-3/CD137L and Fc-CD137L treatment resulted in 30–40% tumor reduction at day 19 post-tumor implantation. At 500 pmol/dose (100, 50, and 75 μg of TNT-3/CD137L, Fc-CD137L, and 2A, respectively), however, the TNT-3/CD137L group showed 70% tumor reduction, whereas the Fc-CD137L-treated mice achieved only 30% tumor reduction. This difference potentially indicates that at this particular dosage, localization of CD137L is more effective. At 1 nmol/dose (200, 100, and 150 μg of TNT-3/CD137L, Fc-CD137L, and 2A, respectively), however, both TNT-3/CD137L and Fc-CD137L treated groups showed 80% tumor reduction, and 2A treated groups continued to demonstrate 95% tumor reduction. All 2A treated groups (except 10 pmol/ dose group) eventually became tumor free and all treated mice were free of signs of toxicity throughout the 140-day observation period.

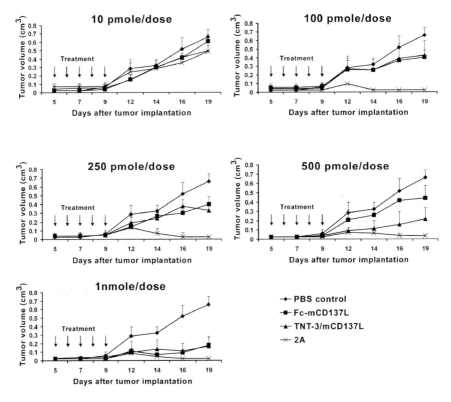

Fig. 11 Dose response of mTNT-3/CD137L, Fc-CD137L, and 2A in COLON 26-bearing BALB/c mice. One pmole is equivalent to 0.2, 0.1, and 0.15 µg of TNT-3/CD137L, Fc-CD137L, and 2A, respectively

3.4.3 GITRL Costimulation

Recently, there have been a number of studies that have attempted to characterize the cell surface of Treg cells to evaluate whether individual proteins play a role in the activation or inhibition of Treg-induced suppression. One such cell surface marker is the 18th member of TNFSF designated GITR (glucocorticoid-induced TNFR-related gene), which is constitutively expressed on $CD4^+CD25^+$ (Treg) cells and is upregulated in $CD4^+$ and $CD8^+$ cells (Nocentini and Riccardi 2005). GITR has a high homology in the cytoplasmic region with other TNFSF members such as CD137, OX40, and CD40L (Rochetti et al. 2004). The ligand for GITR (GITRL) is a type II transmembrane protein that belongs to TNFSF and is normally expressed on APCs such as macrophages, dendritic cells, and B cells (Nocentini and Riccardi 2005). More importantly, GITR activation by GITRL leads to the proliferation of $CD4^+CD25^-$ and $CD8^+$ effector T cells and a reduction of tumor volume in vivo.

Also, an interesting characteristic of GITR activation on Treg cells results in their inability to suppress responding CD4$^+$CD25$^-$ T cells (Zheng et al. 2004). Therefore, GITR engagement by GITRL results in the inhibition of Treg cells and the activation of responding T cells. This dual function of GITR activation may be unique for costimulatory interactions and could be responsible for its highly potent antitumor activity in vivo.

3.4.4 OX40L Costimulation

OX40 (CD134), a membrane-associated glycoprotein, is transiently expressed on the surface of T cells after TCR ligation (Mallet et al. 1990). Its natural ligand, OX40L (TNFSF4, CD134L), is found primarily on APCs such as activated B cells, activated endothelial cells, dendritic cells, and macrophages (Weinberg et al. 1999; Pippig et al. 1999). The OX40L delivers a potent costimulatory signal to OX40$^+$ T cells leading to optimal T cell function. Studies of the primary T cell responses revealed that OX40L is a potent costimulatory molecule for sustaining CD4$^+$T cell response (Maxwell et al. 2000). OX40 signaling strikingly prolongs T cell division initially induced by CD28, and enhances the survival of CD4$^+$ cells during the initial response by promoting Bcl-XL and Bcl-2 expression. OX40-/-T cells fail to maintain high levels of Bcl-XL and Bcl-2 4–8 h after activation and undergo apoptosis (Rogers et al. 2001). In vivo, OX40 signaling would augment tumor-specific priming through stimulating and expanding the natural repertoire of the host's tumor-specific CD4$^+$ T cells (Pippig et al. 1999). Therefore, it is believed that OX40-OX40L interactions are crucial for the survival of effector T cells and the generation of memory T cells. Although the effects of OX40 costimulation on CD4$^+$ T cells were initially studied, more recent work has shown that OX40 signaling also costimulates CD8$^+$ T cells (Wang and Klein 2001). Profound CD8$^+$ T cell clonal expansion and a massive burst of CD8$^+$ T cell effector function were induced by dual costimulation of OX40 and 41BB (Lee et al. 2002). This synergistic response of the specific CD8$^+$ T cells has been shown to last for several weeks, and is sufficient to treat established tumors even under immunocompromised conditions (Lee et al. 2004).

Interestingly, OX40 is also found to be expressed on both naïve and activated CD4$^+$CD25$^+$ Treg cells (Gavin et al. 2002). OX40 signals may abrogate Treg-mediated suppression when they are delivered directly to antigen-engaged naïve T cells (Takeda et al. 2004). Using the agonist antibody, OX86, OX40 signaling on Treg cells inhibited their capacity to suppress, and restored effector T cell proliferation and cytokine production (Valzasina et al. 2005). It has been confirmed that OX40 abrogation of Treg cells occurs in vivo using a graft-versus-host disease model (Valzasina et al. 2005). Because of its potent effects on T cell activation and possible inhibition on Treg cells, fusion proteins with OX40L are currently in progress.

3.5 *Immunoregulatory T Cells (Treg)*

To create more effective immunotherapy for the treatment of cancer, it is important to have a comprehensive understanding of how the immune system is regulated. There is now abundant evidence from a number of diverse experimental systems that a subpopulation of CD4$^+$ T cells, collectively termed Treg cells, are present in normal mice and are essential for both homeostasis and the maintenance of tolerance to tissue-specific antigens (Hill et al. 1989; North and Awwad 1990; Awwad and North 1990; Rakhmilevich and North 1993, 1994; Shevach 2000, 2001, 2002). Although substantial controversy existed regarding their phenotype and their mechanism(s) to mediate suppression, it is now generally agreed that these cells display the CD4$^+$CD25$^+$ phenotype and the FOX3p genotype (Javia and Rosenberg 2003) and that they exert their activity either by cell–cell contact (Sutmuller et al. 2001; Javia and Rosenberg 2003) or by secretion of inhibitory IL-10 or TGFβ cytokines (Hara and Kingsley 2001; Somasundaram and Jacob 2002). With regards to tumor immunity, CD4$^+$ Treg cells were first discovered by North and his colleagues, who published a number of papers on this concept starting from the late-1980s (Hill et al. 1989; North and Awwad 1990; Awwad and North 1990). Although this work was largely ignored, a flurry of papers describing the immunosuppressive effects of CD4$^+$CD25$^+$ Treg cells on tumor growth started to appear by the late 1990s (Onizuka et al. 1999; Shimizu et al. 1999). In these later discoveries, immunocompetent mice bearing syngeneic tumors become tolerant to their tumors by day 9 after transplantation when CD4$^+$CD25$^+$ appeared in the peripheral circulation. If tumor-bearing mice were depleted of Treg cells before or at the time of implantation with the rat monoclonal antibody PC61, tumor growth was arrested (Onizuka et al. 1999). Moreover, tumor suppression could also be produced by low dose whole-body irradiation or chemotherapy, which presumably is also cytotoxic to Treg cells (Awwad and North 1990). In most studies, CD4$^+$ or CD4$^+$CD25$^+$ T cell depletion was tumor suppressive but resulted in either incomplete tumor reduction or a delay in tumor growth. Although CD4$^+$CD25$^+$ cells were first discovered in mice, a population with identical phenotypic and functional properties has been defined recently in humans (Levings et al. 2001; Dieckmann et al. 2001; Jonuleit 2001; Stephens et al. 2001; Ng 2001; Baecher-Allen et al. 2001). Since clinical trials to reduce or delete Treg cells in the setting of cancer immunotherapy have not been performed, the potential of this procedure in humans is currently unknown. Evidence, however, is accumulating that Treg cells are more abundant in the peripheral blood and tumor microenvironment of cancer patients and may be responsible for the observed tolerance displayed in patients (Liyanage et al. 2002).

3.5.1 LEC Fusion Protein Treatment in Combination with Treg Depletion

To evaluate the subpopulation(s) of T cells responsible for the observed tumor destruction, depletion studies were performed in conjunction with the above therapy

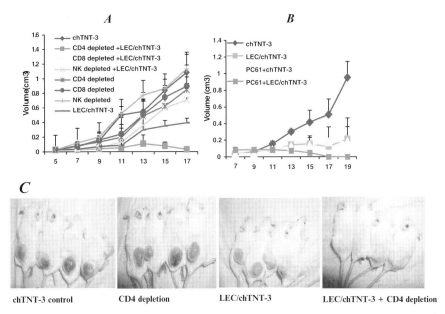

Fig. 12 T-cell depletion studies with LEC/chTNT-3. (**a**) Combination therapy with anti-CD4$^+$, CD8$^+$, and NK cell antisera or (**b**) anti-CD25$^+$ antibody. (**c**) Gross appearance of BALB/c mice bearing COLON 26 tumors on day 25 after tumor implantation, demonstrating complete remission in all the mice treated with combination therapy (fourth panel on right)

studies (Li et al. 2003b). One day after COLON 26 tumor implantation, mice received cytotoxic antisera specific for CD4$^+$, CD8$^+$, or NK cells. Each of these antisera were administered every 5 days, reducing the appropriate cell subpopulation to <2% in the peripheral blood, as demonstrated by flow cytometry. As expected, CD8$^+$ and NK depletion negated the antitumor activity of LEC/chTNT-3 treatment, indicating that these lymphocyte subpopulations are critical to the function of the fusion protein (Fig. 12a). By contrast, mice receiving CD4$^+$ depletion in combination with LEC/chTNT-3 therapy demonstrated 100% regression of tumor and went into lasting remission. These unexpected results were highly significant and turned our attention to the necessity of deleting or suppressing immunoregulatory cells and mechanisms.

To probe this observation further, only the CD4$^+$CD25$^+$ Treg subpopulation was depleted in repeat experiments. Since Treg represents approximately 10% of the CD4$^+$ population in both mice and humans, depletion of this small subpopulation using the rat anti-mouse CD25$^+$ monoclonal antibody PC61 would be highly instructive. As shown in Fig. 12b, depletion of Treg cells in combination with LEC/chTNT-3, did indeed produce complete remissions in COLON 26 tumor-bearing BALB/c mice, suggesting that it is this small population of CD25$^+$ cells that

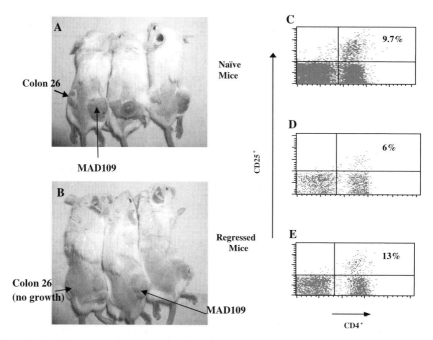

Fig. 13 Rechallenge experiments in combination therapy. The appearance of (**a**) naïve mice and (**b**) 2–3 month COLON 26 tumor-regressed mice challenged with 10^7 COLON 26 (left flank) or MAD109 (right flank) is shown after 2 weeks. The presence of CD4$^+$CD25$^+$ T-cells in tumor draining lymph nodes evaluated by flow cytometry in (**c**) naïve mice, (**d**) 2–3 month tumor-regressed mice, and (**e**) 5–6 month tumor-regressed mice

is responsible minimizing the effects of LEC/chTNT-3. PC61 treatment alone or in combination with control chTNT-3 also produced significant tumor regressions, but never complete responses (Fig. 12c) (Li et al. 2003b).

Rechallenge experiments demonstrated that combining LEC/chTNT-3 treatment with CD25$^+$ depletion produces long-acting memory cells. Tumor-free mice from the experiments described above were again injected subcutaneously with COLON 26 and MAD109 tumor cells in their contralateral flanks, alongside naïve mice injected with each tumor cell line. Two weeks after tumor implantation, all naïve mice had solid tumors growing on their left (COLON 26) and right (MAD109) flanks (Fig. 13a), while the tumor-remission mice (now 60 days after initial tumor implantation) had tumors only on the right flank (MAD109) (Fig. 13b). Interestingly, a second series of rechallenge experiments performed 6 months after the initiation of therapy, however, showed no difference between naïve and remission mice. To determine if regenerated CD4$^+$CD25$^+$ T cells in tumor-draining lymph nodes correlated with the ability of tumor to take in these mice, the percent of Treg cells was measured by flow cytometry in each of these groups of mice. The data showed that CD4$^+$CD25$^+$T cells in naïve mice constituted 9.7% of total T cells

(Fig. 13c), while in 2–3 month tumor-regressed mice they constituted only 6% of total T cells (Fig. 13d) and in 5–6 month tumor-regressed Treg cells constituted 13% of total T cells (Fig. 13e). This increase in Treg cells may explain the failure to reject tumor seen at 6 months. Additionally, these experiments suggest that combination LEC/chTNT-3 treatment and CD25$^+$ depletion does in fact produce long-acting memory cells capable of preventing re-engraftment of the same tumor, so long as Treg regeneration does not suppress the memory response.

3.5.2 Cytokine Fusion Proteins in Combination with Treg Depletion

To show that targeted LEC is critical to the above results, similar combination studies were performed with chTNT-3/cytokine fusion proteins consisting of human IL-2, murine IFN-γ, and murine TNF-α using identical treatment regimens. The results of these studies presented in Table 2, showed only modest improvement indicating that combination therapy with anti-CD25$^+$ antisera requires LEC not cytokine localization to tumor in order to produce complete regression. Of interest, histochemical studies performed on tumor-bearing mice treated with the above fusion proteins showed that only LEC/chTNT-3 treatment produced a coordinated infiltration of lymphoid cells, which started with dendritic cells and neutrophils at the beginning of treatment and ended three days later with a significant T- and B-cell infiltration (Li et al. 2003a). The other cytokine fusion proteins may in fact be more effective at enhancing existing lymphoid responses as opposed to recruiting and initiating a de novo adaptive response resulting in the generation of memory cells.

Table 2 Combination cytokine or chemokine fusion protein immunotherapy and T-cell subset depletion in the treatment of COLON 26 carcinoma

Immunotherapy[a]	T-cell subset depletion[b]	% Tumor reduction (Day 19) (%)
chTNT-3 (control)	–	0
chTNT-3 (control)	CD4$^+$ depletion	33
LEC/chTNT-3	–	60
LEC/chTNT-3	CD4$^+$ depletion	100
chTNT-3/IL-2	–	38
chTNT-3/IL-2	CD4$^+$ depletion	64
chTNT-3/IFN-γ	–	32
chTNT-3/IFN-γ	CD4$^+$ depletion	33
chTNT-3/TNF-α	–	10
chTNT-3/TNF-α	CD4$^+$ depletion	33

[a] Antibodies and fusion proteins (20 μg/dose) were injected i.v. for five consecutive days after tumors reached 0.5 cm in diameter.
[b] CD4$^+$ depletion (0.5 mg per dose of GK1.5) was performed i.p. 1 day after tumor implantation and repeated every 5 days.

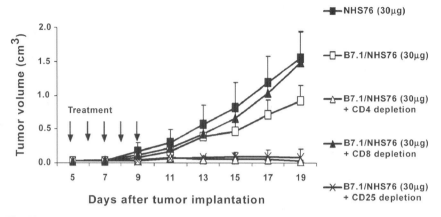

Fig. 14 Combination immunotherapy of tumor-bearing mice by B7.1/NHS76 in MAD109 tumor models of BALB/c mice with anti-CD4, anti-CD8, or anti-CD25 antibodies

3.5.3 B7.1 Fusion Proteins in Combination with Treg Depletion

As shown above (Fig. 8), mice treated with B7.1/NHS76 alone showed a 35–55% reduction in tumor volume. To determine if Treg deletion could enhance the effects of B7.1 fusion proteins, additional tumor-bearing mice were treated with combination therapy using PC61 and B7.1/NHS76. As shown in Fig. 14, combination therapy produced complete regression of established lung tumors (MAD109) and was associated with increased effector T cell tumor infiltration (Liu et al. 2006). When soluble B7.1-Fc was used in combination with Treg depletion PC61 shown in Fig. 15 (Panel a, RENCA model and panel b, MAD109 model), all tumor-bearing mice also went into complete remission and remained so for the observation period of 6 months. Rechallenge experiments performed with these mice showed that they had immunological memory and were able to reject subsequent tumor implantation (Fig. 16).

Using knockout mice, it was determined that the antitumor activity of B7.1-Fc immunotherapy was dependent both on perforin and IFN-γ, but not on IL-4, as demonstrated by the failure of perforin and IFN-γ knockout mice to reject tumors after treatment (Fig. 17). In these studies, anti-IL-4 was found to have no tumor suppressive activity (data not shown). By these experiments, it appears that perforin may not be the exclusive method of tumor cell killing since the activity of the B7.1-Fc was not entirely eliminated as seen in the knock-out experiments. In summary, these data show that B7.1-Fc immunotherapy is dependent upon the induction of IFN-γ, activated CD8[+] T cells, and partially by perforin for tumor cell killing. When used in combination with Treg cell depletion, memory cells are generated to assure the complete destruction of tumor in the host.

A

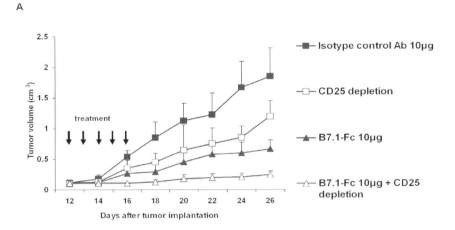

B

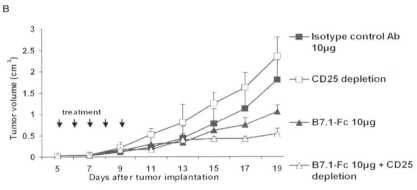

Fig. 15 Combination B7.1 Fc immunotherapy and CD25$^+$ T cell depletion on the growth of (**a**) RENCA and (**b**) MAD109 solid tumors. BALB/c mice were injected with rat anti-mouse CD25 (PC61) antibody on the day of tumor implantation and every 5 days thereafter

3.5.4 CD137L Fusion Proteins Treatment in Combination with Treg Depletion

To assess the role of CD4$^+$ and CD8$^+$ T cells in CD137L mediated immunotherapy, T-subset depletion studies were performed with cytotoxic antibodies against CD4$^+$ and CD8$^+$ cells (Zhang 2007). Anti-CD4 antibody (Clone GK1.5) and anti-CD8 antibody (Clone H35) were injected i.p. on the 5th day after tumor implantation, and these treatments were repeated every 5 days. Depletion was confirmed by flow cytometry. As shown in Fig. 18, panel a, CD8$^+$ T cell depletion completely abrogated TNT-3/CD137L and Fc-CD137L's antitumor effects, indicating that tumor suppression was dependent on this subpopulation of T cells. Like the results shown above for LEC and B7.1, CD137L fusion protein treatment when used in combination

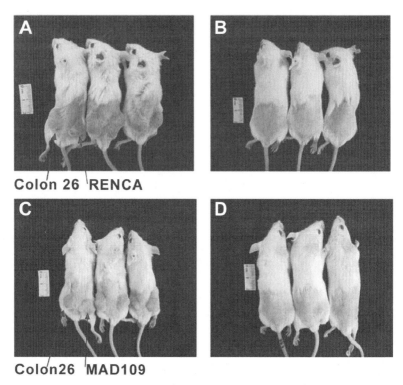

Fig. 16 Rechallenge experiments. (**a**) and (**c**) are naïve mice controls, and (**b**) and (**d**) are tumor-regressed mice from previous studies. (**a**) and (**b**) were s.c. implanted with 10^6 COLON 26 cells on the left flank and 10^6 RENCA cells on the right flank. (**c**) and (**d**) were s.c. implanted with 10^6 COLON 26 cells on the left flank and 10^6 MAD109 cells on the right flank. (**b**) and (**d**) were treated with B7.1-Fc and anti-Treg antibody (PC61) in previous studies and remained tumor-free for 3 month before beginning rechallenge experiments

with anti-CD4$^+$ reagents caused enhanced tumor regression (Fig. 18, panels b and c). Unlike combination therapy with LEC/chTNT-3, the synergy or additive effect of anti-CD4 is not seen in mice co-treated with CD13L fusion proteins.

4 Conclusions

As discussed earlier, the overall objective of this chapter is be to evaluate the efficacy of genetically engineered fusion proteins developed in our laboratory for the

A

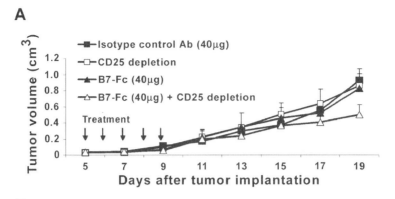

B

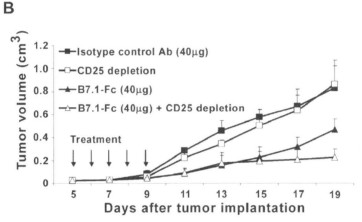

C

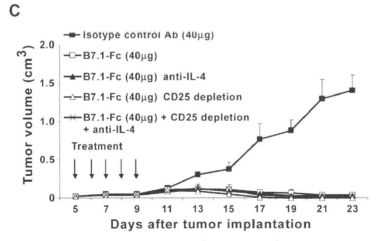

Fig. 17 Combination immunotherapy in (**a**) IFN-$\gamma^{-/-}$, (**b**) perforin$^{-/-}$ mice, and (**c**) IL-4-depleted mice, with CD25$^+$ cell depletion. The antitumor effects of B7.1-Fc were not affected by IL-4 neutralization but were abrogated completely in IFN-γ knockout mice and partially in perforin knockout mice

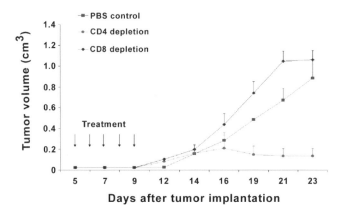

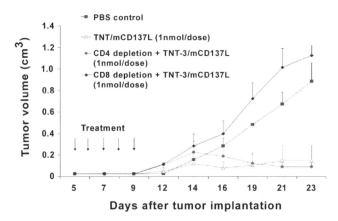

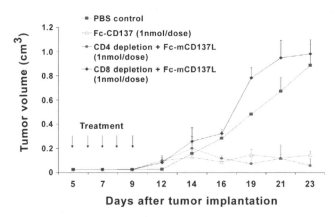

Fig. 18 Combination immunotherapy of CD137L fusion proteins and deleted T-cell subsets. **(a)** Deletion of $CD4^+$ and $CD8^+$ subpopulations only. **(b)** TNT-3/CD137L treatment alone and in combination with T-cell subset deletion. **(c)** Fc-CD137L treatment alone and in combination with T-cell subset deletion. One nmol/dose is equivalent to 200 and 100 μg of TNT-3/CD137L and Fc/CD137L, respectively

immunotherapy of solid tumors. The use of chTNT-3, which targets necrotic areas of solid tumors regardless of the species of origin of the tumor, enabled us to compare by the same targeting antibody, the relative therapeutic potential of selected cytokines, chemokines, and costimulatory molecules in tumor-bearing immuno-competent mice. This point cannot be overemphasized since there are few antibodies available that target murine tumor models. By our studies, it has become clear that the targeting of specific but not all immune modulators to the tumor microenvironment can cause a massive and effective destruction of established tumors. As controls, soluble Fc fusion proteins were also prepared of most of these immunoregulatory molecules, and to our consternation, many of these appear to be as effective as the corresponding antibody fusion proteins that target tumor. It appears that when administered in high enough concentrations, soluble Fc fusion proteins can also reverse immune tolerance to tumor. This is seen clearly in dosing studies in which a threshold amount of soluble Fc is required for the induction of tumor suppression. Threshold amounts were less often seen in those mice receiving antibody fusion proteins. Although very potent in their antitumor action, it remains to be seen if these soluble Fc fusion proteins are more toxic in man than corresponding antibody fusion proteins. The other major finding of these studies, namely the importance of Treg cells in immunotherapy, illustrates the importance of understanding existing mechanisms of immune tolerance in cancer patients. For instance, do all cases of a given tumor type evoke a similar mechanism of tumor escape, and do metastatic lesions display the same mechanism as primary lesions in the same patient? These types of questions should be answered prior to proceeding with the testing of specific immunotherapeutic reagents to maximize the therapeutic potential of a given reagent. We should also be aware that histopathologic diagnosis may not correlate with the immune status of patients and that immunologic phenotyping may be required to identify populations of patients that can respond to immunotherapy. In conclusion, in the last 10 years, we have generated a panel of cytokine, chemokine, and costimulatory fusion proteins and tested them similarly in three solid tumor models of the BALB/c mouse. Cell deletion experiments have identified the importance of NK^+ and $CD8^+$ effector T cells for tumor immunotherapy and the negative influence of $CD25^+$ Treg cells. Both soluble Fc and antibody fusion proteins have been found to be effective agents for the delivery of immunoregulatory molecules that can induce significant tumor regression or cure. In particular, the chemokine LEC and several different costimulatory molecules including B7.1 and CD137L were found to be especially effective in the induction of effective cancer treatment. It is our goal to bring a number of these novel reagents into the clinic in order to test the potential value of immunotherapy as an emerging new treatment of cancer.

Acknowledgements This work was supported in part by grants from the NIH #2R01 CA83001, California Cancer Research Program #00-00749v-20244, the Philip Morris External Research Program, and Cancer Therapeutics Laboratories (Los Angeles, CA).

References

Abken H, Hombach A, Heuser C et al. (2002) Tuning tumor-specific T-cell activation: A matter of co-stimulation? Trends Immunol 23:240–245

Ajani JA, Rios AA, Ende K et al. (1989) Phase I and II studies of the combination of recombinant human interferon-gamma and 5-fluorouracil in patients with advanced colorectal carcinoma. J Biol Response Modifiers 8: 140–146

Alderson MR, Smith CA, Tough TW et al. (1994) Molecular and biological characterization of human 4-1BB and its ligand. Eur J Immunol 24:2219–2227

Aluvaihare VR, Kallikourdis M, Betz AG (2004) Regulatory T-cells mediate maternal tolerance to the fetus. Nature Immunol 5:266–271

Awwad M, North RJ (1990) Radiosensitive barrier to T-cell-mediated adoptive immunotherapy of established tumors. Cancer Res 50:2228–2233

Baecher-Allen C, Brown JA, Freeman GJ et al. (2001) CD4$^+$CD25$^+$ regulatory cells in human peripheral blood. J Immunol 167:1245–1253

Ben-Efraim S (1999) One hundred years of cancer immunotherapy: A critical appraisal. Tumour Biology 20:1–24

Blattman JN, Greenberg PD (2004) Cancer immunotherapy: A treatment for the masses. Science 305:200–205

Bubenik J, Otter W, Huland E (2000) Local cytokine therapy of cancer: Interleukin-2, interferon, and related cytokines. Cancer Immunol Immunother 49:116–122

Cannons JL, Lau P, Ghumman B et al. (2001) 4-1BB ligand induces cell division, sustains survival, and enhances effector function of CD4$^+$ and CD8$^+$ T cells with similar efficacy. J Immunol 167:1313–1324

Chen FM, Hansen EB, Taylor CR et al. (1991) Diffusion and binding of monoclonal antibody TNT-1 in multicellular tumor spheroids. J Natl Cancer Inst 83:200–204

Chen L (2004) Co-Inhibitory molecules of the B7-CD28 family in the control of T-cell immunity. Nature Rev Immunol 4:336–347

Chen S, Yu L, Jiang C et al. (2005) Pivotal study of iodine-131-labeled chimeric tumor necrosis treatment radioimmunotherapy in patients with advanced lung cancer. J Clin Oncol 23:1538–1547

Choi BK, Bae JS, Choi EM et al. (2004) 4-1BB-dependent inhibition of immunosuppression by activated CD4$^+$CD25$^+$ T cells. J Leukoc Biol 75:785–791

DeBenedette MA, Chu NR, Pollok KE et al. (1995) Role of 4-1BB ligand in costimulation of T lymphocyte growth and its upregulation on M12 B lymphomas by cAMP. J Exp Med 181:985–992

Delta-Cruz J, Trinh K, Morriso SL et al. (2000) Recombinant anti-human HER2/neu IgG3-(GM-CSF) fusion protein retains antigen specificity and cytokine fusion and demonstrates antitumor activity. J Immunol 165:5112–5121

Di Cailo E, Forni G, Lollini P et al. (2001) The intriguing role of polymorphonuclear neutrophils in anti-tumor reaction. Blood 97:339–345

Dieckmann D, Plottner H, Berchtold S, et al. (2001) Ex vivo isolation and characterization of CD4$^+$CD25$^+$T cells with regulatory properties from human blood. J Exp Med 193:1303–1310

Dy GK, Adjei AA (2002) Novel targets for lung cancer therapy. J Clin Oncol 20:2881–2894

Epstein AL, Chen FM, Taylor CR (1988) A novel method for the detection of necrotic lesions in human cancers. Cancer Res 48:5842–5848

Epstein AL, Chen D, Ansari A et al. (1991) Radioimmunodetection of necrotic lesions in human tumors using I-131 labeled TNT-1 F(ab')$_2$ monoclonal antibody. Antibody Immunoconjug Radiopharm 4:151–161

Futagawa T, Akiba HK, Jakeda K et al. (2002) Expression and function of 4-1BB and 4-1BB ligand on murine dendritic cells. Int Immunol 14:275–286

Gavin MA, Clarke SR, Negrou E et al (2002) Homeostasis and anergy of CD4$^+$CD25$^+$ suppressor T cells in vivo. Nat Immunol 3:33–41

Gerard C, Rollins BJ (2001) Chemokines and disease. Nature Immunol 2:108–115

Gillis S, Ferm MM, Ward O (1978) T-cell growth factor: Parameters of production and a quantitative microassay for activity. J Immunol 120:2027–2031

Giovarelli M, Cappello P, Forni G et al. (2000) Tumor rejection and immune memory elicited by locally released LEC chemokine are associated with and impressive recruitment of APCs, lymphocytes, and granulocytes. J Immunol 164:3200–3206

Gramaglia I, Cooper D, Miner K et al. (2000) Co-stimulation of antigen-specific CD4 T cells by 4-1BB ligand. Eur J Immunol 30:392–402

Gruss HJ, Duyster J, Herrmann F (1996) Structural and biological features of the TNF receptor and TNF ligand superfamilies: Interactive signals in the pathobiology of Hodgkin's disease. Ann Oncol 7:19–26

Hara M, Kingsley C (2001) IL-10 is required for regulatory T cell to mediate tolerance to alloantigens in vivo. J Immunol 166:3789–3796

Hathcock KS, Laszlo G, Pucillo C et al. (1994) Comparative analysis of B7-1 and B7-2 costimulatory ligands: Expression and function. J Exp Med 180:631–640

Hill JO, Awwad M, North RJ (1989) Elimination of CD4$^+$ suppressor T cells from susceptible BALB/c mice releases CD8$^+$ T lymphocytes to mediate protective immunity against Leishmania. J Exp Med 169:1819–1827

Hisayuki N, Hieshima K, Nakayama T et al. (2001) Human CC chemokine liver-expressed chemokine/CCL16 is a functional ligand for CCR1, CCR2, and CCR5, and constitutively expressed by hepatocytes. Int Immunol 13:1021–1029

Hodge JW, Abrams S, Schlom J et al. (1994) Induction of anti-tumor immunity by recombinant vaccinia viruses expressing B7-1 or B7-2 costimulatory molecules. Cancer Res 54:5552–5555

Hogan MM (1993) Measurement of tumor necrosis factor α and β. In: Colligan JE (ed) Current protocols in immunology. Wiley, New York, pp 6101–6105

Hornick JL, Hu P, Khawli LA, et al. (1998) chTNT-3/B, a new chemically modified chimeric monoclonal antibody directed against DNA for the tumor necrosis treatment of solid tumors. Cancer Biother Radiopharm 13:255–268

Hornick JL, Khawli LA, Hu P et al. (1999) Pretreatment with a monoclonal antibody/ interleukin 2 fusion protein directed against DNA enhances the delivery of therapeutic molecules to solid tumors. Clin Cancer Res 5:51–60

Howard OMZ, Dong HF, Shirakawa A-K et al. (2000) LEC induces chemotaxis and adhension by interacting with CCR1 and CCR8. Blood 96:840–845

Ichihara F, Kono K, Takahashi A et al. (2003) H. Increased populations of regulatory T-cells in peripheral blood and tumor-infiltrating lymphocytes in patients with gastric and esophageal cancers. Clin Cancer Res 9:4404–4408

Javia LR, Rosenberg SA (2003) CD4$^+$CD25$^+$ Suppressor lymphocytes in the circulation of patients immunized against melanoma antigens. J Immunother 26:85–93

Jonuleit H (2001) Identification and functional characterization of human CD4$^+$CD25$^+$ T cells with regulatory properties isolated from peripheral blood. J Exp Med 193:1285–1294

Khawli LA, Miller GK, Epstein AL (1994) Effect of seven new vasoactive immunoconjugates on the enhancement of monoclonal antibody uptake in tumors. Cancer 73:824–831

Khawli LA, Hornick JL, Sharifi J et al. (1997) Improving the chemotherapeutic index of IUdR using a vasoactive immunoconjugate. Radiochimica Acta 79:83–86

Kim Y-M, Son K (1996) A nitric oxide production bioassay for interferon-γ. J Immunol Methods 198:203–209

Leach DR, Krummel MF, Allison JP (1996) Enhancement of antitumor immunity by CTLA-4 blockade. Science 271:1734–1736

LeBerthon B, Khawli LA, Miller GK et al. (1991) Enhanced tumor uptake of macromolecules induced by a novel vasoactive interleukin-2 immunoconjugate. Cancer Res 51:2694–2698

Lee HW, Park SJ, Choi BK et al. (2002) 4-1BB promotes the survival of CD8$^+$ T lymphocytes by increasing expression of Bcl-xL and Bfl-1. J Immunol 169:4882–4888

Lee SJ, Myers L, Muralimohan G et al. (2004) 4-1BB and OX40 dual costimulation synergistically stimulate primary specific CD8 T cells for robust effector function. J Immunol 173:3002–3012

Levings MK, Sangregorio R, Roncarolo MG (2001) Human CD25$^+$CD4$^+$ T cells suppress naïve and memory T-cell proliferation and can be expanded in vitro without loss of suppressor function. J Exp Med 193:1295–1302

Li J, Hu P, Khawli LA et al. (2003a) LEC/chTNT-3 fusion protein for the immunotherapy of experimental solid tumors. J Immunother 26:320–331

Li J, Hu P, Khawli LA et al. (2003b) Complete regression of experimental solid tumors by combination LEC/chTNT-3 immunotherapy and CD25$^+$ T-cell depletion. Cancer Res 63:8384–8392

Liu A, Hu P, Khawli LA et al. (2005) B7-Fc fusion protein treatment induces tumor regressions with long-term memory and is enhanced by Treg cell depletion. Clin Cancer Res 11:8492–8502

Liu A, Hu P, Khawli LA et al. (2006) B7.1/NHS76: A new co-stimulator fusion protein for the immunotherapy of solid tumors. J Immunother 29:425–435

Liyanage UK, Moore TT, Joo HG et al. (2002) Prevalence of regulatory T cells is increased in peripheral blood and tumor microenvironment of patients with pancreas or breast adenocarcinoma. J Immunol 169:2756–2761

Mackay CR (2001) Chemokines: Immunology's high impact factors. Nature Immunol 2:95–101

Maher J, Davies ET (2004) Targeting cytotoxic T lymphocytes for cancer immunotherapy. British J Cancer 91:817–821

Mallett S, Fossum S, Barclay AN (1990) Characterization of the MRC OX40 antigen of activated CD4 positive T lymphocytes – a molecule related to nerve growth factor receptor. Embo J 9:1063–1068

Mapara MY, Sykes M (2004) Tolerance and cancer: Mechanisms of tumor evasion and strategies for breaking tolerance. J Clin Oncol 22:1136–1151

Marshall NA, Christie LE, Munro LR et al. (2004) Immunosuppressive regulatory T-cells are abundant in the reactive lymphocytes of Hodgkin's lymphoma. Blood 103:1755–1762

Maxwell JR, Weinberg A, Prell RA et al. (2000) Danger and OX40 receptor signaling synergize to enhance memory T cell survival by inhibiting peripheral deletion. J Immunol 164:107–112

McHugh RS, Nagarajan S, Wang YC et al. (1999) Protein transfer of glycosyl-phosphatidylinositol-B7-1 into tumor cell membranes: A novel approach to tumor immunotherapy. Cancer Res 59:2433–2437

Melero I, Shuford WW, Newby SA et al. (1997) Monoclonal antibodies against the 4-1BB T-cell activation molecule eradicate established tumors. Nat Med 3:682–685

Miller GK, Naeve GS, Gaffar SA et al. (1993) Immunologic and biochemical analysis of TNT-1 and TNT-2 monoclonal antibody binding to histones. Hybridoma 12:689–698

Miyagishi R, Kikuchi S, Fukazawa T et al. (1995) Macrophage inflammatory protein-1 in the cerebrospinal fluid of patients with multiple sclerosis and other inflammatory neurological diseases. J Neuro Sci 129:223–227

Mizokami MM, Hu P, Khawli LA et al. (2003) Chimeric TNT-3/murine interferon-γ fusion protein for the immunotherapy of solid malignancies. Hybridoma Hybridomics 22:197–207

Mocellin S, Rossi CR, Lise M et al. (2002) Adjuvant immunotherapy for solid tumors: From promise to clinical application. [Review]. Cancer Immunol Immunother 5:1583–1595

Mogi S, Sakurai J, kohsaka T et al. (2000) Tumour rejection by gene transfer of 4-1BB ligand into a CD80$^+$ murine squamous cell carcinoma and the requirements of co-stimulatory molecules on tumour and host cells. Immunology 101:541–547

Morikawa K, Fidler IJ (1989) Heterogeneous response of human colon cancer cells to the cytostatic and cytotoxic effects of recombinant human cytokines: Interferon-alpha, interferon-gamma, tumor necrosis factor, and interleukin-1. J Biol Response Mod 8:206–218

Moro M, Gasparri AM, Pagano S et al. (1999) Induction of therapeutic T-cell immunity by tumor targeting with soluble recombinant B7-immunoglobulin costimulatory molecules. Cancer Res 59:2650–2656

Moser B, Loetscher P (2001) Lymphocyte traffic control by chemokines. Nature Immunol 2:123–128

Naruse K, Ueno M, Satoh T et al. (1996) A YAC contig of the human CC chemokine genes clustered on chromosome 17q11.2. Genomics 34:236–240

Ng WF (2001) Human of CD4$^+$CD25$^+$ cells: A naturally occurring population of regulatory T cells. Blood 98:2736–2744

Nocentini G, Riccardi C (2005) GITR: A multifaceted regulator of immunity belonging to the tumor necrosis factor receptor superfamily. Eur J Immunol 35:1016–1022

North RJ, Awwad, M (1990) Elimination of cycling CD4$^+$ suppressor T cells with an anti-mitotic drug releases non-cycling CD8$^+$ T cells to cause regression of an advanced lymphoma. Immunology 71:90–95

Oppenheim JJ, Feldmann M (2001) Introduction to the role of cytokines in innate host defense and adaptive immunity. In: Oppenhein JJ, Feldmann M (eds) Cytokine reference. pp 3–20

Onizuka S, Tawara I, Shimizu J et al. (1999) Tumor rejection by in vivo administration of anti-CD25 (interleukin-2 receptor alpha) monoclonal antibody. Cancer Res 59:3128–3133

Pardoll D (2003) Does the immune system see tumors as foreign or self? Annu Rev Immunol 21:807–839

Parish CR (2003) Cancer immunotherapy: The past, the present, and the future. Immunol Cell Biol 81:106–113

Parmiani G, Rivoltini L, Andreoda G et al. (2000) Cytokines in cancer therapy. Immunol Lett 74:41–44

Pippig SD, Pena-Rossi C, Long J et al. (1999) Robust B cell immunity but impaired T cell proliferation in the absence of CD134 (OX40). J Immunol 163:6520–6529

Rakhmilevich AL, North RJ (1993) Presence of CD4$^+$ T suppressor cells in mice rendered unresponsive to tumor antigens by intravenous injection of irradiated tumor cells. Int J Cancer 55:338–343

Rakhmilevich AL, North RJ (1994) Elimination of CD4$^+$ T cells in mice bearing an advanced sarcoma augments the antitumor action of interleukin-2. Cancer Immunol Immunother 38:107–112

Rao A, Luo C, Hogan PG (1997) Transcription factors of the Nf-AT family: Regulation and function. Annual Rev Immunol 15:707–747

Rogers PR, Song J, Gramaglia I et al. (2001) OX40 promotes Bcl-xL and Bcl-2 expression and is essential for long-term survival of CD4 T cells. Immunity 15:445–455

Ronchetti S, Zollo O, Bruscoli S et al. (2004) GITR, a member of the TNF receptor superfamily, is costimulatory to mouse T lymphocyte subpopulations. Eur J Immunol 34:613–622

Runyon K, Lee K, Zuberek K et al. (2001) The combination of chemotherapy and systemic immunotherapy with soluble B7-immunoglobulin G leads to cure of murine leukemia and lymphoma and demonstration of tumor-specific memory responses. Blood 97:2420–2426

Sharifi J, Khawli LA, Hu P et al. (2001) Characterization of a phage display-derived human monoclonal antibody (NHS76) counterpart to chimeric TNT-1 directed against necrotic regions of solid tumors. Hybridoma Hybridomics 20:305–312

Sharifi J, Khawli LA, Hu P et al. (2002) Generation of human interferon gamma and tumor necrosis alpha chimeric TNT-3 fusion proteins. Hybridoma Hybridomics 21:421–432

Shevach EM (2000) Suppressor T cells: Rebirth, function and homeostasis. Curr Biol 10:R572–R575

Shevach EM (2001) Certified professionals: CD4$^+$CD25$^+$ suppressor T cells. J Exp Med 193:F41–F46

Shevach EM (2002) CD4$^+$CD25$^+$ suppressor T cells: More questions than answers. Nat Rev Immunol 2:389–400

Shimizu J, Yamazaki S, Sakaguchi S (1999) Induction of tumor immunity by removing CD25$^+$CD4$^+$ T cells: A common basis between tumor immunity and autoimmunity. J Immunol 163:5211–5218

Silagi S, Shaefer A (1986) Successful immunotherapy of mouse melanoma and sarcoma with rIL-2 and cyclophosphamide. J Biol Response Mod 5:411–422

Singh NP, Yolcu ES, Taylor DD et al. (2003) A novel approach to cancer immunotherapy: Tumor cells decorated with CD80 generate effective antitumor immunity. Cancer Res 6:4067–4073

Smith KA (1993) Lowest dose interleukin-2 immunotherapy. Blood 81:1414–1423

Smyth MJ, Godfrey DI, Trapani JA (2001) A fresh look at tumor immunosurveillance and immunotherapy. Nature Immunol 2:293–299

Somasundaram R, Jacob L (2002) Inhibition of cytolytic T lymphocyte proliferation by autologous CD4$^+$CD25$^+$ regulatory T cells in a colorectal carcinoma patient is mediated by transforming growth factor-β. Cancer Res 62:5267–5272

Sone S, Ogura T (1994) Local interleukin-2 therapy for cancer, and its effect induction mechanisms. Oncology 51:170–176

Stephens LA, Mottet C, Mason D et al. (2001) Human of CD4$^+$CD25$^+$ thymocytes and peripheral T cells have immune suppressive activity. Eur J Immunol 31:1247–1254

Sutmuller RP, van Duivenvoorde LM, van Elsas A et al. (2001) Synergism of cytotoxic T lymphocyte-associated antigen-4 blockade and depletion of CD25$^+$ regulatory T cells in antitumor therapy reveals alternative pathways for suppression of autoreactive cytotoxic T lymphocyte responses. J Exp Med 194:823–832

Sturmhoefel K, Lee K, Gray GS et al. (1999) Potent activity of soluble B7-IgG fusion proteins in therapy of established tumors and as vaccine adjuvant. Cancer Res 59:4964–4972

Tanaka H, Tanaka J, Kjaergaard J et al. (2002) Depletion of CD4$^+$CD25$^+$ regulatory cells augments the generation of specific immune T cells in tumor-draining lymph nodes. J Immunother 25:207–217

Takeda I, Ine S, Killeen N et al. (2004) Distinct roles for the OX40-OX40 ligand interaction in regulatory and nonregulatory T cells. J Immunol 172:3580–3589

Thelen M (2001) Dancing to the tune of chemokines. Nature Immunol 2:129–134

Townsend SE, Allison JP (1993) Tumor rejection after direct costimulation of CD8$^+$ T cells by B7-transfected melanoma cells. Science 259:368–369

Valzasina B, Guiducci C, Dislich H et al. (2005) Triggering of OX40 (CD134) on CD4$^+$CD25$^+$ T cells blocks their inhibitory activity: A novel regulatory role for OX40 and its comparison with GITR. Blood 105:2845–2851

Vinay DS, Kwon BS (1998) Role of 4-1BB in immune responses. Semin Immunol 10:481–489

Waldmann TA (2003) Immunotherapy: Past, present, and future. Nature Med 9:269–277

Wang HC, Klein JR (2001) Multiple levels of activation of murine CD8$^+$ intraepithelial lymphocytes defined by OX40 (CD134) expression: Effects on cell-mediated cytotoxicity, IFN-gamma, and IL-10 regulation. J Immunol 167:6717–6723

Weinberg AD, Wegmann KW, Funatake C et al. (1999) Blocking OX40/OX40 ligand interaction in vitro and in vivo leads to decreased T cell function and amelioration of experimental allergic encephalomyelitis. J Immunol 162:1818–1826

Wen T, Bukczynski J, Watts TH (2002) 4-1BB ligand-mediated costimulation of human T cells induces CD4 and CD8 T cell expansion, cytokine production, and the development of cytolytic effector function. J Immunol 168:4897–4906

Yamaguchi N, Hiraoka S-I, Mukai T et al. (2004) Induction of tumor regression by administration of B7-Ig fusion proteins: Mediation by type 2 CD8$^+$ T-cells and dependence on IL-4 production. J Immunol 172:1347–1354

Yu L, Ju D, Chen W et al. (2006) I-131 chTNT Radioimmunotherapy of 43 patients with advanced lung cancer. Cancer Biother Radiopharm 21:5–14

Zhang N, Sadun RE, Arias RS et al. (2007) Targeted and untargeted CD137L fusion proteins for the immunotherapy of experimental solid tumors. Clinical Cancer Res 13:2758–2767

Zheng G, Chen A, Sterner RE et al. (2001) Induction of autitumor immunity via intratumoral tetra-costimulator protein transfer. Cancer Res 61:8127–8134

Zheng G, Wang B, Chen A (2004) The 4-1BB costimulation augments the proliferation of CD4$^+$CD25$^+$ regulatory T cells. J Immunol 173:2428–2434

Zou W (2005) Immunosuppressive networks in the tumor environment and their therapeutic relevance. Nature Rev Cancer 5:263–74

The T-Body Approach: Redirecting T Cells with Antibody Specificity

Z. Eshhar

1 Background 330
2 Optimal Chimeric Receptor Composition 331
   2.1 Combining Costimulatory and Stimulatory Signals 331
   2.2 Signaling Domains 333
3 Preclinical Proof of Concept in Experimental Models 333
4 Clinical Trials... 335
References 338

Abstract "T-bodies" are genetically engineered T cells armed with chimeric receptors whose extracellular recognition unit is comprised of an antibody-derived recognition domain and whose intracellular region is derived from lymphocyte stimulating moiety(ies). The structure of the prototypic chimeric receptor, also known as a chimeric immune receptor, is modular, designed to accomodate various functional domains and thereby to enable choice of specificity and controlled activation of T cells. The preferred antibody-derived recognition unit is a single chain variable fragment (scFv) that combines the specificity and binding residues of both the heavy and light chain variable regions of a monoclonal antibody. The most common lymphocyte activation moieties include a T-cell costimulatory (e.g. CD28) domain in tandem with a T-cell triggering (e.g. CD3ζ) moiety. By arming effector lymphocytes (such as T cells and natural killer cells) with such chimeric receptors, the engineered cell is redirected with a predefined specificity to any desired target antigen, in a non-HLA restricted manner. Chimeric receptor (CR) constructs are introduced ex vivo into T cells from peripheral lymphocytes of a given patient using retroviral vectors. Following infusion of the resulting T-bodies back into the patient, they traffic, reach

Z. Eshhar

Department of Immunology, The Weizmann Institute of Science, P.O. Box 26, Rehovot 76100, Israel

e-mail: zelig.eshhar@weizmann.ac.il

Y. Chernajovsky, A. Nissim (eds.) *Therapeutic Antibodies. Handbook of Experimental Pharmacology 181*.
© Springer-Verlag Berlin Heidelberg 2008

their target site, and upon interaction with their target cell or tissue, they undergo activation and perform their predefined effector function. Therapeutic targets for the T-body approach include cancer and HIV-infected cells, or autoimmune effector cells. To date, the most investigated area is cancer therapy. Here, the T-bodies are advantageous because their tumor recognition is not HLA-specific and, therefore, the same constructs can be used for a wide spectrum of patients and cancers. In addition, they can penetrate and reject not only vascular tumors but also bulky solid tumors. T-bodies have so far been prepared against a variety of tumors using scFv's derived from antibodies specific for tumor associated antigens. Proof of concept for the therapeutical benefit of cancer-specific T-bodies has been provided in animal models, and several phase I clinical trials are in process.

1 Background

The T-body approach, which combines antibody specificity with T cell stimulatory function within the context of a CR, was originally designed to better understand the mode of T-cell receptor (TCR) activation and the physicochemical parameters governing the T cell/antigen interaction (Gross and Eshhar 1992). Shortly thereafter, we and others realized the potential of this approach for cancer immunotherapy, combining the non-HLA restricted specificity of antitumor antibodies with the efficient tissue rejection of T cells (Eshhar et al. 1996).

The first configuration of an antibody-based chimeric receptor was composed of the two TCR chains. Here, the variable regions, Vα and Vβ, of the TCR chains were replaced with the VH and VL of the antibody light and heavy chains (Gross et al. 1989a, 1989b; Eshhar et al. 1996). Upon transfection of T-cell hybridomas and lines with the two chimeric chains (either CαVL and CβVH or CαVH and CβVL), a functional chimeric TCR/CD3 (chTCR) complex with antibody specificity was expressed on the cell surface. This chTCR associated with the CD3 complex and did not mix-assemble with the endogenous TCR chains. The double-chain configuration was instrumental for demonstrating that T cells can undergo activation in a non-MHC dependent or restricted manner (Gross and Eshhar 1992) and to highlight the role that TCR avidity and coreceptors (such as LFA-1, CD4, and CD8) play in T-cell activation (Lustgarten et al. 1991; Gorochov et al. 1993). The two-chain chTCR used in these early studies was directed at haptens and helped delineate the physicochemical parameters for TCR-mediated activation (Gross and Eshhar 1992). For these receptors, two genes were required to be co- or sequentially transferred into T cells to obtain a functional expression. Such double transfections were cumbersome for stable expression in naïve T cells. We therefore adapted the single chain Fv (scFv) unit to serve as an antibody recognition unit, and coupled it, through a hinge sequence, to either the CD3ζ or FCRγ activation chains (Eshhar et al. 1993). Such a single chain chimeric receptor was expressed as a homodimer or monovalent heterodimer associated with the endogenous CD3ζ chain and could, by itself, trigger T-cell activation and stimulate proliferation and effector functions including interleukin release and target cell killing upon antigen encounter (Eshhar et al. 1993).

This prototypic single chain configuration of the chimeric receptor (CR) has served as the template for today's T-body receptors. An additional significant development was the optimization of conditions to enable the transduction of naïve T cells, based on ex vivo activation and the use of retrovirus-mediated transduction (Rosenberg et al. 1990; Culver et al. 1991).

In this Chapter, I focus on the application of the T-body approach for cancer immunotherapy. Adoptive and passive immunotherapy have become a promising therapeutic option based on several clinical trials that demonstrated significant objective responses (and a few complete remissions) in cancer patients receiving tumor-specific T cells (Gomez et al. 2001; Dudley et al. 2002; Rosenberg et al. 2004; Bollard et al. 2004). Because tumor-specific T cells are rare for most human malignancies, the alternative of using genetically redirected, effector cells bearing ectopic receptors has become an attractive option for cancer therapy. Endowing T cells with antitumor specificity by the transduction of the two TCR chains has already proven effective in cancer patients (Morgan et al. 2006). This approach, unlike the T-body approach, is limited to individuals of certain HLA and is not applicable to tumors that escaped the immune system by failing to express surface MHC:peptide complexes.

2 Optimal Chimeric Receptor Composition

To serve as a cancer-specific therapeutic agent able to eliminate the large mass of cells in solid tumors, the T-body receptor must optimally discriminate the tumor from healthy tissue. Following its systemic administration to the patient, the T-body should migrate to the tumor site, interact with the tumor cell, undergo activation, and execute its effector function, culminating in cancer elimination. Optimal performance of this series of events is dependent on predefined, intrinsic properties of the transfected T cell that are triggered and regulated by the CR, and are dependent on its composition. The process of tumor rejection, similar to tissue rejection, is a complex one that requires both CD8 and CD4 cells that can mediate direct target cell killing and induce a local inflammatory response. Apparently, a single CR that interacts with its target antigen at high enough affinity can trigger the activation of both CD8 and CD4 T cells in which it is expressed. Nevertheless, for certain applications and specific targets, fine-tuning of the CR can be achieved by modifying several elements, mainly the activation and costimulatory sequences in its intracellular domain.

2.1 Combining Costimulatory and Stimulatory Signals

For optimal and sustained function of T cells, their development into memory cells and their reactivation, especially by targets lacking the ligands for costimulatory molecules (which are missing on many tumor cells), an added costimulatory signal is advantageous. It has been shown that CR that lack the capacity to provide costimulatory signaling cannot activate resting or naïve lymphocytes, such as T cells derived from genetically modified stem-cells or from CR transgenic mice (Brocker et al. 1995). It is also well established that, in the absence of costimulatory signaling by CD28, resting T lymphocytes typically undergo anergy or apoptosis (Boussiotis et al. 1998).

These obstacles have been resolved by constructing CR in which the scFv is linked to the intracellular part of CD28 or other costimulatory molecules such as OX40 (CD134), CD40L, PD-1, or 4-1BB (CD137) (Finney et al. 1998; Finney et al. 2004). The effect of these costimulatory domains in the context of the CR was compared in unstimulated human CD4 and CD8 T cells and was found that cytokine release and killing activity in response to target cells was dramatically enhanced by all the costimulatory sequences relative to the CR that did not contain any costimulatory signaling moieties. No practical advantage was demonstrated by ICOS, OX40, or 4-1BB over the CD28-based tripartite CR. We designed a novel tripartite CR composed of an scFv recognition moiety, fused to the nonligand binding part of the extracellular and the entire transmembrane and intracellular domains of the CD28 costimulatory molecule, together with the intracellular domain of FcRγ (scFv-CD28-γ). Human PBL transducedwith such a CR gene demonstrate specific stimulation of IL-2 production and target cell killing (Eshhar et al. 2001). Many studies, from different groups, have demonstrated that out of the costimulatory domains, CD28 performed the best in various experimental settings (Gong et al. 1999; Hombach et al 2001; Haynes et al. 2002; Maher et al. 2002; Willemsen et al. 2005; Kowolik et al. 2006). Enhanced tumor rejection in mouse models using human and has been demonstrated (Pinthus et al. 2003, 2004; Westwood et al. 2005; Gade et al. 2005; Vera et al. 2006).To prove the ultimate requirement of CD28 for antigen-specific activation and development of mature naïve T cells, we have recently generated several lines of transgenic mice expressing CR under the control of T-cell-specific regulatory sequences. Unprimed, naïve T lymphocytes from mice transgenic for scFv-CD28-γ tripartite CR undergo high levels of proliferation, IL-2 secretion, and rescue from apoptosis following stimulation by plastic-bound cognate antigen (Friedmann-Morvinski et al. 2005). The rescue from apoptosis by CD28 in the context of T cells stimulation through the antigen-specific CR is an important factor in the persistence of the T-bodies in the patient where they are at the risk of antigen-induced cell death in the absence of B7 on the surface of the tumor target cell. Additional advantage is the recent finding that CD28 costimulation overcomes transforming growth factor (TGF)-β-mediated repression of proliferation of redirected human CD4+ and CD8+ T cells in an antitumor cell attack (Koehler et al. 2007). TGF-β is known for its immunosuppressive activity that is produced by regulatory T cells and some tumors. Along this line is the finding that the inclusion of CD28 to the CR enhances chimeric T-cell resistance to Treg (Loskog et al. 2006).

As to the use of 4-1BB signaling domain in the context of the CR, it was found to elicit potent cytotoxicity against acute lymphoblastic leukemia cells in vitro (Imai et al. 2004). Although the performance to date of CD28 appears quite satisfactory both in vitro and in vivo, the possibility of including additional or alternative moieties, or combinations of costimulatory domains should be further explored, especially to sustain and optimize the anticancer effect of T-bodies in vivo.

2.2 Signaling Domains

In contrast to the costimulatory moieties, only a few stimulatory domains have been used in the CR context. The original studies used both the CD3ζ and FcRγ subunits (Eshhar et al. 1993) and one group used the CD3ϖ domain (Schaft et al. 2006). All these domains signal through the immune T-cell activation motifs (ITAM) that contain a tyrosine, which undergoes phosphorylation as a result of the interaction of the TCR with antigen presenting cells. The phosphorylated ITAM facilitates docking of down stream kinases (such as ZAP70 and Syk) that are involved in signal transduction. FcRγ and CD3ζ contain a single ITAM, while CD3ζ contains three such motifs. No comprehensive comparison has been done so far to identify the most active domain in the context of the CR. We tend to prefer the FcRγ based on early studies showing that phosphorylation of the first ITAM of the CD3ζ leads to anergy (Kersh et al. 1999). Despite the lack of consensus, we have tried to bypass signaling through the ITAM that is impaired in T lymphocytes of tumor-bearing subjects (Mizoguchi et al. 1992). In a series of studies, we found that using the Syk cytoplasmic phosphotyrosine kinase as the signaling domain of the CR instead of an ITAM-containing signaling chain can efficiently induce T-cell activation (Fitzer Attas et al. 1998).

3 Preclinical Proof of Concept in Experimental Models

To date, many antibodies recognizing various tumor antigens have been used to generate CR that target T-bodies to variety of human tumors (for recent reviews see Kershaw et al. 2005; Friedman-Morvinski and Eshhar 2006). In the first preclinical trial (Moritz et al. 1994) of T-body-mediated therapy, mouse T cells expressing HER2-specific CR were injected subcutaneously (s.c.) into nude mice together with a target tumor transfected with the human erbB2 gene. In this model, it was observed that tumor development was significantly delayed. In a more recent study by the same group (Altenschmidt et al. 1997), it was shown that HER2-specific splenic T cells repeatedly administered directly into erbB2-expressing mouse mammary tumors result in total tumor regression. Using murine CTL expressing CEA-specific CR (Haynes et al. 2002), the group in Melbourne showed an in vivo effect against colon carcinoma. The CTL-mediated effect in this study required perforin and IFNγ and was independent of FAS-L or TNF. A more clinically relevant experiment used murine tumor infiltrating lymphocytes transduced with a folate binding protein (FBP)-specific CR (Hwu et al. 1995). The tumor target was a syngeneic metastatic sarcoma, transduced with the human FBP gene. When injected intravenously into mice, together with daily injections of IL-2, FBP-specific T cells induced a significant reduction in the number of lung metastasis.

To test whether human T-bodies (usually from peripheral blood lymphocytes (PBL) derived by retroviral vector transduction) could specifically recognize and eliminate human tumor cells or xenografts, most models used immune deficient

SCID or nude mice. In such a system, we demonstrated the ability of HER/2-specific human T-bodies to reject large established (subcutaneous and orthotopic) prostate cancer human xenografts (Pinthus et al. 2003) and tumors derived from human breast cancer cell lines (Morvinski-Friedman and Eshhar, unpublished). It should be emphasized that in these studies, the T-bodies were injected directly into the tumor; such an administration route is a valid option for primary solid tumors that are accessible. A simpler and more desirable route of effector cell administration is systemic infusion. Here, the redirected T-bodies must circulate in the body and migrate to their tumor target, whether a localized primary tumor, secondary metastases, or disseminated residual tumor cells following conventional therapy. Using systemic administration, most published (and many unpublished) studies showed only a mild and transient effect. On the basis of the experience of Rosenberg's group using either human tumor infiltrating lymphocytes (TIL) for melanoma treatment (Dudley et al. 2002) and results obtained in the murine Pmel system by Restifo and Rosenberg (for recent review see Gattinoni et al. 2006), it was found that treating patients (or mice) with mild lymphodepletion agents (such as cyclophosphamide and fludarabin alone, or together with sublethal irradiation) to create a lymphopaenic environment before T-cell transfer, dramatically improves the antitumor response of the adoptively transferrd cells in the recipient. Indeed, when we treated recipient SCID mice harboring a prostate cancer bone lesion in a similar way, the T-bodies resulted in considerable antitumor respones including complete cure in a significant number of mice (Pinthus et al. 2004). Several mechanisms have been suggested for the effect of lymphodepletion (for reviews see Klebanoff et al. 2005; Wrzesinski et al. 2005) including overcoming homeostatic control, eliminating regulatory cells and cytokine sink (Gattinoni et al. 2005). Because our studies were done in both lympho and myelo deficient strains of SCID mice, in which the homeostatic control and suppressive effects of lymphodepletion do not play a role, we found that at least part of the benefit of lymphoablative preconditioning is due to an increase in SDF-1, which is induced by the regenerative process following the preconditioning treatment. Apparently, the elevation of SDF-1 compensates for the low expression of its receptor, CXCR4, on the ex vivo manipulated cells (Pinthus et al. 2004).

Studies using adoptive cell transfer for the treatment of cancer have been greatly intensified in recent years, mainly due to the lack of success of therapeutic cancer vaccination using active immunization (Rosenberg et al. 2004); these trials have provided many lessons that could be adapted to the T-body approach. Yet, adoptive T-body transfer requiring ex vivo manipulation to introduce the CR genes suffers from the fact that the T cells must be activated to enable the gene transfer process. Such activation, usually induced by anti-CD3 and CD28 antibodies, drives the cells to differentiate into effector cells with modified expression of surface receptors and adhesion molecules, thus resulting in impaired migration patterns and limited persistence in the recipient. Much effort has been invested in recent years in order to improve these key issues that directly affect the therapeutic potency and potential of the T-bodies. Approaches that are currently being tested include the use of nonretroviral vehicles, such as transfection of CTL with naked DNA (Jensen et al. 2000) and RNA-based transfection (Johnson et al. 2006). In addition, cytokines such as IL-2,

IL-7, IL-15, and IL-21 are being tested to support the homeostatic proliferation of T cells in the recipient (Brentjens et al. 2003; Klebanoff et al. 2004; Wang et al. 2005; Hsu et al. 2005; Hwang et al. 2006; Hsu et al. 2007). These interleukins are added during the ex vivo preparation phase and/or as part of the in vivo treatment. One notable example is IL-21, which directs cells to differentiate in vivo into central immune memory cells, rather than into the short-lived effector memory phenotype (Klebanoff et al. 2006). Other variables that are being studied in order to improve and optimize T-body function in vivo are selecting the best costimulatory moiety (as discussed above), not only elimination of regulatory cells from the cancer patient as described above, but also their removal from the lymphocyte population set aside for transduction. Finally, to provide the T-body with growth signals in vivo that will prolong their persistence regardless of the CR signals, several groups have introduced the CR to T cell populations already specific to a common viral antigen (such a EBV (Rossig et al. 2002) or Flu (Cooper et al. 2005)).

A different approach to avoid the need for ex vivo manipulation of T cells is to introduce the CR into hematopoietic stem cells that will eventually differentiate and mature into T cells. Wang et al. (1998) evaluated the potency of murine bone-marrow stem cells, transduced with FBP-specific CR gene, and found that the growth of an FBP-expressing tumor was retarded. Interestingly, T cells are not directly involved in this process, as depletion of CD4 and CD8 cells does not diminish the antitumor activity. It was therefore suggested that NK cells and/or macrophages expressing the anti-FBP CR are responsible for this antitumor effect. More recently, Baltimore's group described a method to genetically program mouse hematopoietic stem cells (HSC) to develop into functional CD8 or CD4 T cells of defined specificity in vivo (Yang et al. 2002 and 2005). To this end, they engineered a bicistronic retroviral vector that efficiently delivers genes for both α and β TCR chains of the TCR to the HSC. By combining cells modified with CD8- and CD4-specific TCRs and boosting with dendritic cells pulsed with cognate peptides, complete suppression of tumor growth was achieved, and even established tumors regress and are eliminated following dendritic cell/peptide immunization. These experiments highlight an extension of the T-body approach through the administration of effector cells into patients undergoing systemic cyto-ablative therapy. Thus, cancer patients treated with bone marrow transplants could be reconstituted with genetically altered stem cells. Immediate possible candidates for such a treatment are leukemic patients receiving stem cell grafts. The tripartite CR is the construct of choice for such treatment, as its built-in costimulatory signaling function supports the priming and activation of naïve T cells to mature specific effector activity.

4 Clinical Trials

As shown in Table 1, several phase-I clinical trials using T-bodies for cancer therapy have been initiated, and several others are on-going or in various stages of planning. Because results from only a few of these studies have been published to date,

Table 1 T-Bodies in clinical trials

Tumor	Antigen	Group	Status[a]
Ovarian	FBP	Hwu, Rosenberg, NCI	Performed
Colorectal ca.	TAG-72	McArthur, Cell Genesys	Performed
Colorectal & breast ca.	CEA	Junghans, Harvard	Performed
Renal ca.	Carboxyanhydrase IX	Gratama, Rotterdam	Ongoing
Neuroblastoma	CD171	Jensen Seattle/City of Hope	Ongoing
Glioblastoma	IL-13 Receptor[b]	Jensen, City of Hope	Ongoing
Neuroblastoma	G(D)2	Brenner, Baylor College of Med.	Ongoing
Gastric ca.	CEA (2nd generation)	Junghans, Roger Williams	Recruiting
Prostate ca.	PSMA	Junghans, Roger Williams	Recruiting
Leukemia	CD19	Jensen, City of Hope	Recruiting
Leukemia	CD19	Hawkins, Manchester	Recruiting
Leukemia	CD19	Sadelain, Sloan Kettering	Recruiting
Leukemia	CD19	Brenner, Baylor College of Med.	Approved
Leukemia	CD19	June, Univ. Pennsylvania	Pending
Pancreatic ca.	Mesothelin	June, Univ. Pennsylvania	Pending
Colorectal ca.	CEA	Hawkins, Manchester	In planning
Prostate ca.	PSMA	Sadelain, Sloan Kettering	In planning
Myeloma	Lewis-Y	Kershaw, Melbourne	In planning
Cutaneous lymphoma	CD30	Abken, Cologne	In planning
Lymphoma	CD20	Cooper, MD Anderson	In planning

[a] Updated to April 2007

[b] Redirected by IL-13 ζ CR (not antibody based)

much of the information in this section is derived from registries and from personal communications. One fully documented phase I trial was conducted in HIV infected subjects receiving autologous lymphocytes bearing the CD4-ζ CR (Mitsuyasu et al. 2000). About half of the patients also received concurrent IL-2 infusions for five days. The treatment was well tolerated with grade 3 or 4 adverse events predominantly associated with the IL-2 infusion. In some patients, a transient decrease of the viral load was observed in the plasma and the rectal mucosa, the tissue reservoir for HIV. All 24 subjects tested negative for replication-competent retrovirus for up to one year after cell infusion. Cell Genesys, which carried out this study, also conducted phase I clinical trials in colorectal patients using the anti-TAG72-ζ CR made from the humanized CC49 mAb (Warren et al. 1998). This trial, however, was terminated due to the identification of anti-idiotypic antibodies in the patient sera, which caused difficulty in interpretation of the results.

The group of Junghans tested 24 doses of CEA-specific CR-bearing lymphocytes, with a total dose of up to 10^{11} cells per patient. The treatment was reported to be adequately tolerated, with only two minor adverse effects observed in two colorectal carcinoma patients (Junghans et al. 2000). Hwu and colleagues (Kershaw et al. 2006) at the NCI conducted a phase I clinical trial in ovarian cancer patients using T-bodies expressing a CR that we generated against human α folate receptor, also known as FBP. This trial demonstrated that large numbers of gene-modified tumor-reactive T cells can be safely given to patients, but these cells do not persist in large numbers in the long term. No reduction in tumor burden was seen in any patient. Tracking ^{111}In-labeled adoptively transferred T cells revealed that the T cells did not localize to the tumor, except in one patient where some signal was detected in a peritoneal deposit. PCR analysis showed that gene-modified T cells were present in the circulation in large numbers for the first two days after transfer, but these quickly declined and became barely detectable one month later in most patients. Five out of eight patients who received a dose escalation of T cells in combination with high-dose IL-2 experienced some grade 3 to 4 treatment-related toxicity that was probably due to IL-2 administration, which could be managed using standard measures. Patients in cohort 2 who received T cells with dual specificity (reactive with both FR and allogeneic cells), followed by immunization with allogeneic peripheral blood mononuclear cells, experienced relatively mild side effects with grade 1 to 2 symptoms. Neutralizing antibodies were found in some of the patient sera, specific to the murine anti-FBP MoV18 mAb.

A group at Daniel den Hoed Cancer Center in Rotterdam reported a phase I clinical trial in renal cell cancer (RCC), using autologous T lymphocytes modified with a CR specific for carboxy anhydrase IX (Lamers et al. 2004, 2006). Infusions of the modified T lymphocytes were initially well tolerated. However, after four to five infusions, all three patients began to develop liver enzyme abnormalities. This was explained by the reactivity of the genetically modified cells with low levels of carboxy anhydrase IX expressed on the bile duct epithelium, limiting treatment to only low doses of CR-expressing T-bodies. The results of this study showed that the T-bodies exert CR-directed functions in vivo. Several patients in the trial also developed antibodies to the murine G250 scFv. Because of these side effects, this trial was put on hold and awaits renewal pending the application of systemic anti-carboxy anhydrase IX antibodies to block antigen expression on the bile duct. The results of a safety/feasibility trial using human CTL clones redirected at metastatic neuroblastoma was recently published (Park et al. 2007). In this trial CD8 | CTL clones were transfected with anti-CD171 CR and the selection suicide expression enzyme HyTK. Six children with recurrent/refractory neuroblastoma received 12 infusions. No overt toxicities to tissues known to express the CD171 adhesion molecule were observed. The persistence of the modified CTL in the circulation was short (1–7 days) in patients with bulky disease, but significantly longer (42 days) in a patient with limited disease burden. The authors suggest this pilot study set the stage for clinical trial in the context of minimal residual disease.

Table 1 also includes clinical trials that are either ongoing or in advanced phases of preparation (e.g., awaiting authorization from regulatory bodies). Many of these trials have been designed based on lessons learned from the preclinical animal models, e.g., use of humanized scFv, inclusion of the CD28 costimulatory domain, use of lentiviral vectors to transduce the PBL, inclusion of homeostatic interleukins in the ex vivo procedures used to prepare the T-bodies, transfection of both CD4 and CD8 T cells, use of T-bodies made from autologous T cells that are also specific to viral antigens such as EBV and influenza. Very importantly, in several of these studies, lymphoablative pretreatments will be used to precondition the patients before the administration of T-bodies. Most of the trials will target blood borne tumors such as lymphoma or leukemia, using anti-CD19 or CD20 scFvs from humanized antibodies. Although less challenging than solid tumors, it is hoped that the results of using T-bodies against these targets will demonstrate some dose-dependent effect, by decreasing the tumor load, and thereby paving the way for applying the T-body approach against more challenging solid tumors. Introduction of genes to T cells using retroviral vectors has been proved safe and it is clear today that the risk of leukemia that occurred in patients receiving retroviral vector-mediated gene transfer into HSC does not exist for mature T cells. Potential severe side effects seen in some patient in the clinical trials reported above are manageable. A careful selection of the antibody whose scFv will serve to redirect the T-bodies, both in terms of specificity and affinity, will diminish the risk of damaging essential healthy tissues and side effects of IL-2 could be controlled and hopefully will be prevented when the persistence of the T-bodies in the body will be improved as discussed above.

Acknowledgements The studies of Prof. Eshhar group were supported in part by EU FP5 and FP6, US Army Prostate Cancer and Breast Cancer Research Program, Prostate Cancer Foundation, Israel Science Foundation, M.D. Moross Institute for Cancer Research, and Benoziyo Center for Cancer Research.

References

Altenschmidt U, Klundt E, Groner B (1997) Adoptive transfer of in vitro-targeted, activated T lymphocytes results in total tumor regression. J Immunol 159: 5509–5515

Bollard CM, Aguilar L, Straathof KC, Gahn B, Huls MH, Rousseau A, Sixbey J, Gresik MV, Carrum G, Hudson M, Dilloo D, Gee A, Brenner MK, Rooney CM, Heslop HE (2004) Cytotoxic T lymphocyte therapy for Epstein-Barr virus+ Hodgkin's disease. J Exp Med 200: 1623–1633

Boussiotis VA, Freeman GJ, Gribben JG, Nadler LM (1998) The role of B7-1/B7-2:CD28/CLTA-4 pathways in the prevention of anergy, induction of productive immunity and down-regulation of the immune response. Immunol Rev 153: 5–26

Brentjens RJ, Latouche JB, Santos E, Marti F, Gong MC, Lyddane C, King PD, Larson S, Weiss M, Riviere I, Sadelain M (2003) Eradication of systemic B-cell tumors by genetically targeted human T lymphocytes co-stimulated by CD80 and interleukin-15. Nat Med 9: 279–286

Brocker T, Karjalainen K (1995) Signals through T cell receptor-zeta chain alone are insufficient to prime resting T lymphocytes. J Exp Med 181: 1653–1659

Cooper LJ, Al-Kadhimi Z, Serrano LM, Pfeiffer T, Olivares S, Castro A, Chang WC, Gonzalez S, Smith D, Forman SJ, Jensen MC (2005) Enhanced antilymphoma efficacy of CD19-redirected influenza MP1-specific CTLs by cotransfer of T cells modified to present influenza MP1. Blood 105: 1622–1631

Culver K, Cornetta K, Morgan R, Morecki S, Aebersold P, Kasid A, Lotze M, Rosenberg SA, Anderson WF, Blaese RM (1991) Lymphocytes as cellular vehicles for gene therapy in mouse and man. Proc Natl Acad Sci USA 88: 3155–3159

Dudley ME, Wunderlich JR, Robbins PF, Yang JC, Hwu P, Schwartzentruber DJ, Topalian SL, Sherry R, Restifo NP, Hubicki AM, Robinson MR, Raffeld M, Duray P, Seipp CA, Rogers-Freezer L, Morton KE, Mavroukakis SA, White DE, Rosenberg SA (2002) Cancer regression and autoimmunity in patients after clonal repopulation with anti-tumor lymphocytes. Science 298: 850–854

Eshhar Z, Bach N, Fitzer-Attas CJ, Gross G, Lustgarten J, Waks T, Schindler DG (1996) The T-body approach: Potential for cancer immunotherapy. Springer Semin Immunopathol 18: 199–209

Eshhar Z, Waks T, Bendavid A, Schindler DG (2001) Functional expression of chimeric receptor genes in human T cells. J Immunol Methods 248: 67–76

Eshhar Z, Waks T, Gross G, Schindler DG (1993) Specific activation and targeting of cytotoxic lymphocytes through chimeric single chains consisting of antibody-binding domains and the gamma or zeta subunits of the immunoglobulin and T cell receptors. Proc Natl Acad Sci USA 90: 720–724

Finney HM, Akbar AN, Lawson AD (2004) Activation of resting human primary T cells with chimeric receptors: Co-stimulation from CD28, inducible costimulator, CD134, and CD137 in series with signals from the TCR zeta chain. J Immunol 172: 104–113

Finney HM, Lawson AD, Bebbington CR, Weir AN (1998) Chimeric receptors providing both primary and co-stimulatory signaling in T cells from a single gene product. J Immunol 161: 2791–2797

Fitzer-Attas, CJ, Schindler DG, Waks T, Eshhar Z (1998) Harnessing Syk family tyrosine kinases as signaling domains for chimeric single chain of the variable domain receptors: Optimal design for T cell activation. J Immunol 160:145–153.

Friedmann-Morvinski D, Bendavid A, Waks T, Schindler D, Eshhar Z (2005) Redirected primary T cells harboring a chimeric receptor require co-stimulation for their antigen-specific activation. Blood 105: 3087–3093

Friedman-Morvinski D, Eshhar Z (2006) Adoptive immunotherapy of cancer using effector lymphocytes redirected with antibody specificity. CCBRM 23

Gade TP, Hassen W, Santos E, Gunset G, Saudemont A, Gong MC, Brentjens R, Zhong XS, Stephan M, Stefanski J, Lyddane C, Osborne JR, Buchanan IM, Hall SJ, Heston WD, Riviere I, Larson SM, Koutcher JA, Sadelain M (2005) Targeted elimination of prostate cancer by genetically directed human T lymphocytes. Cancer Res 65: 9080–9088

Gattinoni L, Finkelstein SE, Klebanoff CA, Antony PA, Palmer DC, Spiess PJ, Hwang LN, Yu Z, Wrzesinski C, Heimann DM, Surh CD, Rosenberg SA, Restifo NP (2005) Removal of homeostatic cytokine sinks by lymphodepletion enhances the efficacy of adoptively transferred tumor-specific CD8+ T cells. J Exp Med 202: 907–912

Gattinoni L, Powell DJ, Jr, Rosenberg SA, Restifo NP (2006) Adoptive immunotherapy for cancer: Building on success. Nat Rev Immunol 6: 383–393

Gomez GG, Hutchison RB, Kruse CA (2001) Chemo-immunotherapy and chemo-adoptive immunotherapy of cancer. Cancer Treat Rev 27: 375–402

Gong MC, Latouche JB, Krause A, Heston WD, Bander NH, Sadelain M (1999) Cancer patient T cells genetically targeted to prostate-specific membrane antigen specifically lyse prostate cancer cells and release cytokines in response to prostate-specific membrane antigen. Neoplasia 1: 123–127

Gorochov G, Gross G, Waks T, Eshhar Z (1993) Anti-leucocyte function-associated antigen-1 antibodies inhibit T cell activation following low-avidity and adhesion-independent interactions. Immunology 79: 548–555

Gross G, Eshhar Z (1992) Endowing T cells with antibody specificity using chimeric T cell receptors. FASEB J 6: 3370–3378

Gross G, Gorochov G, Waks T, Eshhar Z (1989a) Generation of effector T cells expressing chimeric T cell receptor with antibody type-specificity. Transplant Proc 21: 127–130

Gross G, Waks T, Eshhar Z (1989b) Expression of immunoglobulin-T cell receptor chimeric molecules as functional receptors with antibody-type specificity. Proc Natl Acad Sci USA 86: 10024–10028

Haynes NM, Trapani JA, Teng MW, Jackson JT, Cerruti L, Jane SM, Kershaw MH, Smyth MJ, Darcy PK (2002) Rejection of syngeneic colon carcinoma by CTLs expressing single-chain antibody receptors codelivering CD28 co-stimulation. J Immunol 169: 5780–5786

Hombach A, Sent D, Schneider C, Heuser C, Koch D, Pohl C, Seliger B, Abken H (2001) T cell activation by recombinant receptors: CD28 co-stimulation is required for interleukin 2 secretion and receptor-mediated T cell proliferation but does not affect receptor-mediated target cell lysis. Cancer Res 61: 1976–1982

Hsu C, Hughes MS, Zheng Z, Bray RB, Rosenberg SA, Morgan RA (2005) Primary human T lymphocytes engineered with a codon-optimized IL-15 gene resist cytokine withdrawal-induced apoptosis and persist long-term in the absence of exogenous cytokine. J Immunol 175: 7226–7234

Hsu C, Jones SA, Cohen CJ, Zheng Z, Kerstann K, Zhou J, Robbins PF, Peng PD, Shen X, Gomes TJ, Dunbar CE, Munroe DJ, Stewart C, Cornetta K, Wangsa D, Ried T, Rosenberg SA, Morgan RA (2007) Cytokine independent growth and clonal expansion of a primary human CD8+ T cell clone following retroviral transduction with the IL-15 gene. Blood 109(12): 5168–5177

Hwang LN, Yu Z, Palmer DC, Restifo NP (2006) The in vivo expansion rate of properly stimulated transferred CD8+ T cells exceeds that of an aggressively growing mouse tumor. Cancer Res 66: 1132–1138

Hwu P, Yang JC, Cowherd R, Treisman J, Shafer GE, Eshhar Z, Rosenberg SA (1995) In vivo anti-tumor activity of T cells redirected with chimeric antibody/T cell receptor genes. Cancer Res 55: 3369–3373

Imai C, Mihara K, Andreansky M, Nicholson IC, Pui CH, Geiger TL, Campana D (2004) Chimeric receptors with 4-1BB signaling capacity provoke potent cytotoxicity against acute lymphoblastic leukemia. Leukemia 18: 676–684

Jensen MC, Clarke P, Tan G, Wright C, Chung-Chang W, Clark TN, Zhang F, Slovak ML, Wu AM, Forman SJ, Raubitschek A (2000) Human T lymphocyte genetic modification with naked DNA. Mol Ther 1: 49–55

Johnson LA, Heemskerk B, Powell DJ, Jr, Cohen CJ, Morgan RA, Dudley ME, Robbins PF, Rosenberg SA (2006) Gene transfer of tumor-reactive TCR confers both high avidity and tumor reactivity to nonreactive peripheral blood mononuclear cells and tumor-infiltrating lymphocytes. J Immunol 177: 6548–6559

Junghans R, Safa M, Huberman M (2000) Preclinical and Phase I data of anti-CEA designer T cell therapy for cancer: A new immunotherapeutic modality. Proc Am Assoc Can Res 41: 543

Kersh EN, Kersh GJ, Allen PM (1999) Partially phosphorylated T cell receptor zeta molecules can inhibit T cell activation. J Exp Med 190: 1627–1636

Kershaw MH, Teng MW, Smyth MJ, Darcy PK (2005) Supernatural T cells: Genetic modification of T cells for cancer therapy. Nat Rev Immunol 5: 928–940

Kershaw MH, Westwood JA, Parker LL, Wang G, Eshhar Z, Mavroukakis SA, White DE, Wunderlich JR, Canevari S, Rogers-Freezer L, Chen CC, Yang JC, Rosenberg SA, Hwu P (2006) A phase I study on adoptive immunotherapy using gene-modified T cells for ovarian cancer. Clin Cancer Res 12: 6106–6115

Klebanoff CA, Finkelstein SE, Surman DR, Lichtman MK, Gattinoni L, Theoret MR, Grewal N, Spiess PJ, Antony PA, Palmer DC, Tagaya Y, Rosenberg SA, Waldmann TA, Restifo NP (2004) IL-15 enhances the in vivo anti-tumor activity of tumor-reactive CD8+ T cells. Proc Natl Acad Sci USA 101: 1969–1974

Klebanoff CA, Gattinoni L, Restifo NP (2006) CD8+ T cell memory in tumor immunology and immunotherapy. Immunol Rev 211: 214–224

Klebanoff CA, Khong HT, Antony PA, Palmer DC, Restifo NP (2005) Sinks, suppressors and antigen presenters: How lymphodepletion enhances T cell-mediated tumor immunotherapy. Trends Immunol 26: 111–117

Koehler H, Kofler D, Hombach A, Abken H (2007) CD28 co-stimulation overcomes transforming growth factor-beta-mediated repression of proliferation of redirected human CD4+ and CD8+ T cells in an anti-tumor cell attack. Cancer Res 67: 2265–2273

Kowolik CM, Topp MS, Gonzalez S, Pfeffer T et al. (2006) CD28 co-stimulation provided through a CD19-specific chimeric antigen receptor enhances in vivo persistence and anti-tumor efficacy of adoptively transferred T cells. Cancer Res 66: 10995–11004

Lamers CH, Sleijfer S, Willemsen RA, Debets R, Kruit WH, Gratama JW, Stoter G (2004) Adoptive immuno-gene therapy of cancer with single chain antibody [scFv(Ig)] gene modified T lymphocytes. J Biol Regul Homeost Agents 18: 134–140

Lamers CH, van Elzakker P, Langeveld SC, Sleijfer S, Gratama JW (2006) Process validation and clinical evaluation of a protocol to generate gene-modified T lymphocytes for imunogene therapy for metastatic renal cell carcinoma: GMP-controlled transduction and expansion of patient's T lymphocytes using a carboxy anhydrase IX-specific scFv transgene. Cytotherapy 8: 542–553

Loskog A, Giandomenico V, Rossig C, Pule M, Dotti G, Brenner MK (2006) Addition of the CD28 signaling domain to chimeric T cell receptors enhances chimeric T cell resistance to T regulatory cells. Leukemia 20: 1819–1828

Lustgarten J, Waks T, Eshhar Z (1991) CD4 and CD8 accessory molecules function through interactions with major histocompatibility complex molecules which are not directly associated with the T cell receptor-antigen complex. Eur J Immunol 21: 2507–2515

Maher J, Brentjens RJ, Gunset G, Riviere I, Sadelain M (2002) Human T-lymphocyte cytotoxicity and proliferation directed by a single chimeric TCRzeta /CD28 receptor. Nat Biotechnol 20: 70–75

Mitsuyasu RT, Anton PA, Deeks SG, Scadden DT, Connick E, Downs MT, Bakker A, Roberts MR, June CH, Jalali S, Lin AA, Pennathur-Das R, Hege KM (2000) Prolonged survival and tissue trafficking following adoptive transfer of CD4zeta gene-modified autologous CD4(+) and CD8(+) T cells in human immunodeficiency virus-infected subjects. Blood 96: 785–793

Mizoguchi H, O'Shea JJ, Longo DL, Loeffler CM, McVicar DW, Ochoa AC (1992) Alterations in signal transduction molecules in T lymphocytes from tumor-bearing mice. Science 258: 1795–1798

Morgan RA, Dudley ME, Wunderlich JR, Hughes MS, Yang JC, Sherry RM, Royal RE, Topalian SL, Kammula US, Restifo NP, Zheng Z, Nahvi A, de Vries CR, Rogers-Freezer LJ, Mavroukakis SA, Rosenberg SA (2006) Cancer regression in patients after transfer of genetically engineered lymphocytes. Science 314: 126–129

Moritz D, Wels W, Mattern J, Groner B (1994) Cytotoxic T lymphocytes with a grafted recognition specificity for ERBB2-expressing tumor cells. Proc Natl Acad Sci USA 91: 4318–4322

Park JR, Digiust DL, Slovak C, Wright C, et al. (2007) Adoptive transfer of chimeric antigen receptor redirected cytolytic T lymphocyte clones in patients with neuroblastoma. Mol Ther 15: 825–833

Pinthus JH, Waks T, Kaufman-Francis K, Schindler DG, Harmelin A, Kanety H, Ramon J, Eshhar Z (2003) Immuno-gene therapy of established prostate tumors using chimeric receptor-redirected human lymphocytes. Cancer Res 63: 2470–2476

Pinthus JH, Waks T, Malina V, Kaufman-Francis K, Harmelin A, Aizenberg I, Kanety H, Ramon J, Eshhar Z (2004) Adoptive immunotherapy of prostate cancer bone lesions using redirected effector lymphocytes. J Clin Invest 114: 1774–1781

Rosenberg SA, Aebersold P, Cornetta K, Kasid A, Morgan RA, Moen R, Karson EM, Lotze MT, Yang JC, Topalian SL, et al. (1990) Gene transfer into humans – immunotherapy of patients with advanced melanoma, using tumor-infiltrating lymphocytes modified by retroviral gene transduction. N Engl J Med 323: 570–578

Rosenberg SA, Yang JC, Restifo NP (2004) Cancer immunotherapy: Moving beyond current vaccines. Nat Med 10: 909–915

Rossig C, Bollard CM, Nuchtern JG, Rooney CM, Brenner MK (2002) Epstein-Barr virus-specific human T lymphocytes expressing anti-tumor chimeric T cell receptors: Potential for improved immunotherapy. Blood 99: 2009–2016

Schaft N, Lankiewicz B, Drexhage J, Berrevoets C, Moss DJ, Levitsky V, Bonneville M, Lee SP, McMichael AJ, Gratama JW, Bolhuis RL, Willemsen R, Debets R (2006) T cell re-targeting to EBV antigens following TCR gene transfer: CD28-containing receptors mediate enhanced antigen-specific IFNγ production. Int Immunol 18: 591–601

Vera J, Savoldo B, Vigouroux S, Biagi E, Pule M, Rossig C, Wu J, Heslop HE, Rooney CM, Brenner MK, Dotti G (2006) T lymphocytes redirected against the kappa light chain of human immunoglobulin efficiently kill mature B lymphocyte-derived malignant cells. Blood 108: 3890–3897

Warren R, Fisher G, Bergaland E (1998) Studies of regional and systemic gene therapy with autologous CC49-zeta modified T cells in colorecal cancer metastatic to liver. In 7th International Conference on Gene Therapy of Cancer

Wang G, Chopra RK, Royal RE, Yang JC, Rosenberg SA, Hwu P (1998) A T-cell-independent antitumor response in mice with bone marrow cells retrovirally transduced with an antibody/Fc-gamma chain chimeric receptor gene recognizing a human ovarian cancer antigen. Nat Med 4: 168–172

Wang LX, Li R, Yang G, Lim M, O'Hara A, Chu Y, Fox BA, Restifo NP, Urba WJ, Hu HM (2005) Interleukin-7-dependent expansion and persistence of melanoma-specific T cells in lymphodepleted mice lead to tumor regression and editing. Cancer Res 65: 10569–10577

Westwood JA, Smyth MJ, Teng MW, Moeller M, Trapani JA, Scott AM, Smyth FE, Cartwright GA, Power BE, Honemann D, Prince HM, Darcy PK, Kershaw MH (2005) Adoptive transfer of T cells modified with a humanized chimeric receptor gene inhibits growth of Lewis-Y-expressing tumors in mice. Proc Natl Acad Sci USA 102: 19051–19056

Willemsen RA, Ronteltap C, Chames P, Debets R, Bolhuis RL (2005) T cell retargeting with MHC class I-restricted antibodies: The CD28 co-stimulatory domain enhances antigen-specific cytotoxicity and cytokine production. J Immunol 174: 7853–7858

Wrzesinski C, Restifo NP (2005) Less is more: Lymphodepletion followed by hematopoietic stem cell transplant augments adoptive T-cell-based anti-tumor immunotherapy. Curr Opin Immunol 17: 195–201

Yang L, Baltimore D (2005) Long-term in vivo provision of antigen-specific T cell immunity by programming hematopoietic stem cells. Proc Natl Acad Sci USA 102: 4518–4523

Yang L, Qin XF, Baltimore D, Van Parijs L (2002) Generation of functional antigen-specific T cells in defined genetic backgrounds by retrovirus-mediated expression of TCR cDNAs in hematopoietic precursor cells. Proc Natl Acad Sci USA 99: 6204–6209

Intracellular Antibodies (Intrabodies) and Their Therapeutic Potential

A.S.-Y. Lo, Q. Zhu, and W.A. Marasco(⊠)

1   The Structure of Intrabodies and Antibody Fragments 344
   1.1   ScFv and Intracellular Single Variable Domain (IDab) 344
   1.2   Bispecific Tetravalent Intrabody 346
2   The Molecular Mechanism of Intrabodies 346
3   Practical Considerations for Construction and Selection
   of an Intrabody.. 348
   3.1   Intrabody Gene Sources... 348
   3.2   Intrabody Gene Construction 349
   3.3   Recombinant Antibody Selection Methods 352
4   In Vitro or In Vivo Delivery of Intrabody 353
5   Comparison of Intrabodies and RNAi-Mediated Gene Inactivation.................... 358
6   Disease Specific Applications of Intrabodies 359
   6.1   Intrabodies in HIV 359
   6.2   Intrabodies in Cancer 361
   6.3   Intrabodies in Transplantation.. 363
   6.4   Intrabodies in Neurodegenerative Disease 364
   6.5   Intrabodies Targeting Other Viruses 365
7   Conclusion and Future Directions 365
References 366

Abstract Combining exquisite specificity and high antigen-binding affinity, intrabodies have been used as a biotechnological tool to interrupt, modulate, or define the functions of a wide range of target antigens at the posttranslational level. An intrabody is an antibody that has been designed to be expressed intracellularly and can be directed to a specific target antigen present in various subcellular locations including the cytosol, nucleus, endoplasmic reticulum (ER), mitochondria, peroxisomes, plasma membrane and *trans*-Golgi network (TGN) through in frame fusion

W.A. Marasco

Dana-Farber Cancer Institute, Harvard Medical School, 44 Binney Street, Boston MA 02115, USA
e-mail: Wayne_Marasco@dfci.harvard.edu

Y. Chernajovsky, A. Nissim (eds.) *Therapeutic Antibodies. Handbook of*
Experimental Pharmacology 181.
© Springer-Verlag Berlin Heidelberg 2008

with intracellular trafficking/localization peptide sequences. Although intrabodies can be expressed in different forms, the most commonly used format is a single-chain antibody (scFv Ab) created by joining the antigen-binding variable domains of heavy and light chain with an interchain linker (ICL), most often the 15 amino acid linker $(GGGGS)_3$ between the variable heavy (VH) and variable light (VL) chains. Intrabodies have been used in research of cancer, HIV, autoimmune disease, neu-rodegenerative disease, and transplantation. Clinical application of intrabodies has mainly been hindered by the availability of robust gene delivery system(s) includ-ing target cell directed gene delivery. This review will discuss several methods of intrabody selection, different strategies of cellular targeting, and recent success-ful examples of intrabody applications. Taking advantage of the high specificity and affinity of an antibody for its antigen, and of the virtually unlimited diversity of antigen-binding variable domains available for molecular targeting, intrabody techniques are emerging as promising tools to generate phenotypic knockouts, to manipulate biological processes, and to obtain a more thorough understanding of functional genomics.

1 The Structure of Intrabodies and Antibody Fragments

An intracellular antibody or "intrabody" is an antibody or a fragment of an antibody that is expressed within a designated intracellular compartment, a process which is made possible through the in frame incorporation of intracellular trafficking sig-nals. Intrabodies exert their functions upon exquisitely specific interaction with tar-get antigens. This results in interruption or modification of the biological functions of the target protein. An intrabody can be expressed in any shape or form such as an intact IgG molecule or a Fab fragment (Fig. 1). More frequently, intrabodies are used in genetically engineered antibody fragment format and structures of scFv intrabodies, single domain intrabodies, or bispecific tetravalent intradiabodies are discussed below.

1.1 ScFv and Intracellular Single Variable Domain (IDab)

The most commonly used form of intrabodies is a recombinant scFv Ab in which VH and VL segments are held together by a short, flexible interchain linker (ICL), often the 15 amino acid linker $(GGGGS)_3$ (Fig. 1). A scFv antibody can be in either VH–ICL–VL or VL-ICL-VH configuration and longer ICL (20-mer: GGGGSGGGG SGGGGSSGGGS) has been reported with a VL–ICL–VH orientation (Worn et al. 2000). These formats retain essential regions of antigen-binding specificity of its parental antibody consisting approximately 250 amino acids with a molecular mass ∼28 kDa. Because of the extensive sequence and length variation of the comple-mentarity determining region 3 (CDR3), VH domains even have antigen bind-ing activities without their light chain (Ward et al. 1989). An intrabody thus can also be reduced in size to a single functional variable domain. For this designed

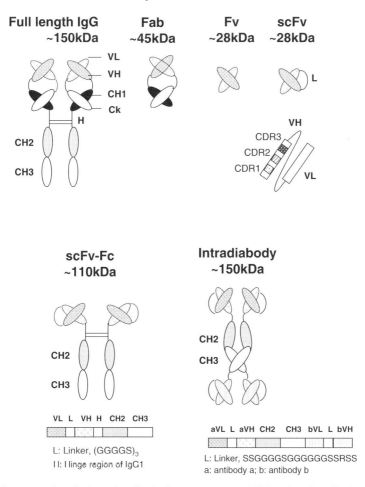

Fig. 1 Structure of antibody and antibody fragments. Intact full length IgG antibody contains heavy chain with variable domain (VH) and three constant domains (CH1, CH2, and CH3), and also the light chain with variable domain (VL) and one constant domain (Cλ or Cκ). One pair of each heavy chain and light chain is held together by interchain disulfide bond within the hinge region (H). Fab fragment is formed without the CH2 and CH3 domain. Single-chain Fv fragment (scFv) is Fv region that contains the variable domains of the heavy and the light chain connected by a linker peptide (L). Complementarity determining regions (CDRs) shape the antigen binding sites and determine the specificity of the antibody. There are three CDRs on each of VH and VL. The CDR1–3 regions of VH domain of scFv are shown. scFv-Fc is an effector antibody, which is composed of scFv and CH2 and CH3 of heavy chain (Fc). Fc domain confers the prolonged half-life of antibody and the Fc-mediated effector functions. The molecular structure is shown as VL–L–VH–H–CH2–CH3. Intradiabody is a bispecific tetravalent antibody with two different scFv antibody fragments (a and b) linked with Fc domain. The molecular structure is shown as aVL–L–aVH–CH2–CH3–bVL–L–bVH

format, a single VH domain, known as an IDab, possesses excellent solubility, stability, and expression within eukaryotic cells. An ideal IDab should exhibit specific antigen recognition and neutralizing activity. IDabs isolated for RAS protein have been shown to inhibit RAS-dependent oncogenic transformation of NIH3T3 cells (Tanaka et al. 2003). In HIV, an important function of viral protein Vif is to suppress the activity of a cytidine deaminase Apobec3G that induces G to A hypermutation in the viral genome and leads to activation of DNA repair mechanisms causing premature degradation of newly synthesized viral DNA. VH single-domain intrabodies against Vif were engineered from rabbit anti-Vif scFv and exhibited a strong neutralization of HIV infectivity and an increase in Apobec3G expression (Goncalves et al. 2002; Aires da Silva et al. 2004). Another format is the Fd fragment (VH-CH1) that has been shown to inhibit glucose-6-phosphate dehydrogenase in the cytoplasm of mammalian cells (Mulligan-Kehoe and Russo 1999). Recently, a VL-Dab and its disulfide bond-free derivative were also successfully utilized as an anti-Huntingtin (htt) intrabody in Huntington's disease (Colby et al. 2004a, 2004b).

1.2 Bispecific Tetravalent Intrabody

Both scFv and IDab are monovalent antibodies. Genetic fusion of scFv or IDab to the IgG Fc region could lead to not only bivalency but also a longer half-life. Multispecific intrabodies have also been engineered. In a recent example, a bispecific tetravalent intradiabody (See Fig. 1, two antivascular endothelial growth factor receptor 2 (VEGF-R2) and two anti-Tie-2 scFv link to the Fc domains of human IgG1) was used to target two endothelial cell receptor-tyrosine kinases: VEGF-R2 and Tie-2. The dual antibody construct simultaneously blocks two independent signaling pathways and affords higher intracellular stability than scFv antibodies. After subtumoral injection of the intradiabody gene carried by a replication incompetent, E1, E3-deleted adenoviral vector and intracellular expression, bispecific intradiabody caused a significant reduction of the growth and angiogenesis of human melanoma M21 in nude mice as compared with a lesser reduction using the monospecific tetravalent intrabody anti-VEGF-R2 over 30 days (Jendreyko et al. 2003; Jendreyko et al. 2005), demonstrating that targeting two different receptors simultaneously yielded an enhanced therapeutic activity.

2 The Molecular Mechanism of Intrabodies

Intrabodies have been used to alter the functions of the target antigens (Marasco, 1995) by modifying related cellular pathways or by redirecting antigen to a new cellular compartment (Zhu et al. 1999; Rajpal and Turi 2001). The unique molecular characteristics of intrabodies allow them to affect protein functions in many ways:

- Sequestration of a target protein from its normal subcellular compartment of action

- Mediating enzyme function through blocking of the active site or modulation of its conformation
- Disrupting biological or signal pathways via interfering normal protein–protein or protein–DNA interactions
- Inducing cell death via activation of the caspase-3-mediated apoptotic pathway
- Selective degradation via the ubiquitin–proteosome pathway

First, intrabodies can be designed to be expressed in different subcellular compartments such as cytoplasm, nucleus, endoplasmic reticulum (ER), Golgi, mitochondria, peroxisomes, plasma membrane, and other locations (Persic et al. 1997). DNA recombinant techniques allow classical intercellular trafficking signals to be genetically fused to the N- or C-termini of antibodies to direct the intrabodies to specific subcellular localizations in order to block or interfere with target antigen function. For instance, ER-retained intrabodies are designed with a signal leader peptide sequence at the N-terminus and a retention peptide, KDEL, at the C-terminus to tether intrabodies within the lumen of the ER. Engineered intrabody can then interact with targeted secretory-pathway proteins, sequestering them within the ER and inhibiting their natural expression. Retention of antibodies in the ER can effectively down regulate its target receptors or signaling molecules (Beerli et al. 1994), such as reduction of cell surface expression of VEGF-R2 and epidermal growth factor receptor (EGFR) (Jannot et al. 1996; Boldicke et al. 2005). Also, ER-targeted intrabody against HIV-1 envelope glycoprotein gp160 blocks HIV-1 envelope processing and virus maturation (Marasco et al. 1993). Similar target protein retention in the *trans*-Golgi has been reported for intrabodies containing a *trans*-Golgi retention signal (Zhou et al. 1998). For expression of cytoplasmic intrabodies, the signal sequences are removed and cytosolic intrabodies are translated on free polysomes. An intrinsically stable amino acid sequence that can fold properly in the absence of disulfide bond formation is required for a cytoplasmic intrabody to function appropriately. Other trafficking signals used to direct antibodies to various specific subcellular locations are listed in Table 1.

Second, intrabodies can modulate enzymatic function by blocking an enzyme active site, by sequestering substrate, or by modulating the conformation of an enzyme catalytic site. It has been shown that cytoplasm-expressed single-domain intrabodies targeting the protein kinase Etk could inhibit its autophosphorylation and ability to phosphorylate its substrate. This resulted in a partial inhibition of cellular transformation in Src-transformed cells (Paz et al. 2005). Third, intrabodies can be used to disrupt biological signaling pathways of target proteins by interfering with normal protein–protein or protein–DNA interactions. For example, a nuclear-targeted intrabody has been used to bind to cyclin-E to inhibit the growth of a breast cancer cell line (Strube and Chen 2002). When genetically fused to caspase-3, intrabodies can be used to promote the death of target cells (e.g. cancer cells) by activating the caspase-3-mediated apoptosis pathway (Tse and Rabbitts 2000). It is also possible for intrabodies to be designed to promote selective degradation of cellular protein targets via the ubiquitin–proteasome pathway by fusion with F-box (Zhou et al. 2000). In addition, intrabodies also have the potential to cause gain-of-function after binding to their target proteins. For example, it has been demonstrated that certain

Table 1 Use of intracellular trafficking signal peptides including leader sequences and retention signal peptides for subcellular compartmental targeting of intrabodies

Subcellular Targeting	The Usage of Leader Sequence and Retention Signal Peptide
Cytoplasm	The immunoglobulin (Ig) leader sequence is removed.
Nucleus	Use of nuclear localization signal (NLS), (T)PPKKK RKV peptide, from the large T antigen of SV40 (Yoneda et al. 1992).
Endoplasmic reticulum (ER)	Use of a signal peptide such as an Ig leader sequence for trafficking to ER and KDEL retention signal for interacting with hERD2 receptor to allow the intrabody effectively tethering within the lumen of ER/Golgi compartment.
Mitochondria	Use of the N-terminal presequence of subunit VIII of human cytochrome C oxidase.
Peroxisomes	Use of the SKL retention signal.
Plasma membrane	Use of the H-Ras or K-Ras CAAX signal to target inner leaflet of the plasma membrane.
Trans-Golgi network (TGN)	scFv fused with 192-bp sequence encoding the trans-membrane domain and cytoplasmic tail of TGN38 protein, including the YQRL retention signal of TGN38 protein.

anti-p53 scFv antibodies restored the transactivating activity of mutant p53 in p53 knockout human tumor cells (Caron de Fromentel et al. 1999). As another example, fusion of an anti-p53 scFv intrabody to the DNA-binding domain of bacterial tetracycline repressor resulted in a protein that acted as a transcription activator and inducer of gene expression (Mary et al. 1999). The unique specificity, affinity, and diversity of antibodies make them useful in a wide variety of basic research and clinical applications. More examples of intrabody applications in cancer, HIV, neurodegenerative disease, and transplantation will be discussed in a later section.

3 Practical Considerations for Construction and Selection of an Intrabody

3.1 Intrabody Gene Sources

An intrabody can be constructed by cloning the V-regions of a mouse monoclonal antibody producing hybridoma cell line with a known specificity or can be selected against a specific antigen from antibody libraries of human or animal sources. Immunogenicity of intrabodies that are derived from nonhuman antibody genes is a concern in applications where long-term intrabody expression is desired (e.g., expression of intrabody based HIV resistance genes in $CD4^+$ T cells) but is less of a concern if the intrabody is acting directly in a tumor cell to induce apoptosis/cell killing. In the former example, one likely has to take steps to "humanize" such antibodies in order to avoid the unwanted immunogenicity as a result of MHC-I presentation of intrabody fragments that may lead to activation of CTL and clearance of the intrabody-expressing cells.

The type and size of recombinant antibody libraries used could also have a direct effect on the success of isolating an intrabody against a specific antigen. "Naïve" or "nonimmune" antibody libraries have been generally built from IgM-V or IgG-V gene pools of B cells of unimmunized individuals, respectively. Rich sources of Ig genes can be from diverse lymphoid organs including bone marrow, peripheral blood, spleen, or tonsils. Early versions of small-size human single-pot libraries with titers of 3×10^7 have been used to isolate antibodies to self-antigens such as thyroglobulin and tumor necrosis factor α (Nissim et al. 1994). However, the antibodies isolated from this library were low in affinity. The larger size library made from over 40 nonimmunized human donors with titer greater than 10^{10} yielded antibodies with higher affinity (Vaughan et al. 1996; Bai et al. 2003). The Marasco laboratory routinely uses the 27 billion member, nonimmune, Mehta I/II libraries that were constructed from peripheral blood B cells from 57 healthy volunteers and have isolated intrabody genes with high affinity and broad epitope diversity (Bai et al. 2003; Gennari et al. 2004). It should be noted that the naïve or nonimmune libraries are biased due to the limited diversity of the Ig repertoire and often unknown exposure history of the B-cell donors. Semisynthetic libraries through CDR randomization, particularly VH CDR3, have been created to address this specific concern (Knappik et al. 2000; Tanha et al. 2001).

In contrast to naïve or nonimmune libraries, the "immune" libraries are constructed from V genes of an immunized animal or human or donors with viral infections, tumors, or autoimmune diseases. Antibodies isolated from these immune sources have been shown to have high affinity and specificity for the antigens under selection since these antibodies have undergone somatic hypermutation leading to their affinity maturation. Using these libraries, antibodies against carcinoembryonic antigen (Chester et al. 1994), major histocompatibility complex/peptide complexes (Yamanaka et al. 1996) and T-cell receptor-Vα (Popov et al. 1996) have been successfully isolated. One limitation of this approach is that this type of library must be newly prepared for each new antigen of interest; however, the approach has been quite useful and has been used for isolating antibodies against self-reactive or toxic antigens (Graus et al. 1997; Wild et al. 2003). For detailed discussion of the types of libraries, their construction and other characteristics, please refer to the reviews cited (Hoogenboom and Chames 2000; Pini and Bracci 2000; Azzazy and Highsmith 2002; Hoogenboom 2005).

3.2 Intrabody Gene Construction

Intrabody constructions, while technically simple to achieve, require a strong understanding of cell biology so that the subcellular compartment that will be used for their translation is properly chosen as this will ultimately effect functional expression, protein folding, solubility, and stability. During the natural secretory process, the Ig leader sequence directs antibodies to rough ER membranes for synthesis. The nascent polypeptides pass through the ER membrane into the lumen where the leader peptides are cleaved cotranslationally. Upon synthesis, antibody peptides pass through the ER/Golgi while being processed/modified and are normally secreted into the extracellular fluid or remain membrane bound on the B-cell surface as antigen receptors. With the help of chaperones and other factors that are active in the ER, efficient intrachain and interchain disulfide bridge formation and H- and L-chain association occurs.

Cytoplasmic expression of intrabodies is more problematic due to unnatural folding of many antibodies in a reducing environment where disulfide bond formation is inefficient or absent. This can result in low solubility, short protein half-life, and a tendency to aggregate with resulting proteosome degradation (Cattaneo and Biocca 1999). Only intrinsically soluble and stable scFv fragments appear to fold correctly in sufficient amounts to be active as functional intrabodies (Cattaneo and Biocca 1999; Worn and Pluckthun 2001).

At present, no consistent rules have been established that reliably predict which intrabodies will fold and function properly in a cytosolic environment based on primary structure (Marasco et al. 1993); however, preselection allows researchers to identify rare, stable scFvs from natural and engineered scFv-phage libraries. One preselection approach has been use of the yeast two-hybrid system (Visintin et al. 1999; Worn et al. 2000). This method had been further developed for the isolation of leucine zipper binding intrabodies from a library with randomized VH CDR3 sequences located in the stable antibody framework (Auf der Maur et al. 2002). A related approach is to employ stringent selection procedures including denaturation under reducing conditions to isolate antibodies with improved stability from phage display libraries (Brockmann et al. 2005); however, positive antibodies obtained under these harsh elution conditions still need to be functionally tested intracellularly to see if they are effective intrabodies.

Gennari and colleagues (2004) investigated whether specific scFvs that were isolated from a human scFv-phage display library could be directly screened in pools as intrabodies without prior knowledge of their individual identity or purity within pools of antigen-specific scFvs. As the target, they used a synthetic transformation effector site 1 (TES1) polypeptide comprising the membrane-most proximal 34 amino acid residues of the carboxy-terminal cytoplasmic tail of the oncogenic latent membrane protein 1 (LMP1) of Epstein Barr virus. Anti-TES1 scFvs, initially identified by phage ELISA screens, were grouped and then transferred as pools into eukaryotic expression vectors and expressed as cytoplasmic intrabodies. Using this direct phage to intrabody screening (DPIS) strategy they were able to identify intrabodies that were able to selectively block LMP1-induced NFκB activity. This should allow investigators to bypass much of the in vitro scFv characterization that is often not predictive of in vivo intrabody function and provide a more efficient use of large native and synthetic scFv phage libraries already in existence to identify intrabodies that are active in vivo.

Several other strategies have also been developed to address these same concerns. For example, stable and functional cytoplasmic cysteine-free scFv have been generated by using DNA shuffling and phage display (Proba et al. 1998). The VH single domain antibody libraries can also be used to avoid disulfide bond requirement (Tanaka et al. 2003). In addition, a known stable framework was created by point mutations and libraries were generated by grafting synthetic CDRs onto the antibody framework (Ewert et al. 2004). Finally, fusion of intrabodies with *E. coli* maltose binding protein (MBP) were shown to enhance their solubility and stability in bacteria and mammalian cell cytoplasm (Bach et al. 2001; Shaki-Loewenstein et al. 2005). Should bacterial components raise immunogenecity problems in a therapeutic application, the MBP could conceivably be replaced with a mammalian chaperon protein in such a fusion construct.

While scFv have been used in many different kinds of applications as the preferable form of intrabodies, in some studies, it has shown that inclusion of the Cκ light chain constant domain at the carboxy-terminus of a scFv could increase the stability and solubility of an intrabody in cytosol by promoting dimerization (Mhashilkar et al. 1995; Cohen et al. 1998). Reinman et al. (2003) using a bidirectional galactose inducible GAL1–10 promoter to express several formats of antibody fragments against Sem1 (the analog of Sem1P in mammalian cells interacts with tumor suppressor BRCA2) in a yeast system and demonstrated that Fabs gave a higher expression level, function, and stability than scFv or scFv containing the lambda constant domain of L chain (scFvCL). Their studies also suggested that addition of constant region of L or H chain to the scFv increased intracellular levels considerably. This may be explained by the observation that while a conserved hydrophobic patch formed at the variable–constant domain interface (v/c interface) is covered by the constant domains in Fab construct, it becomes exposed in scFv format. The resulting antibody is insoluble, nonfunctional protein produced in the periplasm of *E. coli*. Substitution of a key hydrophobic residue (V84D at VH) of antifluorescein antibody 4-4-20 at the v/c interface significantly improved the in vivo folding of the scFv fragment (Nieba et al. 1997).

It should be noted that the functionality of intrabodies in vivo is often nonrelated or poorly related to their in vitro binding affinity. For example, as compared to a higher affinity scFv intrabody, the intrabody with lower binding affinity possessed greater potency due to its ability to (1) transactivate p53 by inducing a favorable conformational change (Caron de Fromentel et al. 1999) or (2) bind the specific activation domain of Rev for efficient blocking (Wu et al. 1996). A study using two anticaspase-7 scFv demonstrated that an extended half-life and high steady state levels of protein accumulation are critical for functional study of an intrabody (Zhu et al. 1999). It is clear that only in vivo studies can ultimately be used to determine which intrabody is most potent. As a result, intrabodies that bind to different epitopes and with different affinities should be examined early and directly through in vivo functional assays.

3.3 Recombinant Antibody Selection Methods

Many methods can be used to obtain antibody genes for the construction of intrabodies and can be used most effectively if the intrabodies are to be directed to the
ER for inhibition of factor secretion or cell surface protein expression. Microbial-
based antibody display methods such on phage, yeast, bacterial, and retroviruses as
well as nonmicrobial-based display methods such as ribosomal display have been
recently reviewed elsewhere by Hoogenboom (2005). During selection, antibodies
are enriched by several rounds of panning, consisting of consecutive cycles of incubation with target antigen (either immobilized, soluble, or on surface of cells or
paramagnetic liposomes), elution, and amplification.

3.3.1 Lentivirus and Mammalian Cell Display

Mammalian cell surface antibody display is a platform that has gained much
attention because its obvious advantage of being able to posttranslationally modify
antibody fragments that may contribute to binding affinity and aid proper folding
leading to a more diversified antibody repertoire (Ho et al. 2006). With the use of
self-inactivating lentiviral vectors, bivalent scFvFc human antibodies were fused in
frame with a transmembrane anchoring moiety to allow efficient high-level expression on surface of human cells and lentivirus particle (Taube, Zhu, and Marasco,
submitted for publication). Both human cells and virus particles bound antigen in a
highly specific manner. FACS sorting in combination with enrichment through magnetic beads allowed isolation of specific scFv expressing cells from a background
cell population with 10^6-fold enrichment in a rapid, single round of selection. If
necessary, the enriched scFv genes could be immediately recovered by PCR rescue, followed by recloning into a lentiviral display vector, generation of viral particles, and additional rounds of transduction and isolation of antigen-specific scFvs
by FACS. Importantly, evidence that the cell surface displayed scFvFc antibodies
could indeed undergo posttranslational modification of the variable regions through
sulfation of CDR tyrosine residues (Choe et al. 2003; Huang et al. 2004), a property
that has been recently shown to markedly broaden the binding affinity and antigen
recognition of variable region genes was obtained (Chen, Sui, Zhu, and Marasco, J.
Immunol. in press). This antibody display platform should be able to complement
existing antibody display technologies by virtue of providing properties unique to
lentiviruses and antibody expression in human cells.

3.3.2 Growth Selection Through Protein Fragment Complementation Assay

Protein fragment complementation assay (PCA) has been adapted to screen for antibody binding by reconstituting the activity of dihydrofolate reductase (DHFR) that
confers a survival advantage on transformed *E. coli*. In this method, antibodies
and antigens are linked with dissected portions of mouse DHFR (mDHFR). The

interaction of antibody and antigen brings the two halves of dissected mDHFR together, thus restoring its enzyme activity and allowing transformed *E. coli* to grow on minimal medium in the presence of antibiotic trimethoprim. Four different target antigens were tested by this system, it was shown that there was about seven orders of magnitude more colonies in antigen pool containing specific antigen as compared with few colonies found in pool with only nonspecific antigen (Mossner et al. 2001). The procedure is relatively simple and fast and only involves transformation of plasmids, functional expression of the fusion proteins, and analysis of the grown bacterial cells. Notably, it gives a very low background of false-positive results. The antigen does not need to be purified and immobilized. However, since the screening is performed in the cytoplasm of *E. coli*, antibodies with inherent stable framework can be isolated under reducing conditions but they would be lack of posttranslational modification.

3.3.3 Growth Selection Through Yeast or Mammalian Two-Hybrid System

Intracellular interaction of antibody with target antigen in yeast could be evaluated by providing conditional cell growth advantage through controlled expression of selected reporter genes (Visintin et al. 1999; Auf der Maur et al. 2002). In such a system, the antigen is usually cloned in frame at C-terminus of the DNA binding domain of Gal 4 (or Lex A) and scFv antibody fused at the N-terminus of a transcription activation domain (AD) of Gal 4 (or VP16). After cotransfection of these plasmids into the yeast cells and upon interaction, the antibody–antigen complex binds to the promoter of reporter genes containing relevant DNA binding sites and activates their transcription. For example, activation of *HIS3* gene controlled by a minimal transcription promoter with Gal 4-binding sites upon antigen–antibody interaction enables the host yeast to grow on plate without histidine and with 3-amino-triazole (3-AT) for selection (Auf der Maur et al. 2002). In addition, Auf der Maur et al. (2001) developed a related procedure in which stable intrabodies could be selected independent of their antigens based on strong correlation between the degree of reporter gene activation and the stability/solubility of the fused antibody. Specifically worth mentioning is a similar system also demonstrated in Hela cells through activation of an integrated luciferase reporter by the strong transcriptional activation domain of the herpes simplex virus type 1 VP16 (VP16-AD) with scFv antibodies fused to its C-terminus and Gal 4 DNA-binding domain at its N-terminus. It should be noted that a library size of 10^7 clones can be screened per assay in these yeast or mammalian systems, which is at disadvantage as compared with $>10^{10}$ clones can be handled with relative ease using phage display.

4 In Vitro or In Vivo Delivery of Intrabody

In vivo and/or clinical applications of intrabody therapy have been limited mainly due to lack of optimal gene transfer vehicles, a common issue in the field of gene

Table 2 In vitro and in vivo expression of intrabodies for intracellular gene targeting

Delivery Method	Intrabody Format and Target (Types of Disease)	Outcome and Reference
Retrovirus	Anti-Tat scFv (HIV)	In retrovirus transduced CD4$^+$-selected, CD8$^+$-depleted, and total PBMC, the anti-Tat scFv expressing cells showed marked inhibition of HIV-1 replication and resistance to HIV-1 infection (Mhashilkar et al. 1999)
Retrovirus	Anti-CCR5 scFv (HIV)	Retrovirus transduced CCR5$^+$ T-cell line, PM1, protected from CCR5-dependent cell fusion and R5 HIV-1 infection (Steinberger et al. 2000)
Retrovirus	Anti-Vif scFv (HIV)	It conferred primary cells highly refractory to challenge with the HIV-1 virus or HIV-1-infected cells and inhibited HIV-1 replication (Goncalves et al. 2002)
Lentivirus	Anti-IL-2Rα scFv Tac (Leukemia)	Using a bicistronic lentivirus vector, the established T-cell line Kit 225 and primary human T cells were shown to have a low or undetectable cell surface expression of IL-2Rα and exhibited a 10-fold reduction of IL-2 responsiveness (Richardson et al. 1998)
Lentivirus pseudotyped with Sindbis envelope	Anti-CCR5 scFv (HIV)	Authors developed lentiviral-derived particles with specificity of gene delivery mediated by pseudotyped Sindbis envelope protein that display scFv recognizing CCR5-expressing cell line and primary lymphocytes in vitro. The nonspecific viral infection was observed by using VSV envelope (Aires da Silva et al. 2005)
Lentivirus	Anti-CXCR4 scFv (HIV)	scFv inhibited infectious entry in primary isolated human brain microvascular endothelial cells (MVECs) and reduced HIV-1 p24 production in postmitotic differentiated human neurons (Mukhtar et al. 2005)
Lentivirus	Anti-CCR5 scFv (HIV)	Lentiviral CCR5 intrabody expression in primary CD4$^+$ T cells were refractory to HIV-1 infection and supported significant growth and enrichment during R5-tropic HIV-1 challenge. Also, thymocytes risen

Table 2 (continued)

Delivery Method	Intrabody Format and Target (Types of Disease)	Outcome and Reference
		from lentivirus transduced CD34$^+$ cells in NOD-SCID-human thymus/liver mice maintained CCR5 intrabody expression and were resistant to HIV-1 challenge (Swan et al. 2006)
Lentivirus	Anti-rat MHC I scFv (Transplantation)	Rat aortic endothelial cells (RAEC) showed a stable expression of the anti-rat MHC I scFv and displayed low MHC I levels. They were protected from killing by allospecific, cytotoxic T cells (CTL) and by allo-antibody/complement-mediated lysis (Doebis et al. 2006)
Adenovirus	Anti-erbB2 scFv (Ovarian cancer)	ER-directed anti-erbB-2 scFv accomplished specific cytotoxicity in erbB-2-overexpressing tumors. Intraperitoneal injection of adenovirus resulted in a reduction of tumor burdens and prolongation of survival (Deshane et al. 1995b)
Adenovirus	Anti-erbB-2 scFv (Ovarian cancer)	Phase I trial was performed using i.p. administration in erbB-2-overexpressing ovarian cancer. 5/13 patients had stable disease and 8/13 had progressive disease. One patient with nonmeasurable disease normalized her CA125 at the 8-week evaluation and one patient had no sign of disease for 6 months (Alvarez et al. 2000)
Adenovirus	Anti-MHC I scFv (Transplantation)	Intrabody achieved a marked reduction of surface MHC I expression in primary human keratinocytes (Mhashilkar et al. 2002)
Adenovirus	Anti-VEGFR-2 (Angiogenesis)	Adenovirus infected HUVEC showed induction of apoptosis and inhibition of tube formation (Wheeler et al. 2003)
Adenovirus	Anti-MHC-1 scFv (Transplantation)	Adenovirus transduced HUVEC showed a reduced cell lysis in a cytotoxicity assay when compared with that of MHC mismatched control. This effect was not reversed by

Table 2 (continued)

Delivery Method	Intrabody Format and Target (Types of Disease)	Outcome and Reference
		stimulation with inflammatory cytokines (Beyer et al. 2004)
Adenovirus	Anti-αV integrin scFv (Cancer)	Virus transduced melanoma cell line caused detachment of cells from extracellular matrix, induced apoptosis, and prevented subcutaneous tumor implantation in SCID mice (Koistinen et al. 2004)
Adenovirus	Intrabdiabody of anti-VEGF-R2 scFv & anti-Tie-2 scFv (Angiogenesis)	Subtumoral injection of adenovirus gave simultaneous blocking of both VEGF-R2 and Tie-2 and resulted in a significant inhibition of tumor growth and tumor-associated blood vessels (Jendreyko et al. 2003; Jendreyko et al. 2005)
Adenovirus	Anti-Tie-2 scFv pAd-2S03 (Angiogenesis)	scFv inhibited human Kaposi's sarcoma (SLK) and human colon carcinoma (SW1222) xenograft growth in mice and also decreased vessel density markedly in both tumor models (Popkov et al. 2005)
AAV	Anti-Amyloid β scFv (Neurophathology)	AAV injection into corticohippocampal regions of Alzheimer disease (AD) mice gave less amyloid deposits than the mice subjected to PBS injection and showed no eliciting inflammation (Fukuchi et al. 2006)
AAV	Anti-Amyloid β scFv Aβ1-16, 40, 42 (Neuropathology)	Intracranial scFv expression in neonatal amyloid precursor protein mice decreased Aβ deposition by 25–50% and attenuated plaque deposition (Levites et al. 2006)
AAV	Anti-death receptor 5 (DR5) scFv rAAV-S3C (Cancer)	A single i.m. injection of rAAV-S3C in nude mice resulted in a stable secretion of S3C scFv in sera for at least 24 days. scFv suppressed the growth and induced tumor cell apoptosis in established s.c. human lung LTEP-sml and liver Hep3B tumor xenografts (Shi et al. 2006)

therapy that is nevertheless making steady advances into the clinic. Viral vectors including retrovirus, lentivirus, adenovirus, and adeno-associated virus (AAV) are currently used to obtain high transduction efficiency and long-term expression of intrabodies (Table 2). While retroviruses produce high transduction level for dividing cells, lentivirus-derived vectors (HIV-1, SIV, EIAV, FIV) can transduce both dividing and nondividing cells including resting T cells, DCs, macrophages, and noncycling hematopoietic stem cells. Lentivirus vectors have been used to express intrabodies against target protein in in vitro studies and result in dramatic reduction of expression and functional activity of target proteins (Table 2). Adenovirus and AAV vectors are also widely used due to their high transduction efficiency, ability to infect a wide variety of cell types, and lack of insertional mutagenesis (Jooss and Chirmule 2003); however, preexisting neutralizing antibodies can significantly reduce the transfer efficiency with these viral vectors. In addition, adenoviral vector induces strong inflammatory responses in vivo. For efficient gene delivery, vectors from different adenovirus serotypes can be used in alternate (Noureddini and Curiel 2005; Bangari and Mittal 2006). Currently, replication incompetent E1, E3-deleted adenoviral vector is the only vector so far used for intrabody gene delivery in a Phase I clinical trial (Alvarez et al. 2000). Compare to adenoviral vectors, although with limited transgene packaging capacity, AAV vectors possess advantages in that they are less immunogenic with a substantially longer lasting gene expression due to their ability to stay extrachoromosomal predominantly as circular concatemers, or in low frequency, to integrate into the host genome (Jooss and Chirmule 2003; Tenenbaum et al. 2003). Originally from rhesus macaques, the new adeno-associated vector rAAV serotype 8 has a very high transduction efficiency by intravenous infusion and avoids the intrinsic immunogenicity against AAV serotypes 1–6 in humans (Gao et al. 2002).

Efficient intravenous targeting to specific cell types is one of the desired gene transfer features for clinical applications. A recent report demonstrated that a Sindbis envelope protein pseudotyped lentiviral vector displaying anti-CCR5 scFv lead to specific targeting to CCR5-expressing cells and primary lymphocytes in vitro (Aires da Silva et al. 2005). P-glycoproteins on metastatic melanoma cells in lung tissue were also successfully targeted by modified lentivirus pseudotyped with a chimeric Sindbis envelope (termed m168) and surface displayed anti-P-glycoprotein antibody through intravenous injection. Unlike other pseudotyped envelope proteins, m168 did not have nonspecific infectivity in the liver and spleen (Morizono et al. 2005). Additionally, by incorporation of an antibody conferring target specificity and a modified influenza hemagglutinin mutant mediating pH-dependent membrane fusion, the lentiviral vector was successfully used to target CD20 in human B cells in vitro and in animals (Yang et al. 2006). Further understanding of envelope tropism and vector trafficking will be important for successful applications of in vivo targeted gene delivery, which, in turn, will accelerate the site-specific expression of therapeutic molecules including intrabodies.

Despite the high transduction efficiency of viral transfer system, viral vectors causes the potential problems including immunogenicity, possibility of insertional mutagenesis, difficulty in large-scale production, and size limitation of exogenous

DNA. Thus nonviral gene delivery systems, although have not been used directly for intrabody delivery, remain as options for the clinical application of intrabody. For example, by linking nucleic acid-binding human protamine to the C-terminus of an anti-erbB2 scFv antibody (Li et al. 2001), exogenous DNA could be selectively delivered into erbB-2 positive cells. Alternatively, an immunoliposome could hold within its lipid bilayer nucleic acids or proteins and has been coupled with antibodies to facilitate targeting and endocytosis to specific cells (Nielsen et al. 2002). Thus immunoliposomes could potentially be utilized for delivery of an intrabody as a gene or a protein. Finally, it is conceivable that an intrabody could also be introduced into cells through protein transduction when fused with short cationic peptide sequences called protein transduction domains (PTD) (Niesner et al. 2002; Lobato and Rabbitts 2003; Joliot and Prochiantz 2004; Heng et al. 2005). This technique eliminates the safety or ethical concerns associated with viral transfer but intrabodies, when delivered as proteins, could be limited in their intracellular level as well as half-life and thus require repeated dosing for an effective treatment.

5 Comparison of Intrabodies and RNAi-Mediated Gene Inactivation

At present, there are two popular technologies for the down-regulation of gene expression – RNA interference (RNAi) and intrabodies. These techniques have shown promising results for biomedical research (Ryther et al. 2005). Researchers choose between these two techniques based on their specific merits and limitations in the context of the desired applications. RNAi is an evolutionarily conserved process of posttranscriptional, sequence-specific gene silencing that uses double-stranded RNA (dsRNA) as an intermediate in the degradation of its homologous mRNA. The silencing effect of dsRNA was first discovered in *Caenorhabditis elegans* and RNAi is now routinely used as a reverse genetics tool in plants (Fire et al. 1998). Gene silencing with RNAi involves two steps. First, long dsRNA are recognized by the ribonuclease III-like enzyme Dicer, which cleaves the dsRNA into small 21–23 bp RNAs. Then these RNAs are associated with helicase and nuclease to form a complex – RNA-induced silencing complex (RISC), which unwinds RNAi and performs sequence-specific degradation of mRNA (Kitabwalla and Ruprecht 2002). It has been reported that RNAi achieves knockdown of gene expression to 10–40% of its normal levels (Coumoul and Deng 2006).

In general, the RNAi strategy follows a simple design with well-defined algorithms and is less technically challenging than intrabody techniques; however, it has nonspecific effects. This nonspecificity takes the form of dsRNA-triggered responses mediated by interferon-associated pathways (Gil and Esteban 2000; Sledz et al. 2003; Sledz and Williams 2004), which do not exist in invertebrates and plants. A gene expression profiling study indicated that $> 1,000$ genes involved in diverse cellular functions are nonspecifically stimulated or repressed in mammalian tissue-culture cells treated with conventional 21-bp RNAi (Sledz et al. 2003; Persengiev et al. 2004). Another limitation of the RNAi technique is the relatively short half-life of the desired knockdown effects unless stimulatory RNAs are expressed via trans-fected recombinant DNA (which delays observation of the knockdown effect). In contrast, it is useful to use intrabodies for a nearly instantaneous and durable effect. Intrabodies can block particular binding interactions of target molecules, by chang-ing their structural conformation or by exerting positive functions including cat-alytic functions, stabilization of protein–protein or protein–DNA interactions, etc. The prominent usages of intrabodies include redirecting target antigen to a particu-lar subcellular location through an appropriate trafficking signal peptide fused with the intrabody (Table 1) and the unique ability to specifically disrupt a specific func-tion of a multifunction protein (Bai et al. 2003). Other molecular mechanisms of intrabodies have been discussed in Sect. 2. Despite the diversity of outcomes elicited through intrabody use, the phage library construction and screening process required to implement intrabody techniques is time consuming and labor intensive. Success in isolation of stable and functional antibody is relatively unpredictable (Sect. 3).

6 Disease Specific Applications of Intrabodies

6.1 Intrabodies in HIV

Intrabodies have important therapeutic potential in microbial pathologies and have been broadly used to interrupt the HIV-1 viral life cycle. ER-directed intrabody F105 targeted to CD4 binding region of HIV envelope protein blocked process-ing of the envelope precursor gp160 and virus-mediated syncytium formation, lead-ing to low infectivity of progeny HIV particles (Marasco et al. 1993). Later, it was shown that both ER- and TGN-retained anti-HIV-1-gp41 scFv intrabodies inhibited HIV replication and syncytial formation, while only the ER-retained form blocked maturation processing of gp160 into gp120 and gp41 (Zhou et al. 1998). When transduced via a MuLV-based vector, an anti-tat scFv intrabody was more effective than an anti-gp120 scFv in stably inhibiting HIV replication in CD4$^+$ T cells iso-lated from patients with HIV-1 infection at different disease stage (Poznansky et al. 1998).

Preintegration blockage of virus replication has been demonstrated by intrabodies against the HIV-1 matrix protein (MA, p17) and reverse transcriptase (RT). A Fab intrabody, directed against a carboxy-terminal epitope of MA, p17 from the Clade B HIV-1 genotype, was shown to inhibit HIV-1 infection when it expressed in the cytoplasm of actively dividing CD4$^+$ T cells (Levin et al. 1997). Anti-HIV-1 RT Fab intrabodies expressed in the cytoplasm were shown to block early stage HIV-1 replication in human T-lymphoid cells SupT1. By targeting to a common structural fold of different DNA polymerases, intrabody neutralized RT activity from avian and murine retroviruses, prokaryotic polymerases, and human DNA polymerase α (Gargano et al. 1996).

Postintegration blockage of HIV-1 replication can be achieved by inhibiting critical HIV-1 regulatory protein functions such as Tat-mediated viral transcriptional transactivation or Rev-mediated nuclear export of singly spliced or genomic viral RNA. A cytosolic scFvC$_k$ directed against the N-terminal-activation domain of Tat efficiently inhibited Tat-mediated transactivation of the HIV-1 LTR and resistance to HIV-1 infection in lymphocytes (Mhashilkar et al. 1995). Mhashilkar et al. (1997) demonstrated cooperative down-regulation of HIV LTR-driven gene expression and more durable inhibition of HIV-1 replication in cells with stably expressed anti-tat scFv intrabody when treated with a combination of NF-κB inhibitors pentoxi-fylline and Gö-6976. Tat binds cooperatively with hCyclin T1, a regulatory partner of cyclin-dependent kinase 9 (cdk9) in the positive transcription elongation factor (P-TEFb) complex, to the transcription response element and is required for HIV transcription elongation. Expression of hCyclin T1-specific scFv intrabodies in SupT1 cells was shown to disrupt the interaction between Tat and hCyclinT1 leading to inhibition of Tat-mediated transactivation and HIV replication. Importantly, the presence of P-TEFb complex indicated that anti-hCyclinT1 intrabody did not disrupt the heterodimerization between hCyclinT1 and Cdk9 (Bai et al. 2003), a prime example to demonstrate intrabody's ability to selectively disrupt a specific function of a multifunction protein while leaving other functions intact. The Rev protein shuttles between the nucleus and cytoplasm of infected cells and is required for the nuclear export of a subset of HIV-mRNAs that encode the structural proteins. A cytosolic directed anti-Rev scFv has been demonstrated to inhibit HIV-1 replication in HeLa-T4 cells (Duan et al. 1994). Wu et al. (1996) showed that a lower binding affinity anti-Rev D8 antibody mapped to activation domain in the C-terminus of Rev had a more potent inhibition of HIV-1 replication in HeLa-T4 cells, human T-cell lines, and PBMC than the higher affinity anti-Rev D10 bound downstream from activation domain in the nonactivation region of the C terminus, demonstrating importance and specificity of an antibody binding site.

Integrase (IN) mediates integration of viral dsDNA into the host genome during early stage of retroviral life cycle. Cytoplasmic or nuclear localized anti-HIV IN scFvs expressed in human T lymphocytes were shown to be resistant to HIV-1 infection by neutralizing IN activity prior to integration (Levy-Mintz et al. 1996). Specific VH single-domain intrabody from immunized rabbit against HIV-1 Vif protein was used to neutralize Vif-mediated enhanced infectivity by reducing late reverse transcripts and proviral integration in nonpermissive cells specifically (Goncalves et al. 2002).

HIV infection requires a coreceptor for entry into permissive cells. CCR5 and CXCR4 are two major coreceptors used by macrophage-tropic and T-cell-tropic HIV strains, respectively. Lentivirus expression of an anti-CXCR4 scFv inhibited infectious entry in primary isolated human brain microvascular endothelial cells (MVECs) and postmitotic differentiated human neurons (Mukhtar et al. 2005). An ER-retained CCR5-specific scFv was shown having a superior effect to RANTES in blocking CCR5 surface expression and cell-to-cell infection in CCR5$^+$ T cell line PM1. Besides, the intrabody ST6 recognizes the conserved region of the first extracellular domain of CCR5 in human and nonhuman primate, thus it could be used to prevent infection by CCR5-dependent viral infection (Steinberger et al. 2000). In another study, the combinational therapy using anti-CCR5 scFv and hammerhead CCR5 specific ribozyme had an additive effect on both abrogation of the CCR5 cell surface expression and inhibition of higher dose HIV infection (Cordelier et al. 2004). Finally, it is proposed that using a combination of different targeting intrabodies that have a role in different phases of HIV life cycle may achieve additional effects of inhibition. It has been demonstrated that using scFv intrabodies against CXCR4, RT, and IN in combination had a synergistic reduction on HIV-1 infection as compared to the results of using individual scFv (Strayer et al. 2002).

6.2 Intrabodies in Cancer

Intrabodies have been widely used in cancer gene therapy to alter the neoplastic phenotype of cancer cells. This includes knockdown of growth-factor receptors, angiogenesis-related receptors, oncogenic proteins (cell cycle and apoptosis-related), transcription factors, and cancer resistance related proteins.

6.2.1 Growth Factor Receptors and Angiogenesis-Related Receptors

ErbB2 is a member of the type I/epidermal growth factor receptor (EGFR)-related family of receptor tyrosin kinases that include erbB/EGFR, erbB2, erbB3, and erbB4. ErbB2 becomes rapidly phosphorylated and activated following ligand treatment of many cell lines. It is amplified in multiple tumors such as breast and ovarian carcinoma, in which it correlated with a poor prognosis. Expressing ER-retained anti-erbB2 scFv in T47D mammary carcinoma cells resulted in selective reduction of erbB2 cell surface expression and functional inactivation of the receptor by reduction in the phosphorylation of Shc. It also inhibited activation of mitogen-activated protein kinase (MAPK) and p70/p85S6K, and impaired induction of c-*fos* expression in response to natural ligands epidermal growth factor (EGF) and Neu differentiation factor (NDF) (Graus-Porta et al. 1995). No tumor growth was detected and complete tumor eradication was found in mice receiving ER directed anti-erbB-2 scFv 80 days after subcutaneous transplant of human ovarian carcinoma cell line SKOV3 (Deshane et al. 1995a). Treatment with intraperitoneal administration of adenovirus encoding anti-erbB-2 scFv in tumor transplanted mice had shown tumor regression and a prolonged survival as compared with control groups (Deshane et al. 1995b). Phase I clinical trial using this anti-erbB-2 encoding adenovirus (Ad21) for intraperitoneal treatment of ovarian cancer patients demonstrated that 5 out of 13 patients (38%) had stable disease and 8 out of 13 patients (61%) had progressive status of disease. It also showed after the treatment, one patient with nonmeasurable disease remained without clinical evidence of disease for 6 months. Patients generally experienced virus vector related fever without Ad21-specific dose-limiting toxicity (Alvarez and Curiel 1997; Alvarez et al. 2000). Epidermal growth factor receptor (EGFR) is a member of type I receptor-tyrosine kinase (RTK) family and it is overexpressed in glioblastomas and many epithelial original cancers. ER-targeted scFv against EGFR had been shown to reduce tyrosine phosphorylation of EGFR and cell growth in EGFR transformed NIH3T3 cells (Jannot et al. 1996). Intrabodies were also designed to target a member of the Met RTK family such as Ron (Secco et al. 2004), angiogenesis-related receptors including VEGF-R2 and Tie-2, and another cancer-related folate receptor (Figini et al. 2003).

IL-2Rα (Tac, CD25) plays a key role in T cell-mediated immune response and is constitutively overexpressed in some T- and B-cell leukemias, most notably in adult T-cell leukemia (ATL), which is caused by HTLV-1. An ER-targeted anti-Tac scFv abrogated the cell surface expression completely in PMA-stimulated Jurkat cells (Richardson et al. 1995). IL-2Rα expression was reduced to undetectable levels without affecting cell viability or growth rate (Richardson et al. 1997).

6.2.2 Cell Cycle and Apoptosis-Related Oncogenic Proteins

p21^{ras} is a guanine nucleotide-binding protein, which is involved in the control of cell growth and differentiation. Cytosolic expression of Y259 scFv by removing immunoglobulin leader sequence was shown to perturb p21^{ras} function. Microinjection of mRNA encoding an anti-p21^{ras} scFv intrabody into *Xenopus* oocytes was shown to inhibit insulin-induced meiotic maturation of the cell, a process known to be p21^{ras}-dependent (Biocca et al. 1993; Biocca et al. 1994). In other studies, activation of p42 MAPK by *ras* in *Xenopus* oocytes was also strongly inhibited by scFv antibody (Montano and Jimenez 1995). As two scFv Y259 and Y238 mapped to different epitopes of *ras*, Y259 scFv was shown to block *ras*-mediated functions and to elicit an effective tumor regression of HCT116 colon carcinoma cells in nude mice (Cochet et al. 1998b), whereas Y238 scFv was demonstrated to bind to *ras* in oocytes without adverse effect on *ras*-dependent activation pathway (Cochet et al. 1998a).

6.2.3 Signal Transduction

Etk, the endothelial and epithelial tyrosine kinase, is a member of the Tec family of nonreceptor tyrosine kinases, others include Btk, Itk, and Tec. It is involved in several cellular processes including proliferation, differentiation, and motility. Anti-Etk single domain intrabodies was shown to bind specifically to the Etk kinase domain, inhibit its kinase activity, and partially block v-Src-induced cellular transformation in transformed NIH3T3 cells (Paz et al. 2005). The serine-threonine kinase Akt contributes to tumor cell proliferation and survival, and dysregulated function of the PI3K/Akt pathways is commonly found in several human cancers. Intracellular expression of cell-permeable anti-Akt scFv antibodies inhibited p-Ser^{473} Akt and GSK-3α/β phosphorylation, blocked activities of exogenously expressed Akt2 and Akt3, induced apoptosis in three cancer cell lines, and reduced tumor volume and neovascularization in polyomavirus middle T antigen (PyVmT)-expressing transgenic tumors implanted in mouse dorsal chambers (Shin et al. 2005).

6.2.4 Drug Resistance Proteins

Cancer patients treated with chemotherapy leading to upregulation of cancer multiple drug resistance (MDR) gene. A MDR gene product, P-glycoprotein (P-gp) is an energy dependent drug efflux pump for multiple anticancer agents in human cancers. Anti-MDR1 monoclonal antibody C219 was shown to bind near the ATP binding domain of the cytoplasmic portion of P-gp and inhibit the ATPase activity of P-gp by inhibiting ATP binding. Intracellular expression of anti-MDR1 scFv inhibited the function of P-gp. As a result, the transfected cells exhibited increased Rhodamine123 (Rh123) retention and Adriamycin (ADM) uptake as well as higher sensitivity to ADM (Heike et al. 2001).

6.2.5 Integrins

Integrin heterodimers constituted by αV integrin with one of five different integrin β subunits (β1, β3, β5, β6 and β8) are adhesion receptors for various extracellular matrix proteins including fibronectin, vitronectin, and osteopontin. They are essential for cell anchoring, differentiation, survival, and metastasis. Constructed with KDEL peptide, anti-αV integrin scFv caused a great impairment in cell adhesion to α4β1 ligands and cell spreading on immobilized one of α4β1 ligands – FN40 protein in RD rhabdomyosarcoma cells and Jurkat cells (Yuan et al. 1996). Transfection of anti-αV integrins in osteosarcoma cells resulted in 70–100% reduction in cell surface expression of αVβ3 and αVβ5 leading to reduced cell spreading on fibronectin and vitronectin, induced expression of osteoblast differentiation markers alkaline phosphatase and osteopontin, and suppressed synthesis of gelatinase matrix metalloproteinase-2 (MMP-2) (Koistinen et al. 1999). Finally, expression of anti-αV integrin scFv by adenovirus in melanoma cell lines depleted αV integrins, detached cells from extracellular matrix, and induced apoptosis. Subcutaneous implantation of one of melanoma cell lines transduced with anti-αV adenovirus prevented tumor formation in SCID mice (Koistinen et al. 2004).

6.3 Intrabodies in Transplantation

Major histocompatibility complex (MHC)-restricted antigen presentation is responsible for the rejection of allogeneic cell and tissue transplants. Transplantation of allogeneic MHC class I expressing keratinocytes induces CTL-mediated lysis in response to alloantigen. ER-directed antihuman MHC I scFv intrabody effectively blocked MHC I cell surface expression on monkey and human cell lines with different HLA-A, B, C haplotypes (Mhashilkar et al. 2002; Busch et al. 2004). Upon transduction by antihuman MHC I scFv encoding adenovirus, susceptibility of primary human keratinocytes to allorecognition by cytotoxic T cells were reduced (Mhashilkar et al. 2002; Busch et al. 2004). Phenotypic knockout of MHC I by intra-body in human umbilical vein endothelial cells (HUVECs) also increased protection of those intrabody-expressing HUVEC from CTL-mediated lysis (Beyer et al. 2004). Furthermore, in xenotransplantation, the carbohydrate structure Galα1,3Gal expressed on pig cells is the major antigen recognized by human xenoreactive natural antibodies (XNA). This activates complement and coagulation cascades and leads to hyperacute rejection of vascularized pig organs in primates. Intracellular expression of anti-α1,3-galactosyltransferase scFv reduced the intracellular accumulation of Galα1,3Gal and its surface expression, thus increased resistance to complement-dependent cytotoxicity mediated by anti-Gal xenoantibodies (Vanhove et al. 1998; Sepp et al. 1999).

6.4 Intrabodies in Neurodegenerative Disease

Abnormal protein aggregation and inclusions in the nuclei of affected neurons is a hallmark of several central nervous system disorders. Huntington's disease is associated with an expanded CAG repeat located within exon 1 of the *IT-15* gene encoding htt. The CAG repeat is translated into a polyglutamine (polyQ) sequence, and abnormal SDS-resistant aggregates with a fibrillar morphology appears when polyQ exceeds more than 37 glutamines (Busch et al. 2003). Intrabodies has been applied to target the proteins related to Huntington's (anti-htt scFv) (Lecerf et al. 2001; Wolfgang et al. 2005) and Parkinson's disease (anti-α-Synuclein scFv) (Zhou et al. 2004) to prevent the misfolding of glutamine-expanded protein and formation of high molecular-weight oligomers, protofibrils and aggregates respectively (Miller and Messer 2005). Lecerf et al. (2001) reported that using nuclear localizing scFv specific to the N-terminal 17 residues adjacent to the polyglutamine of htt successfully reduced length-dependent htt aggregation in cellular and organotypic slice culture models of Huntington's disease. In addition, different domain targeting intrabodies were used to dissect the functional domains of htt. Mouse intrabodies recognized the polyproline region, flanking the polyglutamine on the carboxyl-terminal side, prevented aggregation and apoptosis while intrabodies targeted to expanded polyglutamine stimulated htt aggregation, and induced cell death (Khoshnan et al. 2002). Recently, a single variable light chain (VL)12.3, derived from an scFv against the N-terminal 20 amino acids of htt, was isolated with improved affinity and functional activity by yeast surface-display library (Colby et al. 2004a; Colby et al. 2004b). Another usage of intrabody is targeting to substrate production rather than association with enzyme. ER-targeted intrabody was used to target amyloid β-peptide (Aβ), which is produced as a result of endoproteolysis of the β-amyloid precursor protein by β- and γ-secretases in the brain of Alzheimer's disease patient. (Paganetti et al. 2005). In addition, antiprion intrabodies targeted at ER were shown to prevent abnormal scrapie isoform PrP^{Sc} accumulation and antagonize scrapie infectivity in mice brain (Cardinale et al. 2005; Vetrugno et al. 2005).

6.5 Intrabodies Targeting Other Viruses

ER-directed anti-hepatitis C virus (HCV) C7-50 scFv bound to the HCV core protein specifically in vitro (Heintges et al. 1999) and this intrabody could be used to study its effect on HCV-replication and virus assembly in hepatocytes. Maedi-visna virus (MMV) is a retrovirus that causes pneumonitis, encephalomyelitis, and arthritis in sheep. Two cytosolic scFv against the transmembrane envelope glycoprotein gp46 of the MMV had been isolated and recognized gp46 peptide in ELISA. These intrabodies have the potential to be used for prevention of the maturation process of the gp150 precursor envelope glycoprotein into gp135 and gp46 in infected cells leading to virus particles with less infectivity (Blazek et al. 2004). Hepatitis B virus X protein (HBx) triggers oncogenesis by transactivating various genes such as *c-fos* and *c-myc*, activating Ras-raf-MAP kinase signaling pathway and promoting cell cycle progression in quiescent mouse fibroblasts. Expression of a scFv targeting to HBx was shown to inhibit HBx-stimulated transactivation in vitro and suppression of tumorigenicity in soft agar and nude mice (Jin et al. 2006).

7 Conclusion and Future Directions

Intrabody technology has been used as a promising tool to achieve a variety of purposes in gene therapy for HIV, cancer, neurodegenerative disease, and transplantation. As gene delivery systems become mature and more sophisticated, intrabody techniques will be used more effectively to achieve phenotypic knockout, neutralization of pathogens, or positive functions. Since intrabody methods operate at the protein level, avenues of research and therapy are possible that would not otherwise have been available through RNA interference (RNAi). Intrabodies also could avoid the RNAi-mediated nonspecific immunologic response that elicits IFN-α signaling pathways. Intrabodies can be expressed inside the cell at defined cellular compartments or to interact with specific structural or functional motifs of a target protein. Moreover, an intrabody method may be the only option in situations where the target molecule has not been cloned or is nonprotein in nature (sugars, DNA, or soluble metabolites). A thorough examination of intrabody stability characteristics or the building of stable phage-display libraries will be of key interest in the field of intrabody engineering. The quality of produced antibody will be dependent on its expression, solubility, and stability. Finally, the single domain intrabody, IDab, which has the most versatile antigen-binding domain, good membrane penetration, and reasonable stability, is becoming an important format for future use.

For future clinical applications, intrabodies could be used therapeutically for ex vivo treatment to suppress MHC molecules in tissue transplants or to down regulate the immunogenicity of adult stem cells for allogenic transplantation. Intrabodies could also be used to alleviate the alloimmune response via $CD8^+$ T cells and infiltrating recipient APC's after transplantation and to purge marrow populations of cancer cells before reinfusion into the patients (Heng et al. 2005). Furthermore, intrabody-mediated gene inactivation will be continuously useful in the investigation of signal transduction of the essential pathologic pathways in diseases or of lineage commitment in cell differentiations. At the time of this writing, high levels of intrabody expression have not been reported to have caused cell death or deteriorated metabolic state. Human or humanized antibodies could be used to circumvent the immune recognition problems. The development of an efficient gene delivery system in conjunction with direct intravenous targeting using viral particles will accelerate the prominent outcomes of intrabody technology.

Acknowledgements We would like to thank David Cook for his help with this manuscript. This work was supported by the National Foundation For Cancer Research (W.A.M), by NIH DK072282 (W.A.M.), and by NIH AI058804 (Q.Z.)

References

Aires da Silva F, Santa-Marta M, Freitas-Vieira A, Mascarenhas P, Barahona I, Moniz-Pereira J, Gabuzda D, Goncalves J (2004) Camelized rabbit-derived VH single-domain intrabodies against Vif strongly neutralize HIV-1 infectivity. J Mol Biol 340: 525–542

Aires da Silva F, Costa MJ, Corte-Real S, Goncalves J (2005) Cell type-specific targeting with sindbis pseudotyped lentiviral vectors displaying anti-CCR5 single-chain antibodies. Hum Gene Ther 16: 223–234

Alvarez RD, Curiel DT (1997) A phase I study of recombinant adenovirus vector-mediated delivery of an anti-erbB-2 single-chain (sFv) antibody gene for previously treated ovarian and extraovarian cancer patients. Hum Gene Ther 8: 229–242

Alvarez RD, Barnes MN, Gomez-Navarro J, Wang M, Strong TV, Arafat W, Arani RB, Johnson MR, Roberts BL, Siegal GP, Curiel DT (2000) A cancer gene therapy approach utilizing an anti-erbB-2 single-chain antibody-encoding adenovirus (AD21): A phase I trial. Clin Cancer Res 6: 3081–3087

Auf der Maur A, Escher D, Barberis A (2001) Antigen-independent selection of stable intracellular single-chain antibodies. FEBS Lett 508: 407–412

Auf der Maur A, Zahnd C, Fischer F, Spinelli S, Honegger A, Cambillau C, Escher D, Pluckthun A, Barberis A (2002) Direct in vivo screening of intrabody libraries constructed on a highly stable single-chain framework. J Biol Chem 277: 45075–45085

Azzazy HM, Highsmith WE, Jr. (2002) Phage display technology: Clinical applications and recent innovations. Clin Biochem 35: 425–445

Bach H, Mazor Y, Shaky S, Shoham-Lev A, Berdichevsky Y, Gutnick DL, Benhar I (2001) *Escherichia coli* maltose-binding protein as a molecular chaperone for recombinant intracellular cytoplasmic single-chain antibodies. J Mol Biol 312: 79–93

Bai J, Sui J, Zhu RY, Tallarico AS, Gennari F, Zhang D, Marasco WA (2003) Inhibition of Tat-mediated transactivation and HIV-1 replication by human anti-hCyclinT1 intrabodies. J Biol Chem 278: 1433–1442

Bangari DS, Mittal SK (2006) Current strategies and future directions for eluding adenoviral vector immunity. Curr Gene Ther 6: 215–226

Beerli RR, Wels W, Hynes NE (1994) Intracellular expression of single chain antibodies reverts ErbB-2 transformation. J Biol Chem 269: 23931–23936

Beyer F, Doebis C, Busch A, Ritter T, Mhashilkar A, Marasco WM, Laube H, Volk HD, Seifert M (2004) Decline of surface MHC I by adenoviral gene transfer of anti-MHC I intrabodies in human endothelial cells-new perspectives for the generation of universal donor cells for tissue transplantation. J Gene Med 6: 616–623

Biocca S, Pierandrei-Amaldi P, Cattaneo A (1993) Intracellular expression of anti-p21ras single chain Fv fragments inhibits meiotic maturation of xenopus oocytes. Biochem Biophys Res Commun 197: 422–427

Biocca S, Pierandrei-Amaldi P, Campioni N, Cattaneo A (1994) Intracellular immunization with cytosolic recombinant antibodies. Biotechnology (NY) 12: 396–399

Blazek D, Celer V, Navratilova I, Skladal P (2004) Generation and characterization of single-chain antibody fragments specific against transmembrane envelope glycoprotein gp46 of maedi-visna virus. J Virol Methods 115: 83–92

Boldicke T, Weber H, Mueller PP, Barleon B, Bernal M (2005) Novel highly efficient intrabody mediates complete inhibition of cell surface expression of the human vascular endothelial growth factor receptor-2 (VEGFR-2/KDR). J Immunol Methods 300: 146–159

Brockmann EC, Cooper M, Stromsten N, Vehniainen M, Saviranta P (2005) Selecting for antibody scFv fragments with improved stability using phage display with denaturation under reducing conditions. J Immunol Methods 296: 159–170

Busch A, Engemann S, Lurz R, Okazawa H, Lehrach H, Wanker EE (2003) Mutant huntingtin promotes the fibrillogenesis of wild-type huntingtin: A potential mechanism for loss of huntingtin function in Huntington's disease. J Biol Chem 278: 41452–41461

Busch A, Marasco WA, Doebis C, Volk HD, Seifert M (2004) MHC class I manipulation on cell surfaces by gene transfer of anti-MHC class I intrabodies – A tool for decreased immunogenicity of allogeneic tissue and cell transplants. Methods 34: 240–249

Cardinale A, Filesi I, Vetrugno V, Pocchiari M, Sy MS, Biocca S (2005) Trapping prion protein in the endoplasmic reticulum impairs PrPC maturation and prevents PrPSc accumulation. J Biol Chem 280: 685–694

Caron de Fromentel C, Gruel N, Venot C, Debussche L, Conseiller E, Dureuil C, Teillaud JL, Tocque B, Bracco L (1999) Restoration of transcriptional activity of p53 mutants in human tumour cells by intracellular expression of anti-p53 single chain Fv fragments. Oncogene 18: 551–557

Cattaneo A, Biocca S (1999) The selection of intracellular antibodies. Trends Biotechnol 17: 115–121

Chester KA, Begent RH, Robson L, Keep P, Pedley RB, Boden JA, Boxer G, Green A, Winter G, Cochet O, et al. (1994) Phage libraries for generation of clinically useful antibodies. Lancet 343: 455–456

Choe H, Li W, Wright PL, Vasilieva N, Venturi M, Huang CC, Grundner C, Dorfman T, Zwick MB, Wang L, Rosenberg ES, Kwong PD, Burton DR, Robinson JE, Sodroski JG, Farzan M (2003) Tyrosine sulfation of human antibodies contributes to recognition of the CCR5 binding region of HIV-1 gp120. Cell 114: 161–170

Cochet O, Kenigsberg M, Delumeau I, Duchesne M, Schweighoffer F, Tocque B, Teillaud JL (1998a) Intracellular expression and functional properties of an anti-p21Ras scFv derived from a rat hybridoma containing specific lambda and irrelevant kappa light chains. Mol Immunol 35: 1097–1110

Cochet O, Kenigsberg M, Delumeau I, Virone-Oddos A, Multon MC, Fridman WH, Schweighoffer F, Teillaud JL, Tocque B (1998b) Intracellular expression of an antibody fragment-neutralizing p21 ras promotes tumor regression. Cancer Res 58: 1170–1176

Cohen PA, Mani JC, Lane DP (1998) Characterization of a new intrabody directed against the N-terminal region of human p53. Oncogene 17: 2445–2456

Colby DW, Chu Y, Cassady JP, Duennwald M, Zazulak H, Webster JM, Messer A, Lindquist S, Ingram VM, Wittrup KD (2004a) Potent inhibition of huntingtin aggregation and cytotoxicity by a disulfide bond-free single-domain intracellular antibody. Proc Natl Acad Sci USA 101: 17616–17621

Colby DW, Garg P, Holden T, Chao G, Webster JM, Messer A, Ingram VM, Wittrup KD (2004b) Development of a human light chain variable domain (V(L)) intracellular antibody specific for the amino terminus of huntingtin via yeast surface display. J Mol Biol 342: 901–912

Cordelier P, Kulkowsky JW, Ko C, Matskevitch AA, McKee HJ, Rossi JJ, Bouhamdan M, Pomerantz RJ, Kari G, Strayer DS (2004) Protecting from R5-tropic HIV: Individual and combined effectiveness of a hammerhead ribozyme and a single-chain Fv antibody that targets CCR5. Gene Ther 11: 1627–1637

Coumoul X, Deng CX (2006) RNAi in mice: A promising approach to decipher gene functions in vivo. Biochimie 88: 637–643

Deshane J, Cabrera G, Grim JE, Siegal GP, Pike J, Alvarez RD, Curiel DT (1995a) Targeted eradication of ovarian cancer mediated by intracellular expression of anti-erbB-2 single-chain antibody. Gynecol Oncol 59: 8–14

Deshane J, Siegal GP, Alvarez RD, Wang MH, Feng M, Cabrera G, Liu T, Kay M, Curiel DT (1995b) Targeted tumor killing via an intracellular antibody against erbB-2. J Clin Invest 96: 2980–2989

Doebis C, Schu S, Ladhoff J, Busch A, Beyer F, Reiser J, Nicosia RF, Broesel S, Volk HD, Seifert M (2006) An anti-major histocompatibility complex class I intrabody protects endothelial cells from an attack by immune mediators. Cardiovasc Res 72: 331–338

Duan L, Bagasra O, Laughlin MA, Oakes JW, Pomerantz RJ (1994) Potent inhibition of human immunodeficiency virus type 1 replication by an intracellular anti-Rev single-chain antibody. Proc Natl Acad Sci USA 91: 5075–5079

Ewert S, Honegger A, Pluckthun A (2004) Stability improvement of antibodies for extracellular and intracellular applications: CDR grafting to stable frameworks and structure-based framework engineering. Methods 34: 184–199

Figini M, Ferri R, Mezzanzanica D, Bagnoli M, Luison E, Miotti S, Canevari S (2003) Reversion of transformed phenotype in ovarian cancer cells by intracellular expression of anti folate receptor antibodies. Gene Ther 10: 1018–1025

Fire A, Xu S, Montgomery MK, Kostas SA, Driver SE, Mello CC (1998) Potent and specific genetic interference by double-stranded RNA in *Caenorhabditis elegans*. Nature 391: 806–811

Fukuchi K, Tahara K, Kim HD, Maxwell JA, Lewis TL, Accavitti-Loper MA, Kim H, Ponnazhagan S, Lalonde R (2006) Anti-Abeta single-chain antibody delivery via adeno-associated virus for treatment of Alzheimer's disease. Neurobiol Dis 23: 502–511

Gargano N, Biocca S, Bradbury A, Cattaneo A (1996) Human recombinant antibody fragments neutralizing human immunodeficiency virus type 1 reverse transcriptase provide an experimental basis for the structural classification of the DNA polymerase family. J Virol 70: 7706–7712

Gao GP, Alvira MR, Wang L, Calcedo R, Johnston J, Wilson JM (2002) Novel adeno-associated viruses from rhesus monkeys as vectors for human gene therapy. Proc Natl Acad Sci USA 99: 11854–11859

Gennari F, Mehta S, Wang Y, St Clair Tallarico A, Palu G, Marasco WA (2004) Direct phage to intrabody screening (DPIS): Demonstration by isolation of cytosolic intrabodies against the TES1 site of Epstein Barr virus latent membrane protein 1 (LMP1) that block NF-kappaB transactivation. J Mol Biol 335: 193–207

Gil J, Esteban M (2000) Induction of apoptosis by the dsRNA-dependent protein kinase (PKR): Mechanism of action. Apoptosis 5: 107–114

Goncalves J, Silva F, Freitas-Vieira A, Santa-Marta M, Malho R, Yang X, Gabuzda D, Barbas C, 3rd (2002) Functional neutralization of HIV-1 Vif protein by intracellular immunization inhibits reverse transcription and viral replication. J Biol Chem 277: 32036–32045

Graus YF, de Baets MH, Parren PW, Berrih-Aknin S, Wokke J, van Breda Vriesman PJ, Burton DR (1997) Human anti-nicotinic acetylcholine receptor recombinant Fab fragments isolated from thymus-derived phage display libraries from myasthenia gravis patients reflect predominant specificities in serum and block the action of pathogenic serum antibodies. J Immunol 158: 1919–1929.

Graus-Porta D, Beerli RR, Hynes NE (1995) Single-chain antibody-mediated intracellular retention of ErbB-2 impairs Neu differentiation factor and epidermal growth factor signaling. Mol Cell Biol 15: 1182–1191

Heike Y, Kasono K, Kunisaki C, Hama S, Saijo N, Tsuruo T, Kuntz DA, Rose DR, Curiel DT (2001) Overcoming multi-drug resistance using an intracellular anti-MDR1 sFv. Int J Cancer 92: 115–122

Heintges T, zu Putlitz J, Wands JR (1999) Characterization and binding of intracellular antibody fragments to the hepatitis C virus core protein. Biochem Biophys Res Commun 263: 410–418

Heng BC, Cao T (2005) Making cell-permeable antibodies (Transbody) through fusion of protein transduction domains (PTD) with single chain variable fragment (scFv) antibodies: Potential advantages over antibodies expressed within the intracellular environment (Intrabody). Med Hypotheses 64: 1105–1108

Heng BC, Kemeny DM, Liu H, Cao T (2005) Potential applications of intracellular antibodies (intrabodies) in stem cell therapeutics. J Cell Mol Med 9: 191–195

Ho M, Nagata S, Pastan I (2006) Isolation of anti-CD22 Fv with high affinity by Fv display on human cells. Proc Natl Acad Sci USA 103: 9637–9642

Hoogenboom HR, Chames P (2000) Natural and designer binding sites made by phage display technology. Immunol Today 21: 371–378

Hoogenboom HR (2005) Selecting and screening recombinant antibody libraries. Nat Biotechnol 23: 1105–1116

Huang CC, Venturi M, Majeed S, Moore MJ, Phogat S, Zhang MY, Dimitrov DS, Hendrickson WA, Robinson J, Sodroski J, Wyatt R, Choe H, Farzan M, Kwong PD (2004) Structural basis of tyrosine sulfation and VH-gene usage in antibodies that recognize the HIV type 1 coreceptor-binding site on gp120. Proc Natl Acad Sci USA 101: 2706–2711

Jannot CB, Beerli RR, Mason S, Gullick WJ, Hynes NE (1996) Intracellular expression of a single-chain antibody directed to the EGFR leads to growth inhibition of tumor cells. Oncogene 13: 275–282

Jendreyko N, Popkov M, Beerli RR, Chung J, McGavern DB, Rader C, Barbas CF, 3rd (2003) Intradiabodies, bispecific, tetravalent antibodies for the simultaneous functional knockout of two cell surface receptors. J Biol Chem 278: 47812–47819

Jendreyko N, Popkov M, Rader C, Barbas CF, 3rd (2005) Phenotypic knockout of VEGF-R2 and Tie-2 with an intradiabody reduces tumor growth and angiogenesis in vivo. Proc Natl Acad Sci USA 102: 8293–8298

Jin YH, Kwon MH, Kim K, Shin HJ, Shin JS, Cho H, Park S (2006) An intracellular antibody can suppress tumorigenicity in hepatitis B virus X-expressing cells. Cancer Immunol Immunother 55: 569–578

Joliot A, Prochiantz A (2004) Transduction peptides: From technology to physiology. Nat Cell Biol 6: 189–196

Jooss K, Chirmule N (2003) Immunity to adenovirus and adeno-associated viral vectors: Implications for gene therapy. Gene Ther 10: 955–963

Khoshnan A, Ko J, Patterson PH (2002) Effects of intracellular expression of anti-huntingtin antibodies of various specificities on mutant huntingtin aggregation and toxicity. Proc Natl Acad Sci USA 99: 1002–1007

Kitabwalla M, Ruprecht RM (2002) RNA interference – A new weapon against HIV and beyond. N Engl J Med 347: 1364–1367

Knappik A, Ge L, Honegger A, Pack P, Fischer M, Wellnhofer G, Hoess A, Wolle J, Pluckthun A, Virnekas B (2000) Fully synthetic human combinatorial antibody libraries (HuCAL) based on modular consensus frameworks and CDRs randomized with trinucleotides. J Mol Biol 296: 57–86

Koistinen P, Pulli T, Uitto VJ, Nissinen L, Hyypia T, Heino J (1999) Depletion of αV integrins from osteosarcoma cells by intracellular antibody expression induces bone differentiation marker genes and suppresses gelatinase (MMP-2) synthesis. Matrix Biol 18: 239–251

Koistinen P, Ahonen M, Kahari VM, Heino J (2004) αV integrin promotes in vitro and in vivo survival of cells in metastatic melanoma. Int J Cancer 112: 61–70

Lecerf JM, Shirley TL, Zhu Q, Kazantsev A, Amersdorfer P, Housman DE, Messer A, Huston JS (2001) Human single-chain Fv intrabodies counteract in situ huntingtin aggregation in cellular models of Huntington's disease. Proc Natl Acad Sci USA 98: 4764–4769

Levin R, Mhashilkar AM, Dorfman T, Bukovsky A, Zani C, Bagley J, Hinkula J, Niedrig M, Albert J, Wahren B, Gottlinger HG, Marasco WA (1997) Inhibition of early and late events of the HIV-1 replication cycle by cytoplasmic Fab intrabodies against the matrix protein, p17. Mol Med 3: 96–110

Levites Y, Jansen K, Smithson LA, Dakin R, Holloway VM, Das P, Golde TE (2006) Intracranial adeno-associated virus-mediated delivery of anti-pan amyloid beta, amyloid beta40, and amyloid beta42 single-chain variable fragments attenuates plaque pathology in amyloid precursor protein mice. J Neurosci 26: 11923–11928

Levy-Mintz P, Duan L, Zhang H, Hu B, Dornadula G, Zhu M, Kulkosky J, Bizub-Bender D, Skalka AM, Pomerantz RJ (1996) Intracellular expression of single-chain variable fragments to inhibit early stages of the viral life cycle by targeting human immunodeficiency virus type 1 integrase. J Virol 70: 8821–8832

Li X, Stuckert P, Bosch I, Marks JD, Marasco WA (2001) Single-chain antibody-mediated gene delivery into ErbB2-positive human breast cancer cells. Cancer Gene Ther 8: 555–565

Lobato MN, Rabbitts TH (2003) Intracellular antibodies and challenges facing their use as therapeutic agents. Trends Mol Med 9: 390–396

Marasco WA (1995) Intracellular antibodies (intrabodies) as research reagents and therapeutic molecules for gene therapy. Immunotechnology 1: 1–19

Marasco WA, Haseltine WA, Chen SY (1993) Design, intracellular expression, and activity of a human anti-human immunodeficiency virus type 1 gp120 single-chain antibody. Proc Natl Acad Sci USA 90: 7889–7893

Mary MN, Venot C, Caron de Fromentel C, Debussche L, Conseiller E, Cochet O, Gruel N, Teillaud JL, Schweighoffer F, Tocque B, Bracco L (1999) A tumor specific single chain antibody dependent gene expression system. Oncogene 18: 559–564

Mhashilkar AM, Bagley J, Chen SY, Szilvay AM, Helland DG, Marasco WA (1995) Inhibition of HIV-1 Tat-mediated LTR transactivation and HIV-1 infection by anti-Tat single chain intrabodies. Embo J 14: 1542–1551

Mhashilkar AM, Biswas DK, LaVecchio J, Pardee AB, Marasco WA (1997) Inhibition of human immunodeficiency virus type 1 replication in vitro by a novel combination of anti-Tat single-chain intrabodies and NF-kappa B antagonists. J Virol 71: 6486–6494

Mhashilkar AM, LaVecchio J, Eberhardt B, Porter-Brooks J, Boisot S, Dove JH, Pumphrey C, Li X, Weissmahr RN, Ring DB, Ramstedt U, Marasco WA (1999) Inhibition of human immunodeficiency virus type 1 replication in vitro in acutely and persistently infected human CD4+ mononuclear cells expressing murine and humanized anti-human immunodeficiency virus type 1 Tat single-chain variable fragment intrabodies. Hum Gene Ther 10: 1453–1467

Mhashilkar AM, Doebis C, Seifert M, Busch A, Zani C, Soo Hoo J, Nagy M, Ritter T, Volk HD, Marasco WA (2002) Intrabody-mediated phenotypic knockout of major histocompatibility complex class I expression in human and monkey cell lines and in primary human keratinocytes. Gene Ther 9: 307–319

Miller TW, Messer A (2005) Intrabody applications in neurological disorders: Progress and future prospects. Mol Ther 12: 394–401

Montano X, Jimenez A (1995) Intracellular expression of the monoclonal anti-ras antibody Y13-259 blocks the transforming activity of ras oncogenes. Cell Growth Differ 6: 597–605

Morizono K, Xie Y, Ringpis GE, Johnson M, Nassanian H, Lee B, Wu L, Chen IS (2005) Lentiviral vector retargeting to P-glycoprotein on metastatic melanoma through intravenous injection. Nat Med 11: 346–352

Mossner E, Koch H, Pluckthun A (2001) Fast selection of antibodies without antigen purification: Adaptation of the protein fragment complementation assay to select antigen–antibody pairs. J Mol Biol 308: 115–122

Mulligan-Kehoe MJ, Russo A (1999) Inhibition of cytoplasmic antigen, glucose-6-phosphate dehydrogenase, by VH-CH1, an intracellular Fd fragment antibody derived from a semisynthetic Fd fragment phage display library. J Mol Biol 289: 41–55.

Mukhtar M, Acheampong E, Khan MA, Bouhamdan M, Pomerantz RJ (2005) Down-modulation of the CXCR4 co-receptor by intracellular expression of a single chain variable fragment (SFv) inhibits HIV-1 entry into primary human brain microvascular endothelial cells and post-mitotic neurons. Brain Res Mol Brain Res 135: 48–57

Nieba L, Honegger A, Krebber C, Pluckthun A (1997) Disrupting the hydrophobic patches at the antibody variable/constant domain interface: Improved in vivo folding and physical characterization of an engineered scFv fragment. Protein Eng 10: 435–444

Nielsen UB, Kirpotin DB, Pickering EM, Hong K, Park JW, Shalaby MR, Shao Y, Benz CC, Marks JD (2002) Therapeutic efficacy of anti-ErbB2 immunoliposomes targeted by a phage antibody selected for cellular endocytosis. Biochim Biophys Acta 1591: 109–118

Niesner U, Halin C, Lozzi L, Gunthert M, Neri P, Wunderli-Allenspach H, Zardi L, Neri D (2002) Quantitation of the tumor-targeting properties of antibody fragments conjugated to cell-permeating HIV-1 TAT peptides. Bioconjug Chem 13: 729–736

Nissim A, Hoogenboom HR, Tomlinson IM, Flynn G, Midgley C, Lane D, Winter G (1994) Antibody fragments from a 'single pot' phage display library as immunochemical reagents. EMBO J 13: 692–698

Noureddini SC, Curiel DT (2005) Genetic targeting strategies for adenovirus. Mol Pharm 2: 341–347

Paganetti P, Calanca V, Galli C, Stefani M, Molinari M (2005) beta-site specific intrabodies to decrease and prevent generation of Alzheimer's Abeta peptide. J Cell Biol 168: 863–868

Paz K, Brennan LA, Iacolina M, Doody J, Hadari YR, Zhu Z (2005) Human single-domain neutralizing intrabodies directed against Etk kinase: A novel approach to impair cellular transformation. Mol Cancer Ther 4: 1801–1809

Persengiev SP, Zhu X, Green MR (2004) Nonspecific, concentration-dependent stimulation and repression of mammalian gene expression by small interfering RNAs (siRNAs). RNA 10: 12–18

Persic L, Righi M, Roberts A, Hoogenboom HR, Cattaneo A, Bradbury A (1997) Targeting vectors for intracellular immunisation. Gene 187: 1–8

Pini A, Bracci L (2000) Phage display of antibody fragments. Curr Protein Pept Sci 1: 155–169

Popkov M, Jendreyko N, McGavern DB, Rader C, Barbas CF, 3rd (2005) Targeting tumor angiogenesis with adenovirus-delivered anti-Tie-2 intrabody. Cancer Res 65: 972–981

Popov S, Hubbard JG, Ward ES (1996) A novel and efficient route for the isolation of antibodies that recognise T cell receptor V α(s). Mol Immunol 33: 493–502

Poznansky MC, Foxall R, Mhashilkar A, Coker R, Jones S, Ramstedt U, Marasco W (1998) Inhibition of human immunodeficiency virus replication and growth advantage of CD4+ T cells from HIV-infected individuals that express intracellular antibodies against HIV-1 gp120 or Tat. Hum Gene Ther 9: 487–496

Proba K, Worn A, Honegger A, Pluckthun A (1998) Antibody scFv fragments without disulfide bonds made by molecular evolution. J Mol Biol 275: 245–253

Rajpal A, Turi TG (2001) Intracellular stability of anti-caspase-3 intrabodies determines efficacy in retargeting the antigen. J Biol Chem 276: 33139–33146

Reinman M, Jantti J, Alfthan K, Keranen S, Soderlund H, Takkinen K (2003) Functional inactivation of the conserved Sem1p in yeast by intrabodies. Yeast 20: 1071–1084

Richardson JH, Sodroski JG, Waldmann TA, Marasco WA (1995) Phenotypic knockout of the high-affinity human interleukin 2 receptor by intracellular single-chain antibodies against the α subunit of the receptor. Proc Natl Acad Sci USA 92: 3137–3141

Richardson JH, Waldmann TA, Sodroski JG, Marasco WA (1997) Inducible knockout of the interleukin-2 receptor α chain: Expression of the high-affinity IL-2 receptor is not required for the in vitro growth of HTLV-I-transformed cell lines. Virology 237: 209–216

Richardson JH, Hofmann W, Sodroski JG, Marasco WA (1998) Intrabody-mediated knockout of the high-affinity IL-2 receptor in primary human T cells using a bicistronic lentivirus vector. Gene Ther 5: 635–644

Ryther RC, Flynt AS, Phillips JA, 3rd, Patton JG (2005) siRNA therapeutics: Big potential from small RNAs. Gene Ther 12: 5–11

Secco P, Ferretti M, Gioia D, Cesaro P, Bozzo C, Marks JD, Santoro C (2004) Characterization of a single-chain intrabody directed against the human receptor tyrosine kinase Ron. J Immunol Methods 285: 99–109.

Sepp A, Farrar CA, Dorling T, Cairns T, George AJ, Lechler RI (1999) Inhibition of expression of the Gal-α1-3Gal epitope on porcine cells using an intracellular single-chain antibody directed against α1,3galactosyltransferase. J Immunol Methods 231: 191–205

Shaki-Loewenstein S, Zfania R, Hyland S, Wels WS, Benhar I (2005) A universal strategy for stable intracellular antibodies. J Immunol Methods 303: 19–39

Shi J, Liu Y, Zheng Y, Guo Y, Zhang J, Cheung PT, Xu R, Zheng D (2006) Therapeutic expression of an anti-death receptor 5 single-chain fixed-variable region prevents tumor growth in mice. Cancer Res 66: 11946–11953

Shin I, Edl J, Biswas S, Lin PC, Mernaugh R, Arteaga CL (2005) Proapoptotic activity of cell-permeable anti-Akt single-chain antibodies. Cancer Res 65: 2815–2824

Sledz CA, Holko M, de Veer MJ, Silverman RH, Williams BR (2003) Activation of the interferon system by short-interfering RNAs. Nat Cell Biol 5: 834–839

Sledz CA, Williams BR (2004) RNA interference and double-stranded-RNA-activated pathways. Biochem Soc Trans 32: 952–956

Steinberger P, Andris-Widhopf J, Buhler B, Torbett BE, Barbas CF, 3rd (2000) Functional deletion of the CCR5 receptor by intracellular immunization produces cells that are refractory to CCR5-dependent HIV-1 infection and cell fusion. Proc Natl Acad Sci USA 97: 805–810

Strayer DS, Branco F, Landre J, BouHamdan M, Shaheen F, Pomerantz RJ (2002) Combination genetic therapy to inhibit HIV-1. Mol Ther 5: 33–41

Strube RW, Chen SY (2002) Characterization of anti-cyclin E single-chain Fv antibodies and intrabodies in breast cancer cells: Enhanced intracellular stability of novel sFv-F(c) intrabodies. J Immunol Methods 263: 149–167

Swan CH, Buhler B, Tschan MP, Barbas CF, 3rd, Torbett BE (2006) T-cell protection and enrichment through lentiviral CCR5 intrabody gene delivery. Gene Ther 13: 1480–1492

Tanaka T, Lobato MN, Rabbitts TH (2003) Single domain intracellular antibodies: A minimal fragment for direct in vivo selection of antigen-specific intrabodies. J Mol Biol 331: 1109–1120

Tanha J, Xu P, Chen Z, Ni F, Kaplan H, Narang SA, MacKenzie CR (2001) Optimal design features of camelized human single-domain antibody libraries. J Biol Chem 276: 24774–24780

Tenenbaum L, Lehtonen E, Monahan PE (2003) Evaluation of risks related to the use of adeno-associated virus-based vectors. Curr Gene Ther 3: 545–565

Tse E, Rabbitts TH (2000) Intracellular antibody-caspase-mediated cell killing: An approach for application in cancer therapy. Proc Natl Acad Sci USA 97: 12266–12271

Vanhove B, Charreau B, Cassard A, Pourcel C, Soulillou JP (1998) Intracellular expression in pig cells of anti-α1,3galactosyltransferase single-chain FV antibodies reduces Gal α1,3Gal expression and inhibits cytotoxicity mediated by anti-Gal xenoantibodies. Transplantation 66: 1477–1485

Vaughan TJ, Williams AJ, Pritchard K, Osbourn JK, Pope AR, Earnshaw JC, McCafferty J, Hodits RA, Wilton J, Johnson KS (1996) Human antibodies with sub-nanomolar affinities isolated from a large non-immunized phage display library. Nat Biotechnol 14: 309–314

Vetrugno V, Cardinale A, Filesi I, Mattei S, Sy MS, Pocchiari M, Biocca S (2005) KDEL-tagged anti-prion intrabodies impair PrP lysosomal degradation and inhibit scrapie infectivity. Biochem Biophys Res Commun 338: 1791–1797

Visintin M, Tse E, Axelson H, Rabbitts TH, Cattaneo A (1999) Selection of antibodies for intracellular function using a two-hybrid in vivo system. Proc Natl Acad Sci USA 96: 11723–11728

Ward ES, Gussow D, Griffiths AD, Jones PT, Winter G (1989) Binding activities of a repertoire of single immunoglobulin variable domains secreted from *Escherichia coli*. Nature 341: 544–546

Wheeler YY, Kute TE, Willingham MC, Chen SY, Sane DC (2003) Intrabody-based strategies for inhibition of vascular endothelial growth factor receptor-2: Effects on apoptosis, cell growth, and angiogenesis. FASEB J 17: 1733–1735

Wild MA, Xin H, Maruyama T, Nolan MJ, Calveley PM, Malone JD, Wallace MR, Bowdish KS (2003) Human antibodies from immunized donors are protective against anthrax toxin in vivo. Nat Biotechnol 21: 1305–1306

Wolfgang WJ, Miller TW, Webster JM, Huston JS, Thompson LM, Marsh JL, Messer A (2005) Suppression of Huntington's disease pathology in Drosophila by human single-chain Fv antibodies. Proc Natl Acad Sci USA 102: 11563–11568

Worn A, Auf der Maur A, Escher D, Honegger A, Barberis A, Pluckthun A (2000) Correlation between in vitro stability and in vivo performance of anti-GCN4 intrabodies as cytoplasmic inhibitors. J Biol Chem 275: 2795–2803

Worn A, Pluckthun A (2001) Stability engineering of antibody single-chain Fv fragments. J Mol Biol 305: 989–1010

Wu Y, Duan L, Zhu M, Hu B, Kubota S, Bagasra O, Pomerantz RJ (1996) Binding of intracellular anti-Rev single chain variable fragments to different epitopes of human immunodeficiency virus type 1 rev: Variations in viral inhibition. J Virol 70: 3290–3297

Yamanaka HI, Inoue T, Ikeda-Tanaka O (1996) Chicken monoclonal antibody isolated by a phage display system. J Immunol 157: 1156–1162

Yang L, Bailey L, Baltimore D, Wang P (2006) Targeting lentiviral vectors to specific cell types in vivo. Proc Natl Acad Sci USA 103: 11479–11484

Yoneda Y, Semba T, Kaneda Y, Noble RL, Matsuoka Y, Kurihara T, Okada Y, Imamoto N (1992) A long synthetic peptide containing a nuclear localization signal and its flanking sequences of SV40 T-antigen directs the transport of IgM into the nucleus efficiently. Exp Cell Res 201: 313–320

Yuan Q, Strauch KL, Lobb RR, Hemler ME (1996) Intracellular single-chain antibody inhibits integrin VLA-4 maturation and function. Biochem J 318: 591–596

Zhou C, Emadi S, Sierks MR, Messer A (2004) A human single-chain Fv intrabody blocks aberrant cellular effects of overexpressed α-synuclein. Mol Ther 10: 1023–1031

Zhou P, Goldstein S, Devadas K, Tewari D, Notkins AL (1998) Cells transfected with a non-neutralizing antibody gene are resistant to HIV infection: Targeting the endoplasmic reticulum and trans-Golgi network. J Immunol 160: 1489–1496

Zhou P, Bogacki R, McReynolds L, Howley PM (2000) Harnessing the ubiquitination machinery to target the degradation of specific cellular proteins. Mol Cell 6: 751–756

Zhu Q, Zeng C, Huhalov A, Yao J, Turi TG, Danley D, Hynes T, Cong Y, DiMattia D, Kennedy S, Daumy G, Schaeffer E, Marasco WA, Huston JS (1999) Extended half-life and elevated steady-state level of a single-chain Fv intrabody are critical for specific intracellular retargeting of its antigen, caspase-7. J Immunol Methods 231: 207–222

Index

Abciximab, 70
Acceptor framework, 63
ACR criteria, 167
Active specific immunotherapy, 206
Acute transplant rejection, 5
Adalimumab, 87, 103, 110, 118
    markers, inflammation and angiogenesis,
        118
    pharmacokinetics, 113
ADCC, 28, 198
ADCP, 28
Affinity, 4, 10, 27
    maturation, 9
Age-related macular degeneration (AMD),
        134, 140
Alanine-scanning mutagenesis, 139, 142
Alemtuzumab, 239
Alloantigen-specific tolerance, 225
American Food and Drug Administration
        (FDA), 4, 40
Anaphylactic shock, 48
Anatomic pathology, 32
Angiogenesis, 132, 133, 139
Ankylosing spondylitis (AS), 103, 112
Anti-CD20 monoclonal antibody rituximab,
        163
Anti-human CD3 antibodies, 222
Anti-humanized antibody (HAHA), 4
Anti-T cell antibodies, 225
Anti-VLA4, 231
Antibodies, 133, 134, 137, 140, 142, 143, 145,
        330, 333, 336, 338
    antitumor, 330
    scFv, 330, 338
Antibody libraries
    human phage Mehta I/II libraries, 349
    immune libraries, 349

naïve or nonimmune antibody libraries, 349
synthetic libraries, 350
Antibody screening
    E. coli maltose binding protein (MBP), 351
    direct phage to intrabody screening (DPIS),
        350
    DNA shuffling, 351
    lentivirus and mammalian cell display, 352
    phage display, 351
    protein fragment complementation assay
        (PCA), 352
    ribosomal display, 350, 352
    yeast two-hybrid system, 353
Antibody toxicities, 41
Antibody-dependent cytotoxicity (ADCC), 11
Antibody-directed enzyme prodrug therapy
        (ADEPT), 11
Antigen density, 27
Approved mAbs, 20
Arming mAb, 11
Asthma, 9, 258, 260, 262, 272, 277–280
Athymic mouse models, 194, 201
    anti-tumor activity, 193, 198, 202
    tumor localization, 195, 197, 199
    whole body autoradiography, 200
Autoantigen presenting cells, 224

B cells, 166, 174, 259, 262, 263, 281
    chronic lymphocytic leukaemia, 5
    lymphoma, 4
B Lymphocyte Stimulator (BLys), 177
B7 costimulation, 305
B7.1 fusion protein, 306, 307, 318, 323
Basophil, 268
Belimumab, 178
β cell antigens, 224
Beta-agonists, in treatment of asthma, 261

Bevacizumab, 134, 136–138, 140, 142, 144, 145, 239, 244, 250
  clinical studies, 244
  harmacokinetics, 139
  humanization, 134, 137
  immunogenicity, 134
  side effects, 140
  structure, 138
  Xenograft models, 244
Bexxar, 205, 206
Bi-specific, 11
BILAG index, 176
Bio-breeding (BB) rat, 223
Biodistribution, 27, 37, 311
Bispecific tetravalent intrabody
  anti VEGF-R2 scFv, 346, 356
  anti-Tie-2 scFv, 346, 356
  structure, 344
Breast cancer, 5, 193, 195, 199, 203, 204, 206, 209, 211
Bridging toxicity study, 24, 25

C_{max} and C_{min}, 29
c-Met, 188, 190
Cancer therapy, 238
Carcinogenic, 34
Carcinogenicity, 36
$CD4^+CD25^+FoxP3^+$ T cells, 224
$CD4^+CD25^-$ precursors, 225
CD137L fusion proteins, 293, 309, 310, 319, 323
CD22 molecule, 177
CD3-specific, 221
CDC, 28
CDR
  donor, 63
  graft, 61
  shuffling, 10
Certolizumab pegol, 103, 111, 113, 118
  markers, inflammation and angiogenesis, 117, 118
  pharmacokinetics, 111–113
  specificity, 111
Cetuximab, 79, 80, 239, 240, 242
  clinical studies, 243
  Xenograft models, 243
ChAglyCD3, 229
Charge cluster, 65
Chemokine, 299, 323
  fusion proteins, 301
Chemotherapy, 192, 196, 202, 204, 211
  cisplatin, 198, 201, 202
  doxorubicin, 198, 199, 204
  fluorouracil, 184, 204

Childbearing, 35
Chimeric, 22
  antibodies, 4
Chimeric receptor, 330, 331
  co-stimulation, 332
  composition, 331
  signaling, 333
Chinese hamster ovary, 7
chTNT-3, 295
Circular dichroism spectroscopy, 58
Clinical trials, 23, 201, 203
Comparability, 25
Complement-dependent cytotoxicity (CDC), 11
Complementarity-determining regions (CDRs), 4
Complications, 168
Corticosteroids, in treatment of asthma, 261, 270, 278, 281
Costimulatory, 323
  molecule B7.1, 293
  pathway, 225
Crohn's disease (CD), 102, 103
Cross-reactivity, 30, 31
CTLA-4, 249
  clinical studies, 249
  MAbs, 249
Cytokine fusion proteins, 296, 305, 317, 323

DANCER, 172
DAS28, 167
Dendritic cell, 259, 263–265, 268
Denosomab, 81, 82
Developmental immunotoxicity, 36
Developmental toxicity, 27
Diabetic retinopathy, 134, 140
Diabetogenic T cells, 229
Diabodies, 13, 50
Differential scanning calorimetry (DSC), 58
Disease
  incidence, 223
  remission, 226
Disulfide bond, 49
Dose–response relationship, 28
Drug conjugates, 30

E. coli HB2151 and TG-1, 8
Effector function, 10
EGFR, 242, 243
  expression, 242, 243
Embryo–fetal, 35
Embryonic development, 35
Embryonic stem cells, (ES), 72, 73
Enbrel, 209
Endocrinopathies, 224

Endothermic transition, 58
Epratuzumab, 177
ER retention peptide, KDEL, 347, 348
Experimental allergic encephalomyelitis
    (EAE), 226
Experimental inflammatory bowel disease, 227
Exposure, 26, 28, 31
Exposure–response relationships, 29

Fab, 7
FACS, 31
Fc
    mutation, 222
    portion, 7
FcεRI and RII receptor, 259, 262, 263, 265,
    268
FDA, see American Food and Drug
    Administration
Fertility, 35
Flu-like syndrome, 222
Folding efficiency, 48

Gemtuzumab, 240
Gene knockout, 73, 75
Generic grafting strategy, 62
Genotoxicity, 34
Germline
    diversity, 55
    family, 51
GITRL, 312
Glycosuria, 223
Golimumab, 82, 86, 87

Haemolytic anemia, 223
Half-lives, 28, 37
Hapten binding pocket, 60
Haptens, 60
Health-related quality of life, 269, 271, 272
Hematology, 32
HER family members, 192, 208, 211
    antibody therapeutics, 194, 201
    canonical ligands, 207, 208, 210
    overexpression (in cancer), 190, 208, 212
HER2, 240
    dimerization, 241
    expression, 241
    gene amplification, 240
Hermodulins, 209, 211
Histoincompatible, 226
HNSTD, 29
hOKT3γl Ala-Ala, 229
Human anti-chimeric antibodies (HACA), 166
Human anti-mouse antibody (HAMA), 4, 195,
    197, 200

Human antichimeric antibodies, 4
Humanized, 22
    antibody, 366
Hyperglycemia, 223
Hypervariable regions, 4

Ibritumomab tiuxetan, 240
IGF-1, 190, 208
IGF-IR, 245
    clinical studies, 245
    expression, 245
    MAbs, 245
    Xenografts models, 245
IL-4, 228
Immune libraries, 9
Immune-mediated inflammatory disease, 102,
    110, 114, 118, 119
Immunoconjugate, 30, 39
Immunocytokines, 12
Immunogenicity, 26, 31
Immunoglobulin
    fold, 49
    loci, 5
Immunoglobulin E receptor (IgE receptor),
    259, 262, 265
Immunohistochemisty, 30
Immunophenotyping, 38
Immunoregulatory T cells (Treg), 314
Immunotherapy, 292–294, 321–323
    in treatment of asthma, 273, 276
in vitro and in vivo affinity maturation, 5, 7
in-vitro evolution, 64
Inclusion bodies, 58
IND-enabling, 30
Infliximab, 110–112, 114–117, 119
    markers, bone and cartilage turnover, 117
    markers, inflammation and angiogenesis,
        114
    pharmacokinetics, 112
    specificity, 110
Initial study, 167
Insulin
    dependent diabetes, 222
    independency, 230
    usage, 230
Insulitis, 224
Interleuin-4, -5, -13, 280, 281
Interleukin-6 (IL-6)
    IL-6 receptor, 152, 155
Interspecies, 29
Intrabody application
    in bone marrow transplantation, 349
    in cancer, 361

cell cycle and apoptosis-related oncogenic
    protein, 362
drug resistance proteins, 363
growth factor receptors and angiogenesis-
    related receptors, 361
integrins, 363
HIV-1 envelope glycoprotein gp160, 347
in HIV, 359
in neurodegenerative disease, 364
target other viruses, 365
in transplantation, 363
signal transduction, 362
Intrabody clinical trial
    adeno-associated virus (AAV), 357
    adenovirus (Ad21), 361
    anti-erbB2 scFv, 355, 358
    ovarian cancer, 361
Intrabody delivery system
    adeno-associated virus (AAV), 357
    adenovirus, 355–357
    immunoliposome, 358
    lentivirus, 352, 354, 355
    lentivirus with Sindbis envelope protein, 354
    membrane fusion by influenza hemagglu-
        tinin mutant, 357
    protamine mediated delivery, 358
    protein transduction domains (PTD), 358
    retrovirus, 354, 357
Intrabody gene construction
    ER targeted intrabody, 347
    Ig leader sequence, 348, 350
    intrabody cytoplasmic expression, 350
Intrabody gene source
    B cells, 349
    hybridoma cell line, 348
    lymphoid organs, 349
Intrabody library, 62
Intrabody stability
    anticaspase-7 scFv, 351
Intrabody structure
    complementarity determining regions
        (CDRs), 345
    Fab fragment, 344, 345
    Fd fragment (VH-CH1), 346
    immunoglobular (IgG), 346
    interchain linker (ICL), 344
    intracellular single variable domain (IDab),
        344
    intradiabody, 345
    scFv-Fc, 345
    VH single-domain intrabody, 360
Intrabody subcellular targeting, 348
Intrinsic thermodynamic stability, 47
Investigational new drug (IND), 185

Ipilimumab, 82, 85, 86
Irreversible aggregation, 56
Islets of Langerhans, 223

Kappa, 51
Kinetic stabilization, 47

Lambda, 51
Late autoimmune diabetes of adult, 223
LEC fusion protein, 300, 302, 305, 314, 323
Leucine zipper, 62
Leukocyte counts, 37
Libraries, 7
Ligand trap, 201, 209, 210
Light chains, 51
Linker length, 13
Long-term follow-up data, 176
Lower core residue H55, 64
Lupus nephritis, 176
Lymphocytes, 38
Lymphopenia, 228

Macrophage, 188–190, 192
Macroscopic, 32
Marketing, 34
Mast cells, 259, 262–265, 268, 277, 281
Maximum tolerated dose, 39
Metabolic reconstitution, 226
Metabolism, 37
MHC haplotype, 223
Microcell-mediated chromosome transfer, 73,
    74
Microscopic, 32
Minibodies, 13
Minilocus, 75, 76
Minimizing immunogenicity, 10
Mitogenic potential, 222
Molecular mechanism of intrabody action, 346
Monkey anti-mouse antibody (MAMA), 196
Monoclonal antibodies
    fully human, 240
    humanized, 239–241
    naked, 239, 240, 242
    radiolabelled, 247
Mouse hybridomas, 4
Multimerization domains, 50
Multiple sclerosis, 231
Multiple-dose, 33
Muromonab-CD3, 70
Muromonomab-CD3, 69, 70
Mutual stabilization, 56

NOAEL, 29
Non Fc binding, 228

Non insulin-dependent diabetes, 223
Nonmitogenic CD3-specific MAbs, 229
Nonobese diabetic (NOD) mouse, 223

Ofatumumab, 82, 88
OKT3, 221
Omalizumab, 275, 276
Omalizumab, humanization of, 265–267, 269,
    270, 272–276
Open trials, 167
Organ transplantation, 231
OX40L, 313

p185^{HER2}
    antibody, 195, 197–200, 202, 205
    extracellular domain (ECD), 185, 190, 201,
        206, 209
    receptor, 185, 197
    shed antigen, 201
Panitumumab, 70, 72, 79, 80, 82, 89, 240, 243
    clinical studies, 243
    Xenograft models, 243
Pathogen environment, 223
Pathogenic T cells, 224
Payload, 38
PDB databank, 59
PEGylated antibody, 14
Peptidic tags, 50
Periplasmic expression, 58
Pertuzumab, 191, 192, 209, 211, 241, 242
Phage coat protein, 8
Phage display, 50, 142, 145, 146
    libraries, 8
Pharmacokinetics, 12, 23, 37
Pharmacology, 36
Phase 1, 23
Phase I trials, 33
Phase I/II trial of rituximab, 175
Phase II, 24, 33
Phase IIa trial, 169
Phase IIb trial, 172
Phase III trial, 24, 34, 172
Postnatal development, 35
Posttranslational modification, 9
Prenatal, 35
Prodrug, 12
Pronuclear microinjection, 72, 73, 75, 77
Prostate Cancer, 238, 240, 246
    hormone-refractory/androgen-independent,
        238, 244
    MAb products, 239, 251
    metastatic disease, 238, 246
    therapy, 238
Protooncogene, 185, 186, 188, 189

PSCA, 247
    clinical studies, 248
    expression, 247
    MAbs, 248
    Xenograft models, 247
Pseudomonas aeruginosa exotoxin A, 50
PSMA, 246
    clinical studies, 247
    expression, 246
    MAbs, 246
    Xenograft models, 246
Psoriasis, 103, 109, 113, 116
Psoriatic arthritis, 103, 112, 116, 117

RA pathogenesis, 166
Radioimmunodiagnosis (RAID), 205
Radioimmunotherapy (RAIT), 194, 196, 205,
    211
Radiolabeled, 198, 201, 205, 206
    mAbs, 11
Ranibizumab, 137, 140, 141, 143, 144, 146
    humanization, 140, 141
    immunogenicity, 144
    pharmacokinetics, 143
    side effects, 141
    structure, 143
Receptor tyrosine kinase, 185, 188–190, 206
Rechallenge, 320
REFLEX, 172
Relapse, 168
Renal allograft, 229
    rejection, 221
Reproductive, 27
Rheumatoid arthritis (RA), 4, 102, 103, 163
Ribosome display, 9, 50
Rituximab, 80, 88, 164, 239
RNA interference (RNAi)
    comparison with intrabody, 358
    gene expression knockdown, 358
    nonspecific interferon response, 358

Safety, 23
scFv, 8
Self-tolerance, 221
Semisynthetic libraries, 9
Serum chemistry, 32
Single-domain V_H, 50
SLE, 175
Somatic hypermutation, 51
Species, 26
Specific pathogen-free (SPF), 223
Stability, 25
STEAP-1, 249
    expression, 249

MAbs, 249
 Xenograft models, 249
Structure–function of antibody, 4
Super-agonist, 41
Suppressor CD4$^+$CD25$^+$ cells, 229
Surrogate antibody, 27
Syngeneic islet grafts, 226
Synthetic repertoire, 9
Systemic lupus erythematosus, 163, 174

T cell
 anergy and depletion, 228
T cells, 259, 263, 265, 330–333, 335, 337
 T cell receptor, 330
 tumor specific, 331
T-body immunotherapy, 330, 331
 clinical trials, 335
 experimental models, 333
Targets, 238
 antigen, 28
 Established, 240
 Novel, 240, 246
 organs, 23
TDAR, 38
Telemetry, 36
Tetrabodies, 13
Tetramers, 50
Therapeutic, 20, 22
Thermodynamic stability, 55
Thymus weight, 38
Tissue microarrays, 31
TNF antagonists, 231
TNFSF ligands, 309
Tocilizumab
 efficacy, 158
 pharmacokinetics, 154
 safety, 155
 structure, 152
Tomoregulin, 250
Tositumomab, 240
Toxicity, 23, 41
Toxicokinetics, 26
Transgenes, 74, 75, 78
Transgenic, 75, 76, 79, 86
 animals, 5, 27
 mice, 74–78, 80, 89
 mouse, 74, 78, 79, 87–89

Trastuzumab, 198, 239, 241
 clinical trials, 241
 Xenograft models, 241
Treg, 225, 317–319
 cells, 294
Triabody, 13, 50
Trials of Rituximab in Rheumatoid Arthritis,
  167
Tumor necrosis factor (TNF-α), 102, 186, 260,
  277
 apoptosis, 105, 109
 arthritis, 108
 cancer, 107
 cell proliferation, 105
 characterization, 103
 expression, 104, 107
 inflammatory bowel disease, 108, 115, 119
 psoriasis, 116
 receptor signaling, 103, 104
 sepsis, 107
 in vitro studies, 105
Tumor necrosis therapy, 292
Turmor necrosis factor-alpha (TNF)
 arthritis, 108
 cancer, 107
 psoriasis, 109
 sepsis, 107
 in vitro studies, 105
Type I diabetes, 222

Ulcerative colitis, 108, 114

V_L/V_H pseudodimer, 60
v-erb-B, 185
Vascular endothelial growth factor (VEGF),
  132, 134, 138, 140, 243
 antibodies to, 144, 145
 expression, 132, 244
 isoforms, 132, 133
 receptors, 144, 145
Verteporfin, 143, 144

WAM antibody modeling, 65

Yeast display, 9

Zalutumumab, 79–82, 87
Zevalin, 205